D0041389

Adrenal Fatigue

The 21st Century Stress Syndrome©

What It Is and How You Can Recover Your

- Energy
- Immune Resistance
- Vitality and
- Enjoyment of Life

By

James L. Wilson ND, DC, Ph.D.

ADRENAL FATIGUE THE 21ST CENTURY STRESS SYNDROME©

By James L. Wilson ND, DC, Ph.D.

Published by:
Smart Publications™
PO Box 4667
Petaluma, CA 94955

Fax: 707 763 3944
www.smart-publications.com

Eleventh Printing 2007
Printed in the United States of America
First Edition

ISBN: 1-890572-15-2 $14.95   Softcover

Warning - Disclaimer

Smart Publications™ has designed this book to provide information in regard to the subject matter covered. It is sold with the understanding that the publisher and the author are not liable for the misconception or misuse of the information provided. Every effort has been to make this book as complete and as accurate as possible. The purpose of this book is to educate. The author and Smart Publications™ shall have neither liability nor responsibility to any person or entity with respect to any loss, damage, or injury caused or alleged to be caused directly or indirectly by the information contained in this book. The information presented herein is in no way intended as a substitute for medical counseling.

Acknowledgments

This book would not have been written without the help and encouragement of many people. My deepest gratitude goes out to all those who as patients, friends, colleagues, students and family showed me how much a book like this was needed. I would like to gratefully acknowledge the following people for their roles in making this book a reality.

Thanks to Dr. Ward Dean who first prompted me to write this book. His inspiration and encouragement provided the spark and the decision to write it.

I would also like to thank the American College for Advancement in Medicine (ACAM), with a special thanks to ACAM's Dr. Jack Young and Dr. Michael Hanson, for repeatedly inviting me back to speak on the diagnosis and treatment of adrenal fatigue. Through the continual gathering of material for these lectures, the book took much of its form.

Finding a publisher is often the most difficult task for an author. Fortunately for me Smart Publications was willing to take the risk of publishing this book based primarily on a tentative outline, an audio cassette of one of my lectures and my reputation.

Next, I would like to thank Neera Jain who helped compile many of the references used in this book and thousands that do not appear, but were researched in the preparation of its writing. Thanks also to the University of Arizona Medical Library staff, especially Na Nguyen, Hanna Fisher, Fred Heidenreich, Mary Riordan and Cathy Wolfson who were always more than willing to help.

I am grateful to Dr. Gary Gordon who provided many of the historical texts and research papers that added substance, filled in many of the historical gaps and answered many of the questions about the early research and clinical reports of adrenal fatigue.

My appreciation and thanks also goes out to Dr. Jonathan Wright whose keen interest in this area prompted him to offer to write the foreword to this book.

I would also like to thank my many, many patients who have shared personal information and been dedicated enough to their health to follow through with my suggestions. It has been so wonderful to see their lives turn around. Some of their stories appear in this book.

Susan Nickol had the onerous task of transcribing my writing into readable text. She worked tirelessly on the initial copy and various revisions without complaint. Her cheerful presence in my office while managing to expertly type the book around her other duties was greatly appreciated.

After eating, breathing and living a book, a writer becomes blind to the writing. I am very grateful to Florencia Patterson, Marie Wagner, Dr. Tim Lohman, Dr. Michael Stone and Deborah Mitchell who very generously agreed to review this book and to point out needed changes.

Every Thursday morning I meet with a group of 7 men. These men have given their continual support for me to write this book. Thanks to: Joe Breck, Michael, Kiropatkin; John Eisele, Tim Lohman, James Hamilton, Jack Halstead and Bill Mawhinney.

My wife Vivien's constant encouragement and belief in the importance of bringing this information to light were essential. Over the past 2 years, she has been my staunchest supporter as well as my greatly valued editor who helped write and rewrite the entirety of the book. She also contributed her expertise as a hypnotherapist and meditation instructor to the meditation and reframing sections of the book.

Thanks also to my 4 children who have faithfully cheered me on and sacrificed many hours of our time together so that this book could be written. I was especially touched when my 13-year-old son told me that what he wanted for his birthday was for my book to be finished. This book was indeed a family affair.

The user friendliness of this book has been enormously enhanced by the wonderful cartoons and illustrations done by Richard Capener. Richard's exceptional talents as an artist have perceptively and sympathetically captured the essence of adrenal fatigue.

I owe so much to people I have never met, especially the pioneering doctors of the 1920-40s who organized the various manifestations of adrenal fatigue into a recognizable syndrome. Their writings continue to inspire. I hope that this book will be true to their fine example and bring relief to the many who are suffering from this distressing but often hidden disorder.

Dedication

This book is dedicated to the late Dr. Leo Roy, my friend and mentor, who first brought my attention to the significance of the subtle functioning of the endocrine glands and how important they are in health and illness. Leo showed me the power of natural therapies and the importance of nutrition in health and disease. Many times I watched him take people on their last legs and rehabilitate them to full health, primarily using food concentrates and glandular extracts. He was a uniquely gifted physician whose absence is sorely felt.

About the Author

Dr. Wilson has helped hundreds of people with adrenal fatigue regain their health and vitality during his 24 years of private practice. For the past 10 years he has also lectured extensively to physicians and is acknowledged as an expert on adrenal function and other endocrine imbalances, and their impact on health. With a researcher's grasp of the science behind adrenal function and a clinician's understanding of its human impact, he has helped many understand the physiology behind the condition.

One of the few people to hold 3 doctorate degrees and 2 master's degrees, all from different disciplines, he received his Ph.D. in Human Nutrition from the University of Arizona, with minors in immunology, microbiology, pharmacology and toxicology. In addition, he holds degrees as a Doctor of Chiropractic and Doctor of Naturopathic Medicine. His master's degrees are in bio/nutrition and experimental psychology. Dr. Wilson was also one of 14 founding fathers of the Canadian College of Naturopathic medicine (CCNM) in Toronto, Ontario. He is listed in *The International Who's Who in Medicine* (Cambridge, England) and currently resides in Tucson, Arizona.

About the illustrator- Richard Capener is a graphic artist, cartoonist and video producer living on his 50 acre farm in rural Ontario, Canada. E-mail: capenerrichard@hotmail.com.

Foreward

Tired, worn-out, just can't regain your normal energy no matter what you do or how many doctors you visit? You're about to read an important and badly-needed book. Despite an absolute flood of "health books" in the last decade, there have been none that describe the not-uncommon but mostly-overlooked problem of weak adrenal gland function in such a thorough but understandable way. The answers you're looking for may well be here.

Adrenal fatigue (technically called "hypoadrenia" and "hypoadrenalism") has been one of our most prevalent yet rarely diagnosed conditions for the last fifty years. Despite being described in medical texts in the 1800s, and despite the development of the first really effective treatment in the 1930s, most "conventional" physicians are unaware that the problem exists!

At Tahoma Clinic, our physicians work with several individuals every week who suffer from adrenal fatigue. Many have "made the rounds" to multiple physicians; most have had one or more recommendations to "see a psychiatrist, there's nothing the matter". Others have diagnoses that include chronic fatigue syndrome, fibromyalgia, and serious food and/or inhalant allergies. Others have been "congratulated" about their unusually low blood pressure. All have one thing in common: fatigue that 'simply can't be overcome'.

As Dr. Wilson explains so well, there is hope! Adrenal fatigue can be overcome, and energy restored. As with so many problems, recovery starts with making the right diagnosis, and uncovering as many of the factors that caused it to occur as we possibly can. Only then can we make and carry out a plan that'll help us recover.

Why is help for adrenal fatigue so hard to find? Many readers may have already guessed at "the usual suspects": money and politics. Money: there are no patentable treatments for adrenal fatigue produced by patent-medicine ("pharmaceutical") companies. There's just no "big money" to be made. Politics: Since the 1970s, the Food and Drug Administration (FDA) has "outlawed" and actively persecuted one of the chief natural remedies for adrenal fatigue, an extremely safe remedy called adrenal cortical extract (ACE). [However, when ACE was produced by major patent medicine companies, from the 1930s through the 1960s, FDA had no problem with it.]

But back to Dr. Wilson's book: very few physicians have read and understood the entire range of medical journal reports (one hundred years, and more!) about adrenal fatigue as he does. More importantly, very few have taken that kind of study and put it to use for over twenty years, helping patient after patient recover, while using entirely natural means. And he's now taken his efforts even further, bringing all of his knowledge and experience to a public audience, reaching many more people than any one physician could personally see in many lifetimes.

But there is a warning: if you discover through reading this book that you may suffer from adrenal fatigue, you will need to do most of the work to achieve a recovery. As Dr. Wilson explains, there are lifestyle changes to be made, diets to alter forever (sometimes in a major way), vitamins, minerals, and herbs to swallow, tests to take and understand, and much patience required. Even 'attitude' and relationships sometimes need to be adjusted. While a knowledgeable physician can give guidance and coaching, she or he can't do all of that for us! But all that effort will be worth it. If you have adrenal fatigue and 'follow the program', it's extremely likely you'll recover.

Fortunately, we now have this book to help with the recovery program. There's more practical information here about "what to do about adrenal fatigue" than I've ever seen printed in one place. If you can't get in to see Dr. Wilson personally, and want to work with a physician well-informed about adrenal fatigue, contact the American College for Advancement in Medicine (1-800-532-3688, **www.acam.org**), the American Association of Naturopathic Physicians (1-703-610-9037, **www.naturopathic.org**), or the International College of Integrative Medicine (1-866-464-5226, **www.icimed.com**).

Just one more note: As Dr. Wilson writes, the pioneers in researching and bringing information about adrenal fatigue to the public were John Tintera, M.D., and William Jeffries, M.D.. Dr. Jeffries book (Safe Uses of Cortisol) is in print, available in many natural food stores, compounding pharmacies, and through "on-line" sources. Dr. Tintera's book (Hypoadrenocorticism) is long out of print, but photocopies may be obtained through Meridian Valley Labs, 1-253-859-8700. Readers interested in more technically-oriented information may wish to refer to these books.

Thank you, Dr. Wilson, for bringing us this book, and letting us all know that adrenal fatigue is a very real and not-uncommon problem, but most importantly, that complete recovery is very possible!

———Jonathan V. Wright, M.D.
Medical Director, Tahoma Clinic
Kent, Washington,
Author: Natural Hormone Replacement for Women over 45
Maximize Your Vitality and Potency for Men over 40
The Patient's Book of Natural Healing (with Alan R. Gaby, M.D.)

Table of Contents

Part One — *Your Adrenal Glands and You*

Part Two — *Do I Have Adrenal Fatigue?*

Part Three — *Helping Yourself Back To Health*
Treatment of Adrenal Dysfunction

Prologue

A Sorry Story of Adrenal Fatigue

Erica was an up-and-coming computer whiz, or at least she used to be. She loved the challenge of working in a field that was always changing. Her goal was to head her own software company within 10 years and, as a rising star in the industry, she took pride in her expertise and dedication. She already worked 12-hour days and most weekends and never said no to new projects. There was a reason the company facilities included showers, a free breakfast bar and even a few beds to crash in.

In February Erica caught the flu and was home for over a week. After that she had a hard time getting back up to speed and was sick with colds or flu several times during the next few months. None of the illnesses were serious but each time she seemed to be left with a little less energy.

Even when she wasn't sick, work felt like it required more effort than it used to. Her head often seemed cloudy and her concentration and memory were not as sharp as they had been. Even after a full night's sleep she still felt tired. Instead of rushing eagerly out of the door in the morning, she now had to drink two and sometimes three cups of coffee before she was ready to go. Despite the extra coffee, it was usually close to noon before she really woke up, and by around 3:00 in the afternoon she was often so lethargic and tired that she wanted to lie down. Erica noticed she had become more irritable and impatient with everyone and everything, including herself.

After 6:00 PM she usually felt better than she had all day, especially if she ate a decent supper. This energy surge lasted until around 9:00 to 9:30 PM when she began slowing down again. However, if she drank some coffee or just pushed on, by 11:00 PM she seemed to catch a second wind and could continue working quite easily until 1:00 or 2:00 AM. She often found she did her best work during those early morning hours.

Her food habits had changed as well. By mid morning, she was nearly always ravenously hungry and craved sweet snacks like doughnuts with her coffee. Often during the afternoon low she wanted really salty foods. If she skipped meals, as she had done easily in the past, her focus and concentration suffered. Regular meals definitely decreased the mental fuzziness, fatigue and other disturbing symptoms she was experiencing but, with her workload, she seldom put aside time for regular meals.

Sometimes by the end of the day, even when she had not been very productive, she felt utterly exhausted. She was also mildly depressed. Where she used to be optimistic, she was now discouraged, and instead of having goals to set the world on fire, she was now just trying to make it through each day.

Concerned about her deteriorating energy level and mental lows, she consulted her family doctor. Her doctor gave her a thorough check-up and ran some blood tests. At the follow-up visit he told Erica the test results were normal and that there was nothing wrong with her. His advice was to stop worrying so much and to take it easier. Erica told him that if she took it any easier, she would not have a job. The doctor responded with a prescription for an anti-anxiety medication that only made Erica feel worse. Although she consulted several other doctors, Erica got the same story from all of them - that there was nothing physically wrong. Instead, she ended up with a medicine cabinet full of prescription tranquilizers and anti-depressants, and a referral to a psychiatrist. Discouraged, Erica gave up trying to find an answer. She resigned herself to dragging herself through life, discouraged, depressed and continually fatigued.

Erica's story is a common one, but only one of the many and varied stories of the millions of people suffering from adrenal fatigue. This book is dedicated to people like Erica, to help them recognize and recover from their own adrenal fatigue.

Introduction

Why I Wrote This Book

For over 20 years in my practice I have witnessed the impact of helping people recover from adrenal fatigue, not just in terms their health, but also in their ability to feel happy. Happiness may be a "choice," as far as popular thinking goes, but for those whose adrenal glands are "running on empty," this choice seems almost out of reach.

Talking with other doctors in the United States and abroad, I realized that adrenal fatigue is a common and growing problem of modern life. Although I had suspected it, my conversations, research and clinical experience lead me to believe that we are dealing with a problem of monstrous proportions that is largely unrecognized by the medical establishment. This has left millions of people suffering from an untreated problem that interferes not only with their ability to function but also with their capacity to enjoy life. It is difficult to assess exactly how much money is lost by corporations due to worker absenteeism, poor or clouded decision making, alcoholism, drug abuse, "nervous breakdowns," burnout, employee conflict, acute and chronic illness, loss of employees, and a host of other costly problems that stem from the effects of over-stressed adrenal glands. It is also not possible to estimate the personal cost to people who have to switch to a lower paying job to avoid a total collapse, or to the chronically ill who just do not have the energy to get back on their feet. People suffering from adrenal fatigue are much more likely to develop a host of other common diseases and syndromes in which fatigue is one of the primary symptoms.

Many of us who see this syndrome in our practices, time and time again, knew that a book like this one needed to be written, but I did not really want to be the one to write it. I waited and waited for someone else to do it, but despite my patience, no one did. Then one day, just after I had finished giving a lecture on the adrenal glands at the American College for the Advancement in Medicine (ACAM), a friend and prominent doctor stopped me on my way out and said, "Doctor, when are you going to write a book on adrenal fatigue?" I responded that I didn't have time to write it, but if he could tell me how to do it with my schedule, I would be interested. As he had written several books himself, he put me in touch with a publisher who said he would get someone to help me write the book. However, after going through 5 writers, for various reasons, I finally admitted what I had intuitively known all along; this was my book to write.

My first orientation to the book was to produce a book that documented all the facts to the hilt. It was to be written for physicians and would document once and for all the significant and ongoing problems of adrenal fatigue, first described over 100 years ago. With this intent, I hired a Ph.D. student from the University of Arizona and together we compiled over 2400 scientific references. After collecting these references I began writing.

During the writing of the first few chapters, however, I realized that as deep as my commitment is to physician education, my real commitment is to the many, many people who are suffering from this invisible epidemic of adrenal fatigue. These people often go from doctor to doctor complaining of various signs and symptoms that are frequently ignored by the physicians they consult. Even worse, they find themselves unfairly and inappropriately branded as hypochondriacs, chronic complainers, neurotics or worse. Many have given up, accepting their plight as something they must learn to live with. Others have found ways of coping, to minimize their symptoms and limp through life. At the moment, it is a bleak picture for the person who is experiencing symptoms of what is probably the most widespread, yet unrecognized, health syndrome today, adrenal fatigue.

For these reasons I decided to write this book for the person suffering from adrenal fatigue. It is designed to be a self-help book, both in the diagnosis and the treatment of adrenal fatigue. I write it with the hope that it will provide you with the information, guidance, encouragement and tools you need to recover from this sometimes subtle, yet debilitating, health problem and to be able to make happiness your choice once again.

How to use this book

The book is arranged sequentially so that each section prepares you for the next section.

Part I will give you an overview of adrenal fatigue: what it is; who suffers from it, what causes it, how it progresses and why medicine has not recognized it as a syndrome. At the end of this overview, you will see illustrations of some of the common signs and symptoms of adrenal fatigue. If you find yourself relating to several of these illustrations, then you should go on to Part II.

Part II guides you through a questionnaire and some other simple processes to determine if you have adrenal fatigue and, if you do, what may be causing it. Once you have determined that adrenal fatigue is definitely affecting you, proceed to Part III.

Part III provides a very comprehensive guide to recovering from adrenal fatigue. It contains specific information about which therapies work and exactly what you can do to help yourself feel energized and well again. In Part III you will find descriptions of many of the hidden sources of stress that can drain your adrenals and your vitality. This section of the book ends with a question and answer section that covers many of the questions my patients commonly ask me as they are going through this recovery process.

Part IV explains in relatively plain English what your adrenal glands do and how and why they are so important to just about every process that occurs in your body and mind. It will help you understand why you feel so bad when they are not functioning adequately.

Part One

Your Adrenal Glands and You

Chapter 1

How Adrenal Function Affects Your Everyday Life

"With our present partial knowledge of the function of the endocrine chain of glands, it appears as though the suprarenals were the first to show signs of fatigue, for the simple reason that they seem to have most of the work to do in the auto protective functions." (McNulty, J., New York Medical Journal, 1921, XCIII, pg. 288)

The purpose of your adrenal glands is to help your body cope with stresses and survive. In fact, the adrenals are known as "the glands of stress." It is their job to enable your body to deal with stress from every possible source, ranging from injury and disease to work and relationship problems. Your resiliency, energy, endurance and your very life all depend on their proper functioning.

Just as Napoleon, a small man with great power, mobilized huge forces to make his presence felt in every part of his world, so your adrenal glands command powerful hormones to extend their influence throughout your body and your life. No bigger than a walnut and weighing less than a grape, each of your two adrenal glands sits like a tiny pyramid on top of a kidney. From this central location they not only significantly affect the functioning of every tissue, organ and gland in your body, they also have important effects on the way you think and feel. The forces that these two little Napoleons mobilize largely determine the energy of your responses to every change in your internal and external environment. Whether they signal attack, retreat or surrender, every cell responds accordingly, and you feel the results.

One way to get an overview of the far-reaching extent, variety and depth of the effects of your adrenal hormones is to take a look at the wide range of medical conditions treated with drugs that imitate the actions of the adrenal hormone, cortisol (synthetic corticosteroids). The uses of hydrocortisone (a corticosteroid) listed in <u>The Physicians' Desk Reference</u>

will give you the story. They include treatment of diseases and disorders of the joint mucus membranes, the heart, the blood, the respiratory tract and lungs, the gastrointestinal tract, the skin, the eyes, and the nervous system. Hydrocortisone is also used to control swelling and inflammation as well as symptoms of allergies, cancer, viral infection, and immune and auto-immune disorders. However, the effects of your body's own adrenal hormones on your health and bodily functions are even more varied, profound and extensive.

The hormones secreted by your adrenals influence all of the major physiological processes in your body. They closely affect the utilization of carbohydrates and fats, the conversion of fats and proteins into energy, the distribution of stored fat (especially around your waist and at the sides of your face), normal blood sugar regulation, and proper cardiovascular and gastrointestinal function. The protective activity of anti-inflammatory and anti-oxidant hormones secreted by the adrenals helps to minimize negative and allergic reactions to alcohol, drugs, foods and environmental allergens. After mid-life (menopause in women), the adrenal glands gradually become the major source of the sex hormones circulating throughout the body in both men and women. These hormones themselves have a whole host of physical, emotional and psychological effects, from the level of your sex drive to the tendency to gain weight. Every athlete knows that muscular strength and stamina are acutely affected by the adrenal hormones, more commonly known as steroids.

Even your propensity to develop certain kinds of diseases and your ability to respond to chronic illness is influenced significantly by the adrenal glands. The more chronic the illness, the more critical the adrenal response becomes. You cannot live without your adrenal hormones and, as you can see from this brief overview, how well you live depends a great deal on how well your adrenal glands function.

Chapter 2

What Is Hypoadrenia and Adrenal Fatigue?

Crash and Burn: The Onset of Adrenal Fatigue

Beth was a Wall Street executive, brilliant, beautiful and driven. The classic Type A personality, she had achieved the highest level of success in her field. An over-achiever going at breakneck speed, she would typically work 19-hour days for 10 days straight, rush home for a shower and go right back to work. Once a month, every month, she would fly to 10 countries in 10 days on business. Incredibly, she still found time to work out a lot, and she did it all without caffeine.

Then, over the course of one short year, Beth fell apart. It started with a respiratory illness. She reacted violently to the antibiotics, with seven days of unbearable itching and swollen arms and legs. Three months later she started feeling dizzy all the time, but she kept on working and, after several months, the dizziness went away.

Two and a half months later Beth had an allergic anaphylactic reaction to something on a flight to Aspen. Her bronchial tubes swelled, making it difficult to breathe, and she broke out in intensely itchy hives. Severe untreated anaphylactic reactions are potentially fatal, suffocating the victim or sometimes leading to vascular collapse. Fortunately Beth recovered from this one, although she never discovered what had triggered it.

She was right in the middle of a business meeting two months later when she heard bells ringing, felt dizzy and collapsed. After a week in the hospital, the doctors still couldn't come up with a diagnosis. No one had any idea what was wrong with her.

Beth went back to work, and over the next spring had six more severe anaphylactic reactions and frequent respiratory illnesses. Even when she was "well" she always felt like she had the flu.

Money was no object, and Beth went to eight separate hospitals and clinics looking for answers, but no one knew anything. Even the prestigious Mayo Clinic in Rochester told her there was nothing really wrong with her. The last doctor she saw recommended a psychiatrist.

By the time she found me, Beth had been to some of the most prominent New York doctors. She had never heard of adrenal fatigue. It had been three years since the onset of her illness. Three years of hearing that the constant exhaustion was "just something you'll have to learn to live with", or "all in your head", or "just part of getting older". She was only 37 years old.

Her fiancé had heard my lecture on adrenal fatigue at a 1999 conference of the American College of Advancement in Medicine (ACAM). He set up a phone consultation and when Beth described her symptoms to me, he exclaimed, "She could be reading my notes from your lecture!" Beth had all the classic symptoms of adrenal fatigue; the same ones outlined in my lecture. But like many people who suffer from adrenal fatigue, she had no idea what was wrong, and neither did her doctors.

Although it's estimated that up to 80% of adult Americans suffer some level of adrenal fatigue at some time during their life, it remains one of the most under-diagnosed illnesses in the U.S. That is why I wrote this book, because once recognized, adrenal fatigue can be treated. You can get better.

What is Hypoadrenia?

Hypoadrenia, from the root word "hypo" (lower) and adrenia (related to the adrenals), is a deficiency in the functioning of the adrenal glands. Normally functioning adrenal glands secrete minute, yet precise and balanced, amounts of steroid hormones. But because they are designed to be so very responsive to changes in your inner physical, emotional and psychological environment, any number of factors can interfere with this finely tuned balance. This means that too much physical, emotional, environmental and/or psychological stress can deplete your adrenals, causing a decrease in the output of adrenal hormones, particularly cortisol. This lowered adrenal activity (hypoadrenia), resulting from adrenal fatigue, can range in severity all the way from almost zero to almost normal.

The extreme low end of hypoadrenia, Addison's disease, was named for Sir Thomas Addison, who first described it in 1855. It is life threatening if untreated and can involve actual structural and physiological damage to the adrenal glands. People suffering from Addison's usually have to take corticosteroids for the remainder of their lives in order to function. Luckily, it is the rarest form of hypoadrenia with an occurrence of only about 4 persons per 100,000. Approximately 70% of cases of Addison's disease are the result of auto-immune disease. The other 30% arise from a variety of other causes, including very severe stress.

What is Adrenal Fatigue?

Hypoadrenia more commonly manifests itself within a broad spectrum of less serious, yet often debilitating, disorders that are only too familiar to many people. This spectrum has been known by many names throughout the past century, such as non-Addison's hypoadrenia, sub-clinical hypoadrenia, neurasthenia, adrenal neurasthenia, adrenal apathy and adrenal fatigue. I prefer to use the term adrenal fatigue when referring to this common form of hypoadrenia. Not only does it remind us of the chief symptom of hypoadrenia, but it also most aptly describes this common syndrome in which the paramount symptom is fatigue. Adrenal fatigue affects millions of people in the U.S. and around the world in many ways and for many reasons.

Non-Addison's hypoadrenia (adrenal fatigue) is not usually severe enough to be featured on TV or to be considered a medical emergency. In fact, modern medicine does not recognize it as a distinct syndrome. Nevertheless, it can wreak havoc with your life. In the more serious cases of adrenal fatigue, the activity of the adrenal glands is so diminished that the person may have difficulty getting out of bed for more than a few hours per day. With each increment of reduction in adrenal function, every organ and system in your body is more profoundly affected. Changes occur in your carbohydrate, protein and fat metabolism, fluid and electrolyte balance, heart and cardiovascular system, and even sex drive. Many other alterations take place at the biochemical and cellular levels. Interestingly, even your body shape can transform when your adrenals are fatigued. Your body does its best to compensate for under-functioning adrenal glands, but it does so at a price.

Although fatigue is a universal symptom of low adrenal function, it is such a common complaint and occurs in so many other conditions, that today's medical doctors rarely consider pursuing an adrenal-related diagnosis when someone complains of fatigue. In fact, fifty years ago, physicians were far more likely than their modern counterparts to correctly diagnose this ailment. Information about non-Addison's hypoadrenia has been documented in medical literature for over a hundred years but unfortunately, this milder form of hypoadrenia is missed or misdiagnosed in doctors' offices every day, even though the patient clearly presents its classic symptoms. The anecdote at the beginning of this chapter actually occurred while this book was being written. Adrenal fatigue is all too often the cause of patients' run down feeling and inability to keep up with life's daily demands. The fact that it usually remains undiagnosed does not lessen its debilitating influence on their health and feelings of well being.

Adrenal fatigue is a collection of signs and symptoms, known as a "syndrome." It is not a readily identifiable entity like measles or a growth on the end of your finger. People with adrenal fatigue often look and act relatively normal. They may not have any obvious signs of physical illness, yet they are not well and live with a general sense of unwellness or "gray" feelings. They often use coffee, colas and other stimulants to get going in the morning and to prop themselves up during the day.

Other Conditions Related to Adrenal Fatigue
People who suffer from adrenal fatigue frequently have erratic or abnormal blood sugar levels in the form of hypoglycemia. In fact, people who have functional hypoglycemia are usually suffering from decreased adrenal function. With hypoadrenia there is more of a tendency to experience allergies, arthritic pain and decreased immune response. Most women who have low adrenal function have more premenstrual tension as well as increased difficulty during menopause.

The adrenals also have an effect on mental states. As a result, people with adrenal fatigue show a tendency toward increased fears, anxiety and depression, have intervals of confusion, increased difficulties in concentrating and less acute memory recall. They often have less tolerance than they normally would and are more easily frustrated. When the adrenals are not secreting the proper amount of hormones, insomnia is also one of the likely outcomes.

As their condition worsens, it lays the foundation for other seemingly unrelated conditions such as frequent **respiratory infections**, **allergies**, **rhinitis**, **asthma**, **frequent colds** and a number of other health problems such as **fibromyalgia, chronic fatigue syndrome**, **hypoglycemia, adult onset diabetes, auto-immune disorders** and **alcoholism.** These people may appear to friends and family to be lazy and unmotivated, or to have lost their ambition, when in reality quite the opposite is true; they are forced to drive themselves much harder than people with healthy adrenal function merely to accomplish life's everyday tasks.

Will My Doctor Treat Adrenal Fatigue?
If doctors were to look for and treat adrenal fatigue in their patients, many of the above problems could be avoided. Adrenal fatigue syndrome is a fully recognizable condition. In most cases, it can be alleviated with natural, safe substances, and in some cases it is totally preventable. The tendency of the medical profession to ignore this syndrome results in many unnecessary health problems for millions. Even if you are aware that you have adrenal fatigue, you may not find any sympathy or understanding from your doctor. Medicine only officially recognizes Addison's disease as hypoadrenia.

Generally, people's understanding of hypoadrenia is vague. You might have heard someone sigh and say something like, "My adrenals are shot." These people do, indeed, have some inkling of why they are suffering from fatigue, but if pressed for an explanation, they know very few actual details about how adrenal function is directly related to their feelings of being "dragged out."

With the help of the next few chapters, you will learn to recognize the major signs and symptoms of the most common kinds of adrenal fatigue which occur somewhere on the spectrum of adrenal function between Addison's disease and normal. In Part II you will be able to take a simple paper and pencil questionnaire to determine if you have adrenal fatigue. In Part III you will learn how to help yourself and your loved ones to recover. But now read on to find out what causes adrenal fatigue.

Chapter 3

What Causes Adrenal Fatigue

Adrenal fatigue, in all its mild and severe forms, is usually caused by some form of stress. Stress can be physical, emotional, psychological, environmental, infectious, or a combination of these. It is important to know that your adrenals respond to *every* kind of stress the same, whatever the source.

Life's stresses at their worst come in the form of such cataclysmic events as the death of a loved one, an automobile accident or a serious illness. But stress can also take its toll in less obvious ways, like an abscessed tooth, a bout of the flu, intense physical exertion, a severe quarrel with a loved one, pressure at the workplace, an unhappy relationship, environmental toxins, poor diet, etc. If these smaller stresses occur simultaneously, accumulate or become chronic, and the adrenals have no opportunity to fully recover, adrenal fatigue is usually the result. Its symptoms are clear, distinct and sometimes, uncomfortably familiar.

The illustration "Factors Affecting the Adrenals" gives some examples of common causes of adrenal fatigue. In short, adrenal fatigue occurs when the amount of stress overextends the capacity of the body (mediated by the adrenals) to compensate and recover from that stress or the combined stresses. Once this capacity to cope and recover is exceeded, some form of adrenal fatigue occurs.

FACTORS AFFECTING THE ADRENALS

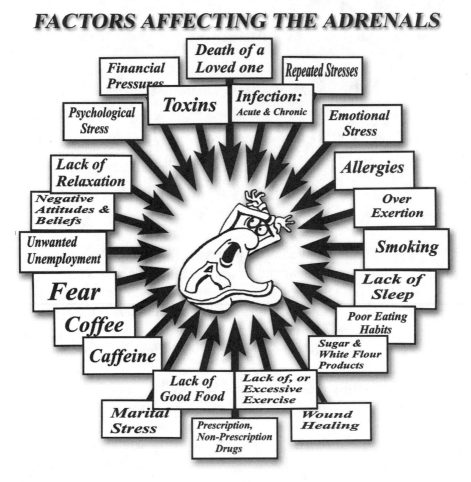

Often the causes of adrenal fatigue are not obvious because the combined stresses look so different. Our bodies may not even tell us when we are under stress. In one study, hospital workers in a pediatric nursing care unit (a workplace noted for its high stress and burnout) were totally unaware of being under stress, but their cortisol levels were elevated by 200-300%. The level of the adrenal stress hormone cortisol is a common measure of stress. It is important to remember that all stresses are additive and cumulative. That is, the number of stresses, whether or not you recognize them as stresses, the intensity of each stress and the frequency with which it occurs, plus the length of time it is present, all combine to form your total stress load.

Although it is impossible to exactly quantify the total stress load, your body does it every day, minute by minute, making instantaneous adjustments as these stresses change. It is when the body becomes unable to make the appropriate changes to these stresses that adrenal fatigue begins. The worse the overload relative to the ability of the body to respond, the worse the adrenal fatigue. Each person has a different capacity to handle the total stress load, and the capacity of each person varies over time and events.

One of the commonly overlooked sources of stress and resistant adrenal fatigue is chronic or severe infection. Adrenal fatigue is often precipitated by recurring bouts of bronchitis, pneumonia, asthma, sinusitis, or other respiratory infections. The more severe the infection, the more frequently it occurs or the longer it lasts, the more likely it is that the adrenals are involved. Adrenal fatigue can occur after just one single episode of a particularly nasty infection, or it can take place over time as the adrenals are gradually fatigued by prolonged or recurrent infections. If there are other concurrent stresses, such as an unhappy marriage, poor dietary habits or a stressful job, the downhill ride is deeper and steeper. The reciprocal is also true; people suffering from low adrenal function often have a propensity toward respiratory illness. The next chapter will show you who is most susceptible to adrenal fatigue, and why.

Chapter 4

Who Suffers From Adrenal Fatigue?

Anyone who does not get enough rest and relaxation to enjoy life, who drives him/herself constantly, who is never satisfied or is a perfectionist, who is under constant pressure (especially with few outlets for emotional release), who feels trapped or helpless, who feels overwhelmed by repeated or continuous difficulties, or who has experienced severe or chronic emotional or physical trauma or illness is probably already suffering from some degree of adrenal fatigue. Do you recognize any of these patterns in your own life? If so, this book is going to help you. Keep reading to find out how at risk you are and what you can do to help yourself.

Anyone Can Experience Adrenal Fatigue
People from every walk of life, every culture, and every age can suffer from adrenal fatigue. The political leader, the university student, the environmentalist, the farmer, the villager in a war torn country, the Hollywood director, the factory worker on a swing shift, the medical doctor with an HMO, and the mother with more than one child and little support probably all have the factors in their lives that can lead to adrenal dysfunction, even though they lead very different lifestyles. The cost is untold in the loss of productive hours, creative ideas, sound business decisions, and other intangibles such as happiness, not to mention good health and long life.

Your Job May Be a Factor
Some professions are harder on the adrenal glands than others. If you look at insurance company actuarial tables of the mortality rates, drug abuse, and number of sick days in different professions, what you are seeing, barring physically dangerous jobs, is largely the amount of adrenal fatigue experienced in those jobs.

The medical profession is a good example of a profession prone to adrenal fatigue. Physicians, on average, die approximately 10 years younger, have higher rates of alcoholism and several times the drug addiction rates of the normal population. Typically medical students go directly to medical school from an undergraduate program. During the first two years of medical school they learn approximately 25,000 new words, staying up many late nights to do so. At the end of the four years of study, they graduate and become residents in a specialized area of study, working between 80 and 110 hours per week, sometimes under a great deal of pressure from superiors and other students. By the time they graduate and finish their residency, they are often up to one hundred thousand dollars in debt and emotionally isolated. Over two-thirds of those who are married, end up divorced by the end of their residency. Because of their experiences during their training they may feel they can trust no one. This makes work and home unsafe places to be. After residency, most new doctors move immediately into a practice. Once in practice, they frequently work long hours with little rest, sometimes resorting to amphetamines or other stimulants in order to keep going. They often have little home life because they are working most of the time, which leads to marital dissatisfaction. Although this is a generalization and is certainly not true for every doctor, it is a description that fits many of the medical students, residents and young doctors recently in practice I have worked with. In fact, I know one doctor who, after collapsing at the end of her residency, decided to make a career of teaching professionals how to deal with stress.

The police force is another profession that is very hard on the adrenals. I have counseled many policemen who are on the verge of collapse because of the stress involved in their job. You might think that it is the danger these people live with day in and day out that produces the stress, but much of their stress comes from the demands placed upon them by their commanding officers. If these people are also involved in a weekly rotating shift, the stress is magnified because their bodies never have a chance to adjust to the new circadian rhythm produced by each sleep change. People on alternating shifts with less than three weeks between shift changes are continually hammering their adrenal glands. Every time the wake/sleep cycle is altered, it takes several days to weeks to establish a normal hormonal pattern for the new wake/sleep cycle.

Middle executives, secretaries, and teachers are examples of professionals who suffer from "sandwich stress." This is stress that comes from having to meet the demands and expectations from above and below without the power or authority to make the necessary changes or to do their job effectively. It is frequently the person in the middle who takes the blame when things go wrong but not the credit when things go right. People in this position commonly have more than their share of health problems. They often suffer from Syndrome X (a complex of signs and symptoms that includes glucose intolerance, increased triglycerides, low HDL cholesterol, insulin resistance, hypertension, central obesity, and accelerated atherosclerosis). These disorders reflect the effects of stresses that produce elevated cortisol levels. However, sometimes this phase is followed in time by a drop in cortisol levels to below normal, as the adrenals fatigue and are less able to respond to the stress.

The Ability To Withstand Stress Varies
One person may withstand a stress quite easily and be ready for more, but another person, or that same person at another time, may find the same stress overwhelming and impossible to bear. It is important to understand that the onset and continuation of adrenal fatigue has great individual variation.

Below are some of the primary lifestyle factors that lead to adrenal fatigue. It is important to note that most of these are within your control.

Primary Components of Lifestyle Leading to Adrenal Fatigue

- Lack of sleep
- Poor food choices
- Using food and drinks as stimulants when tired
- Staying up late even though fatigued
- Being constantly in a position of powerlessness
- Constantly driving yourself
- Trying to be perfect
- Staying in double binds (no-win situations) over time
- Lack of enjoyable and rejuvenating activities

Examples of Lifestyles Leading to Adrenal Fatigue

- University student
- Mother with two or more children and little support from family or friends
- Single parent
- Unhappy marriage
- Extremely unhappy and stressful work conditions
- Self-employed with a new or struggling business
- Drug or alcohol abuser
- Alternating shift work that requires sleep pattern to be frequently adjusted
- All work, little play

Examples of Life Events Leading to Adrenal Fatigue

- Unrelieved pressure or frequent crises at work and/or home
- Any severe emotional trauma
- Death of a close friend or family member
- Major surgery – with incomplete recovery or subsequent persistent fatigue
- Prolonged or repeated respiratory infections
- Serious burns – including severe sunburn
- Head trauma
- Loss of stable job
- Sudden change in financial status
- Relocation without support of friends or family
- Repeated or overwhelming chemical exposure (including drug and alcohol abuse)

Stresses Add Up

Repeated stresses, no matter what their cause, make a person more prone to adrenal fatigue. The effects of stress are cumulative, even when the individual stressors are quite different. For example, you come down with a bronchial infection that has not quite cleared up when your father dies. Six months after your father's death someone younger and newer gets the job promotion you had been expecting and, within a month, you are injured in a car accident. The doctors are concerned by how long it is taking you to recover from the accident. They are puzzled only because they do not recognize that this series of stressors, although seemingly unrelated, has gradually depleted your adrenal reserves. Each of these separate events, emotional and physical, is an insult to your body to which your adrenal glands have had to respond. By the time the accident occurs, your adrenals have nothing left to give. Had the accident been the only major stressor, you would probably recover quickly and without incident.

Physical and Emotional Stresses Interact

Physical traumas (such as infection, physical injury, malnutrition, surgery, extreme cold, extreme heat, dehydration, exhausting physical exertion, exposure to toxic chemicals, allergies, asthma, and lack of sleep) and emotional traumas (such as divorce, separation, serious arguments, loss of a job, financial problems, injury or death of a friend or family member, and significant ridicule or humiliation) cumulatively drain your adrenal reserves, particularly if you cannot or do not do what is necessary to recover between traumas.

Poor Diet Reduces Your Adrenals' Ability to Respond to Stress

In addition to the emotional and physical traumas that can produce hypoadrenia, there are chronic conditions or lifestyles that continually drain the adrenals or prevent them from recuperating properly after a trauma. One of the most common of these chronic factors is poor diet. For example, 62 % of North Americans do not eat even one vegetable per day. Many nutrients not found in typical fast food meals are necessary to make proper hormones in the adrenal glands. If you eat primarily pre-prepared or processed foods and not many vegetables or raw fruits, you can be sure your adrenal glands are not getting the nutrients they need to function optimally and to respond well in a crisis. You will find a complete breakdown of the nutrients required by your adrenals, how to get them and what they do in Chapter 13 titled "Food."

Respiratory Infections Commonly Precede Adrenal Fatigue

Respiratory ailments have an especially devastating effect on the adrenals. Written about in older medical literature and still seen frequently by astute physicians, adrenal fatigue is often precipitated by recurring bouts of bronchitis, pneumonia, asthma, sinusitis, or other respiratory infections. The more severe the infections, the more frequently they occur, or the longer they last, the more likely it is that the adrenals will be over-worked. Adrenal fatigue can occur after even just one single episode of a particularly nasty infection, or it can take place over time as the adrenals are gradually fatigued by prolonged or repeated infections. If there are other concurrent stresses, such as an unhappy marriage, poor dietary habits or stressful job, the downhill ride is deeper and steeper.

Your Adrenals May Be Weak From Birth

As well as these factors of lifestyle and life events, there are also congenital differences in adrenal resiliency. Children born to mothers already suffering from adrenal fatigue and children who experience severe stress in the womb (including those given above) typically have lower adrenal function. Because of this, from birth on, they have less capacity to deal with stress in their own lives and so are more prone to adrenal fatigue throughout their lives.

Some Representative Case Histories of Adrenal Fatigue

Frank was a backslapper of a salesman; a guy who always had a few jokes and a laugh. He was a middle manager in a growing company and over time he hoped to become an executive. With his goals clear, Frank was always at the office. He was the guy everyone wanted to be like. Within 6 years he had been promoted 4 times and had become Vice-president of Sales. His dreams were coming true. Unfortunately the company had expanded too fast just as the market turned against it. Covering its losses, the company began downsizing, asking more of those remaining. Frank was one of the fortunate ones whose job was secure, but he had to dramatically expand his workload. This meant late hours at the office several times per week and taking work home almost every weekend. Frank ate most of his meals in restaurants, the faster, the better because he now had more work to do. By cutting out his exercise time and getting fast food meals on the run, Frank was able to squeeze more hours out of the day. Because he often felt tired during the many evenings he stayed late, he switched from his regular 1 cup of coffee with his evening meal to alternating high caffeine soft drinks with coffee every hour or so to keep going. With all the caffeine, Frank had more trouble sleeping, so he began taking sleeping tablets to help him sleep. More cups of coffee were required to get him going in the morning, but once noon rolled around, he was as good as new. Frank then discovered that he could get even more work done if he could just get past 11:00 at night. Once he got past 11:00, he got a second burst of energy that kept him going until about 2:00. Although he began to look a little ragged around the edges, Frank was able to keep this up for 6 years. One early morning, Frank came home to find his wife's car gone. Going inside he found her clothes gone and a note. Frank was dumbfounded. How could she leave him? The next morning Frank was still sitting in the same chair he'd sat in to read the note she'd left him. In fact he hadn't moved from that chair. At noon he managed to pick up the phone to order some food but, except for the coffee, he just picked at it. Ignoring any phone calls, Frank just sat there, wondering what had gone wrong. Friends finally got Frank to come to the door and check himself into a hospital. He was diagnosed as suffering from post-traumatic depression, but the medications were only partially effective. Frank improved, but dragged himself through life. Soon after taking a leave of absence, he came into my office at the advice of a friend. With time and treatment, Frank made a full recovery. Frank is a good example of someone who has driven himself to adrenal exhaustion through blind ambition, overwork, poor food and no relaxation.

Frank's case is a common story of adrenal fatigue brought on by overwork, poor food, poor lifestyle, over-ambition and lack of perspective. The emotional trauma of his wife leaving him flattened an already depleted man. By the time he read her note he was already running on empty and had no reserve to fall back on.

Jim worked in a full service gas station. He was good at his job and very good with customers. After 2 years, the company representative for one of the major oil companies noticed Jim and offered him a chance to have his own service station. Jim was delighted to be given this opportunity, as he was well aware that his present position was a dead-end job. The company built a new station, outfitted with the latest equipment, and gave him easy terms on its purchase. Jim soon had the business of his dreams. With the combination of his personality and the excellent service he offered, it wasn't long before he had to hire more help to meet the increasing customer volume. Jim loved his work and took pride in running his own successful business. However the demands of building and maintaining a business were taking their toll. His wife was very unhappy about the 70+ hours a week he put in at the station and complained bitterly about how little time he spent with her and their 2 children. So when the oil company offered Jim an additional service station based on his success with the first one, he reluctantly turned them down. Disheartened by his wife's constant dissatisfaction and the long work hours, he began feeling trapped and helpless to change his situation. In order to relieve the stress of these frustrations, Jim began drinking at night. This quickly turned into a daily habit and all too soon his business began to drop off. His drinking problem reached a peak one Tuesday morning when a customer shouted, "Get your drunken hands off my car." An employee called Jim's wife and took him home. Soon after, Jim developed a bleeding ulcer and had to be hospitalized. Having time to reflect and recover in the hospital and at home, Jim saw how he was suffering from too much stress. As a result he gave up drinking, sold the service station and took a job with much less pressure and greater job security. With good nutrition and dietary supplements for adrenal support he was able to recover and find a balance that allowed him to lead a happy, fulfilling life.

Jim is a good example of how continual internal emotional stress and work demands can combine to lead to adrenal fatigue.

Brianna was a mother of 4. She had always wanted children, but also wanted a career. Being self-employed, she had little time to spare, especially when the children became older and had different social activities and sports to attend. Although she had never really had time to recover between the birth of her third child and her fourth, she continued to push herself with constant pep talks, chiding herself for not having the energy she used to, she kept herself going with more coffee, strong tea and constant sweets, especially chocolate. In fact, she was known to her friends as the "chocolate queen." Most of her family's activities still revolved around Brianna, leaving her with almost no free time. What little free time she had was not very relaxing as most of it was spent with the family and there was almost palpable tension between her husband and her. Brianna felt chronically tired and stressed. On the way to work one morning, she was hit from behind while sitting in her car waiting for the light to change. The constant pain she had in her neck tired her even more. At the end of her rope and unable to really function at work or at home due to her constant neck pain, she finally heeded the advice of a friend and sought the help of a chiropractor. Luckily, in addition to being able to get her out of pain, the doctor recognized that she was suffering from adrenal fatigue. He put her on the right nutritional supplements and had her shift more family responsibilities onto her husband, as well as hire 2 people to do much of the work she had been struggling with. Eventually she recovered her long lost energy and was once again a happy woman.

Brianna's case illustrates how an already over-burdened person with unrealistic expectations combined with lack of rest and marital discord produced adrenal fatigue. When a physical trauma was the straw that broke the camel's back, she could no longer compensate and felt the full extent of her adrenal fatigue.

Kevin was a bright chemical engineer who loved his job and his family. A few years ago he was promoted to manage a small chemical plant in the Midwest. Almost as soon as Kevin came on the scene, he saw the need for increased safety at the aging plant. But the plant was not generating the projected profits it should have, so improvements had to be delayed until there was room in the budget to make them. Within the first year of his new job assignment, Kevin's wife noticed that he was changing. He developed allergies for the first time. He began wanting to sleep in instead of rising at 4:00 AM as he used to. He became more short-tempered and intolerant of her and the children. In fact he began having uncharacteristic sudden temper outbursts for which he was always remorseful. Thinking it was probably the pressure of his new job, Kevin asked for and was given an assistant, as he had already increased production considerably. But even with working fewer hours and taking less active responsibility, Kevin continued to deteriorate. His energy dropped lower and lower and he became almost despondent as he just tried to make it through each day. The company doctor diagnosed Kevin as being too tense and prescribed tranquilizers and some "stomach pills" for his constantly upset stomach. When Kevin showed no improvement, his wife demanded a vacation, thinking what he needed was a rest. Not knowing what else to do, Kevin agreed. Within a few days of their vacation Kevin felt like a new man. His old energy returned and he once again became loving and affectionate. He looked forward to returning to his job. Once back, however, it was only a matter of a day before Kevin felt the same old tiredness and cloudy headedness descend on him again. They had only been back for 2 weeks when their family got notice that Kevin's father had died. The family left immediately on the 1000 mile drive to his home. Although Kevin dreaded the stress of the funeral, to his surprise, as they approached his old home, he felt better and better. Even having to drive most of the night to return to work by the following Monday morning didn't bother him. However, by the first evening of work, Kevin was back to his same old symptoms. He struggled on for a few more weeks until one day the previous manager made a brief stop to the plant. As they talked, Kevin learned that the former manager had taken an early retirement for health reasons. The man told him that as soon as he left the plant he felt 20 years younger. Telling the previous manager of his growing problems with handling the job, Kevin described some of his symptoms. The retired manager revealed that he had left because of chemical sensitivities and that while in the plant he had experienced many of the same symptoms as Kevin. He was good enough to meet Kevin at a place outside the plant to discuss what might be done about the situation. Together they approached the company to make the needed safety improvements, including a drastic reduction in chemical fumes collecting in several of the plant buildings. Kevin was transferred to a part of the company away from the fumes, read a book by a clinical ecologist on chemical sensitivities and one of my articles on adrenal fatigue, and slowly recovered his full health.

Kevin's case is an example of adrenal fatigue caused by chemical sensitivity. Any number of 'body burdens' can continually zap your adrenals, often without you being aware of what is happening.

Sandra was never a high-energy person. Frequently sick as a child, she chose to work as a librarian because it made little physical demand on her. However, her first job was not what she expected it to be. Taking a position in a university medical library, she was given a rotating shift that changed weekly. As the library was open 24 hours a day, she hardly had a chance to get used to one schedule before it was time to change. This schedule interrupted her sleeping pattern, which interfered with her concentration at work. Her boss became more and more demanding until one day Sandra simply broke down and started crying for no reason while re-shelving books. Afterwards, she poured out her tortured soul about how she couldn't sleep anymore, how she was constantly fatigued, that her boss expected too much, and how she hated being a librarian, something she thought she would love. She also complained that she felt mildly ill most of the time, her memory and patience were shot, and that she had become even more socially withdrawn. All she wanted to do was get away from everyone, pull the covers up over her head and sleep until she was darn good and ready to get up. Being already somewhat fragile, it didn't take much to push Sandra beyond her limits. After her outbreak she was referred to a staff psychiatrist who diagnosed her as being depressed. Several antidepressants later, when she showed only slight improvement, she was given a series of shock treatments that only made her fragile constitution more vulnerable. After several years on disability, she finally discovered a doctor who understood adrenal fatigue. Slowly she was able to find her way back to health and found a job in a library much more suited to her personality and needs. For Sandra, it was a long, hard journey back to recovery, because no one understood her limited capacity for stress.

Sandra's case is an example of people who have marginal adrenal reserve to begin with. Not much is needed for her to be overwhelmed. Looking at it from the outside, people are often quick to judge these people as weaklings or quitters, when they just do not have the reserve capacity to take on the stresses inherent in many work and social events.

The next chapter contains some of the more common symptoms of adrenal fatigue. If more than 2 or 3 of these sound strangely familiar, complete the questionnaire in Part II of this book to see if you have adrenal fatigue. If the cartoons in the next chapter are simply amusing, but do not strike home at all, pass this book on to someone the cartoons remind you of.

Chapter 5

Signs and Symptoms of Adrenal Fatigue

Listed below are some of the common symptoms of low adrenal function. Please look at them and see if one or more of them sound like you or people you know.

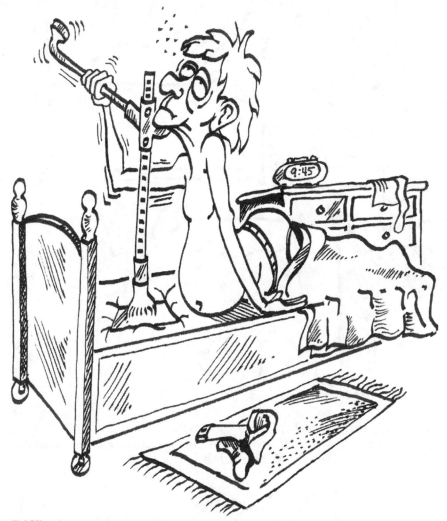

Difficulty getting up in the morning. *Three alarms and you still don't feel awake enough to lift your head off the pillow.*

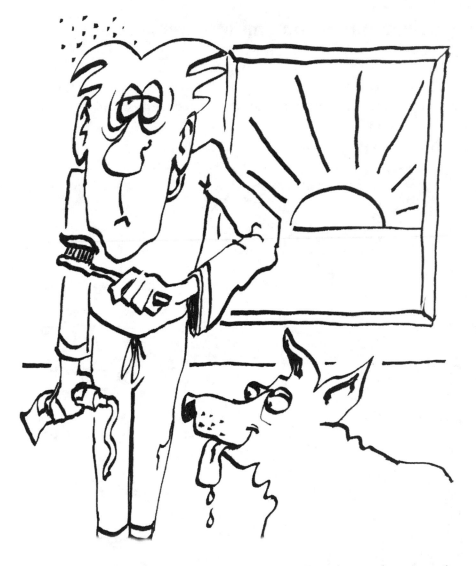

Continuing fatigue not relieved by sleep. Despite getting a good night's sleep, you still feel tired when you wake up. Refreshed is a foreign word to people with adrenal fatigue.

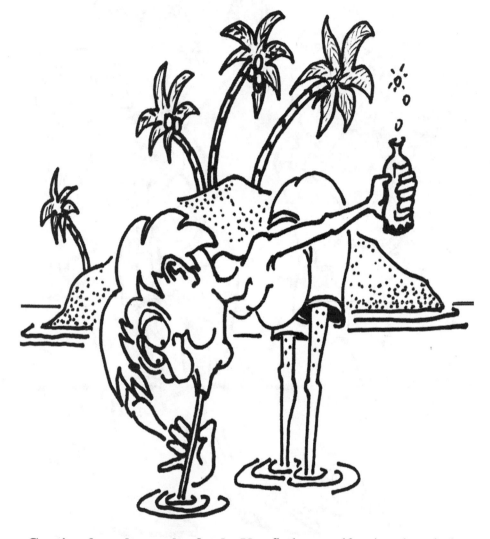

Craving for salt or salty foods. You find yourself eating the whole bag of chips or adding salt to already salted foods.

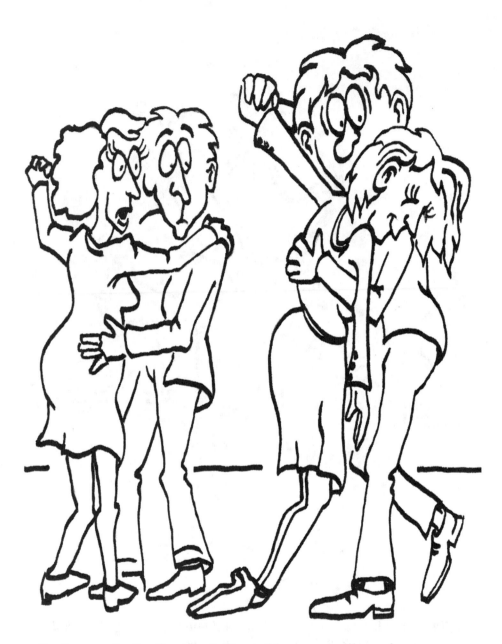

Lethargy (lack of energy). *Everything seems like a chore, even the things you used to enjoy. Frequently, just getting up out of the chair requires too much energy.*

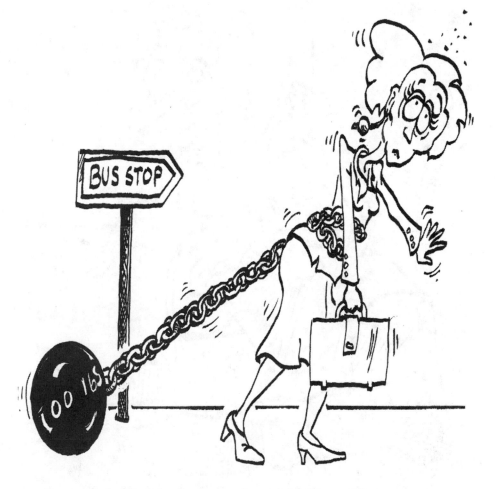

Increased effort to do every day tasks. Everything seems to require ten times as much effort as it should.

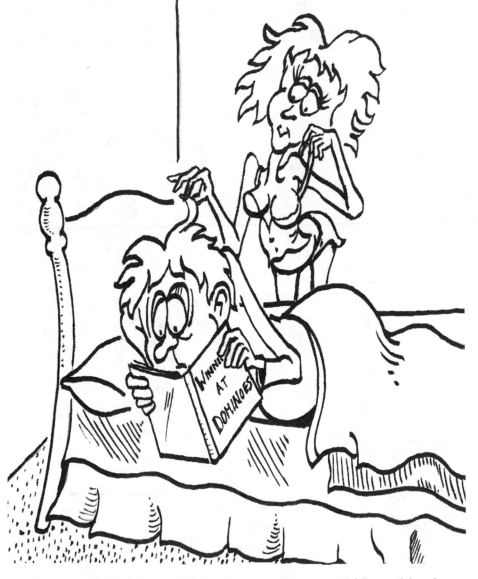

Decreased sex drive. *The hottest movie star could be waiting in your bedroom and you would ask for a rain check. Sex is the last thing on your mind when you hardly have the energy to keep your head up.*

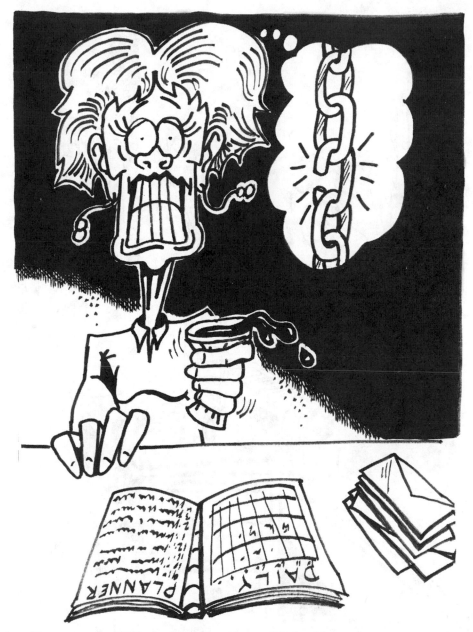

Decreased ability to handle stress. *Little things that never used to bother you get to you. Road rage, constant anxiety, yelling at your kids, and compulsive eating, smoking or drug use let you know your adrenals are crying out for help.*

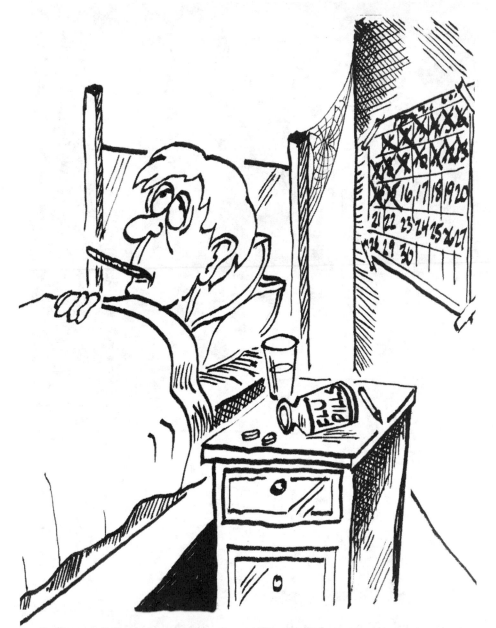

Increased time to recover from illness, injury or trauma.
The cold you got in October is still hanging on in November. The cut on your finger takes weeks to heal. Two years after your father died you are still incapacitated by grief.

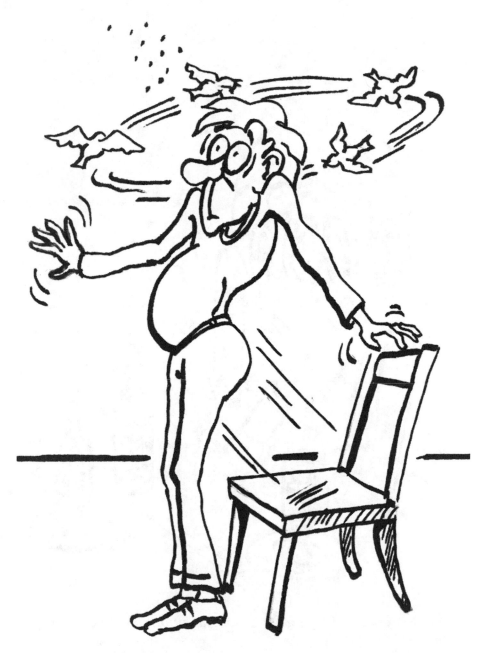

Light-headed when standing up quickly. Sometimes you feel like you are going to pass out when you get up from the bed or a chair.

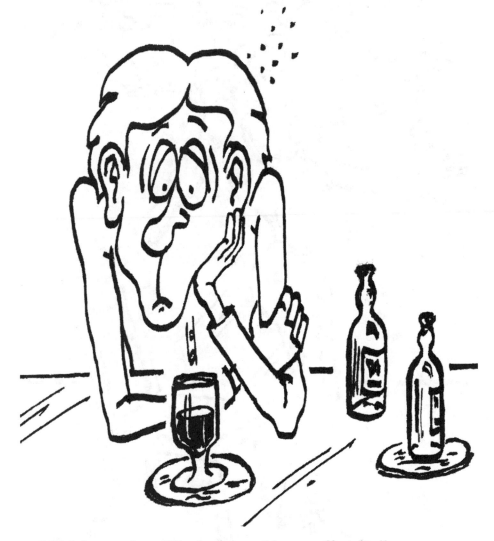

Mild depression. Why bother making an effort, it all seems so pointless?

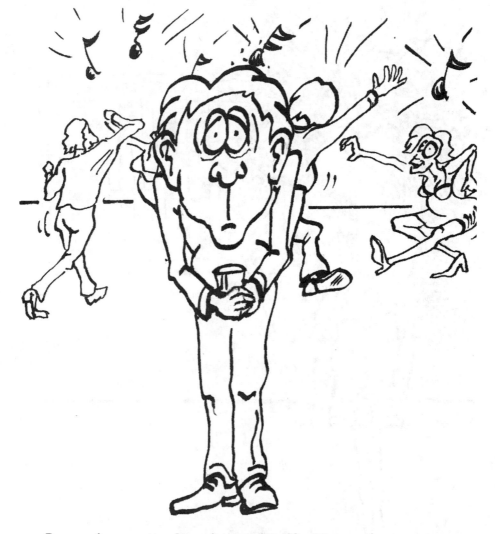

Less enjoyment or happiness with life. Not much seems to interest you any more. Work and relationships feel empty and you almost never do something just for fun.

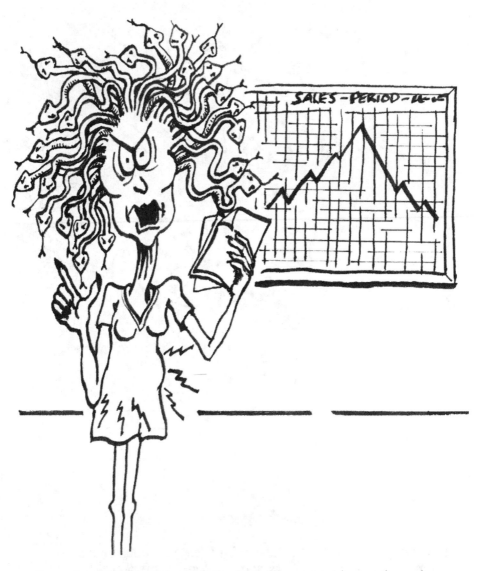

Increased PMS. *Bloated, tired, crabby, cramping and craving chocolate – does it get any worse than this?*

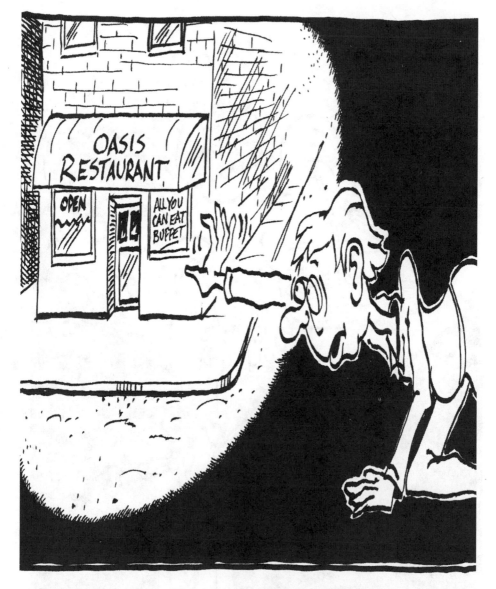

Symptoms increase if meals are skipped or inadequate. You have to drive yourself with snacks, colas and coffee just to keep from collapsing.

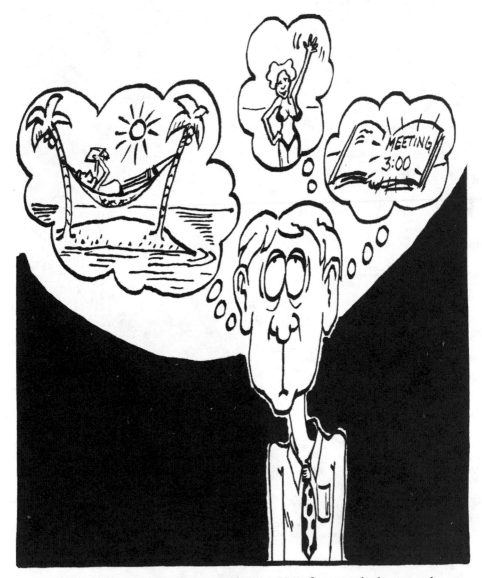

Thoughts less focused, more fuzzy. You frequently lose track of your train of thought and it is harder and harder to make decisions, even about little things like what to wear.

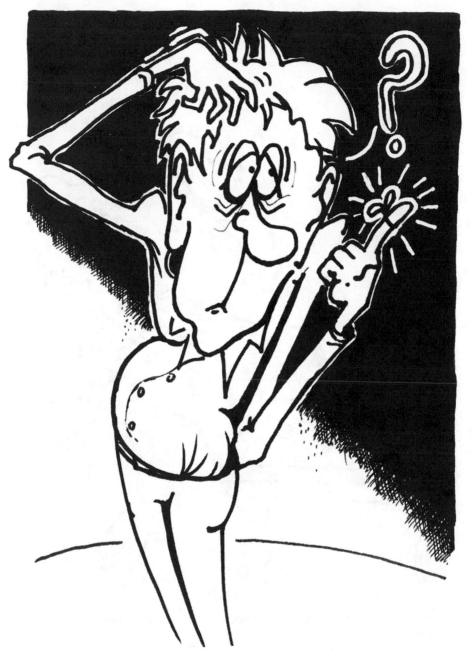

Memory less accurate. *You are so absentminded, you should be a professor.*

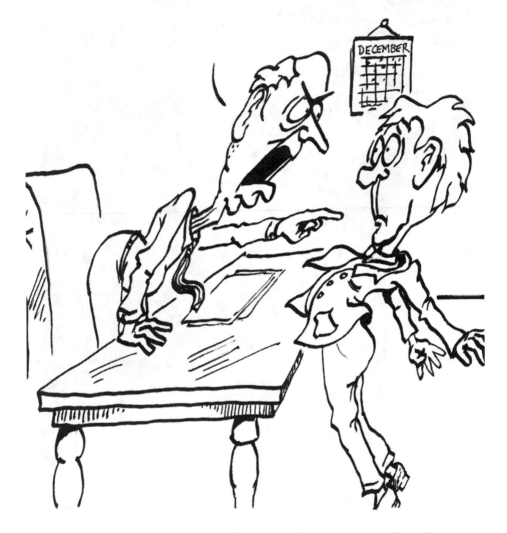

Decreased tolerance. People seem a lot more irritating than they used to.

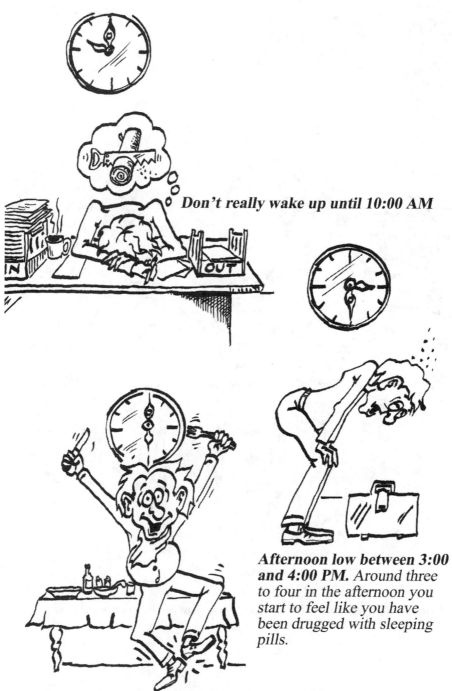

Don't really wake up until 10:00 AM

Afternoon low between 3:00 and 4:00 PM. Around three to four in the afternoon you start to feel like you have been drugged with sleeping pills.

Feels better after evening meal.
After 6:00 PM and supper, you start to feel alive again.

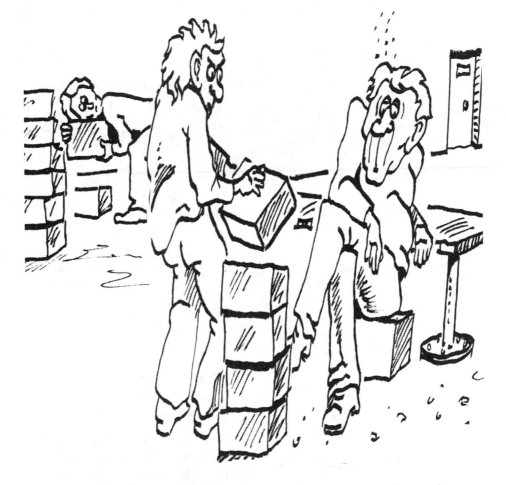

Decreased productivity. *It takes you longer to complete tasks and it is harder to stay on task.*

No single one of these symptoms gives a definitive diagnosis of hypoadrenia (adrenal fatigue), but taken collectively as a syndrome, they strongly suggest its presence. If many of these seem familiar, then you are probably suffering from some level of adrenal fatigue. Although we have come to accept it as such, adrenal fatigue is *not* a part or normal life! The illustrations may be humorous, but the symptoms for adrenal fatigue are not. These symptoms indicate defective adaptation of your adrenal glands to the stresses you are experiencing. They are warnings that something needs to change if you want to feel well again.

If you are experiencing more than three of these symptoms, read the next section on "Progression of Adrenal Fatigue" and then go on to complete the questionnaire and exercises in Part II to assess your level of adrenal fatigue.

Chapter 6

The Progression of Adrenal Fatigue

Adrenal fatigue can come on suddenly or gradually, depending upon the circumstances. It can be precipitated by a single, easily identifiable event such as a serious car accident, head injury, infection, toxic exposure, emotional shock, or life crisis. When an incident such as this is the decisive factor in producing adrenal fatigue, signs of adrenal fatigue are usually present after the event occurs which were not present before. In many cases people had been experiencing some degree of adrenal fatigue before the event but afterwards it became much more pronounced.

Because of our generally stressful lifestyles, adrenal fatigue frequently develops gradually. When this happens, the *symptoms* (what we sense and feel in our body) usually precede the *signs* (visible changes, and laboratory or clinical test findings). As the problems progress, these symptoms and signs accumulate to form a *syndrome*, which is a collection of signs and symptoms attributable to a known medical condition. Unfortunately medicine does not often recognize a condition until it has progressed to a full-blown syndrome. By that time you have probably already suffered considerable disruption to your life and well being. A syndrome may require much more extensive treatment to reverse than early symptoms. With the help of this book you will be able to detect early symptoms before they turn into a full-blown adrenal fatigue syndrome. You will learn what you can do to prevent those symptoms from becoming more severe and to reduce or eliminate them. I also hope that you will gain the understanding needed to protect yourself from adrenal fatigue in the future.

Disease and Health Conditions Associated with Hypoadrenia

Because the adrenals are the glands of stress, they are involved in the processes of and recovery from most chronic diseases. The reason for this is simple. Most chronic disease is stressful. The processes that take place in chronic diseases from arthritis to cancer pull on the adrenals as

more and more demand is made upon the body by the disease. Therefore, take it as a general rule that if someone is suffering from a chronic
disease and morning fatigue is one of their symptoms, the adrenals are
likely involved. In any disease or disease process in which the medical
treatment includes the use of corticosteroids, diminished adrenal function is most likely a component of that disease process. All corticosteroids are designed to imitate the actions of cortisol, a hormone secreted
by the adrenals, and so the need for them arises primarily when the
adrenals are not providing the required amounts of cortisol. If the cortisol response is appropriate, there is little need for the external synthetic
drugs that imitate its action, except in extreme instances.

**There are a few diseases that particularly stand out as having an
adrenal component.** Chronic fatigue syndrome, fibromyalgia,
alcoholism, ischemic heart disease, hypoglycemia, rheumatoid arthritis
and chronic and recurrent respiratory infections all usually involve
decreased adrenal function. In the cases of chronic fatigue syndrome
and fibromyalgia, substantial evidence is now emerging that these
syndromes may result from unusual infectious microorganisms that are
not detected by the typical laboratory tests. Special, sophisticated lab
tests such as polymerase chain reaction (PCR) tests can, however, detect
these invaders. A growing number of peer reviewed papers are now
confirming the presence of these microorganisms in these particular
illnesses. Once they have been detected, the proper treatment can be
given. Often there are two or more microorganisms associated with the
same syndrome and both have to be eliminated before recovery can be
expected. These pathogenic microorganisms act as a tremendous body
burden, draining adrenal resources. Simultaneously eradicating these
infectious agents from the body, while providing adequate adrenal support
will greatly facilitate recovery in these often profoundly debilitating cases.

Adrenal fatigue often precedes a syndrome such as chronic fatigue,
fibromyalgia and some cases of alcoholism. The immune weakness that
results from altered adrenal function sets the stage for easier infection or
greater debilitation. In many alcoholics, adrenal fatigue and the resulting
hypoglycemia predispose the person to a compulsive desire for alcohol.
In other cases of alcoholism, the adrenals become fatigued by the continual
use of alcohol. In either case, adrenal fatigue is an intimate component
of most alcoholism. Adrenal support greatly enhances the treatment

protocol for alcoholism. See the section entitled "Drinks To Avoid" for more detail.

Chronic and recurrent bronchitis, pneumonia and other chronic lung and bronchial diseases typically have an adrenal fatigue component. This includes many cases of asthma, influenza and allergies. This relationship appears to be both causal and resultant. That is, frequent respiratory ailments can lead to adrenal fatigue and adrenal fatigue leaves a predilection toward developing respiratory problems. The association between adrenal function and respiratory infection was first written about in 1898, but by the mid 1930's physicians apprised of the importance of the adrenals in resistance to infection and to overall health were also aware of the relationship of the adrenals to chronic and recurrent respiratory problems. Later it became known that even the proper development of the lungs in the fetus is dependent upon an adequate amount of adrenal hormones, especially cortisol. If there is a lack of cortisol from the adrenals in the fetus during development, the lungs don't develop properly and early problems in the lungs are more frequent and more serious.

The tip-off that there is a low adrenal component to any of these illnesses is a longer than normal recovery period with decreased stamina and excess fatigue. When these symptoms are present, adrenal fatigue is likely a component of the symptom picture, no matter the cause.

If the number of health conditions given above seems long and several of the symptoms seem familiar, you are getting the picture. Adrenal fatigue is a generally unrecognized component in many types of health problems ranging from bothersome to life threatening. To close this chapter, here is a quote from one of the most recognized authorities on clinical manifestations of adrenal dysfunction, Dr. John Tintera. "For the sake of credibility, we have previously stated that about 16% of the population has some moderate-to-severe degree of hypoadrenocorticism [adrenal fatigue] with hypoglycemia but in actuality, the figure should read 67% if all the arthritics, asthmatics and hay fever sufferers, alcoholics and all other related groups are included." (Tintera'69)

Chapter 7

Why Medicine Has Not Recognized Adrenal Fatigue

"Doctor, I think I have hypoadrenia," the patient said. *"I'm exhausted all the time, I'm depressed, and I've had several major traumas in the last four years – a serious car accident plus two surgeries, one for ovarian cancer and one for an Achilles tendon rupture. I haven't been the same since. The least little thing just flattens me." "Hypoadrenia?"* the doctor replied. *"What's hypoadrenia? I've had 12 years of medical school and I've never heard of it. Let me do the diagnosing here."* – Quote from a patient recalling her first encounter with a doctor concerning her adrenal fatigue.

Diagnoses of Low Adrenal Function Lost to Modern Medicine

Adrenal fatigue, under many different names, has been recognized, written about, discussed and treated for over one hundred years. It has been dealt with by thousands of doctors, both personally and clinically. Yet today, it is still not taught in medical schools. The average physician is therefore unaware of its presence and so, not surprisingly, seldom looks for it. Even endocrinologists (specialists in treating disorders of the endocrine glands, which include the adrenal glands) rarely recognize adrenal fatigue as a distinct condition or are prepared to treat it. This is why it is important that you become informed yourself. You may not find help in the places you would usually expect to. Low adrenal function is one of those problems that have become invisible to modern medicine. Despite the fact that subclinical hypoadrenia was recognized as a distinct syndrome earlier in the 20th century, there is little acknowledgment of it today. With only a few rare exceptions, the only form of hypoadrenia recognized by medicine is Addison's disease. Addison's disease and Cushing's disease (extremely high levels of cortisol caused mostly by steroid drugs) are covered in medical texts and lectures, but adrenal fatigue, a condition that affects many more people than Addison's and Cushing's combined, is rarely, if ever, mentioned.

The Influence of the Pharmaceutical and Insurance Industries on Medicine

It provides interesting, albeit disturbing, insight into the orientation of modern health care systems to look at why conventional medicine has forgotten or dismissed this low adrenal syndrome as non-existent. In fifty years the tremendous influence of pharmaceutical and insurance companies has completely altered the practice of medicine and, as a result, the emphasis in physician training and health care has changed radically. A doctor's acute skills of observation, physical examination and deductive reasoning, which used to be considered his most essential diagnostic tools, have now been replaced by reliance on narrowly interpreted lab tests and lists of numerical diagnoses allowable by insurance plans. The health insurance industry has forced the entire practice of medicine to restrict itself to pre-approved numbered codes for both the diagnosis and the treatment of all health conditions. Drugs or surgery are usually the only therapies offered by modern medicine, even when they are inappropriate. So if an illness does not show up clearly on a lab test or fit a diagnostic code, and if there is no known surgical or drug treatment for the symptoms, then it is as though the problem is not real.

Medical doctors of today are constricted by medical licensing boards, the health insurance and pharmaceutical industries, and their patients' expectations of quick recovery. As a result of these influences and a certain bias in their training, they think and practice primarily pharmaceutical medicine, seeking to prescribe the appropriate drug for the condition. Because of the ever-present threat of a malpractice suit and the conservative influence of peer review boards, medical doctors have become much less willing and able to try something different to help their patients. Malpractice is not decided just on the basis of the harm suffered by the patient, but on the consensus of the medical profession about what would be "proper" procedure in that particular situation. So, to protect themselves, most doctors have become much more orthodox in their practice of medicine. Their training no longer prepares them to explore beyond lab tests or routine signs and symptoms, nor do they often, if ever, consider truly alternative therapies. It has become unrewarding and down right dangerous to do any real thinking when it comes to diagnosis and treatment.

In addition to the fact that medical training is now dependent on huge pharmaceutical corporations for funding, modern medicine is currently in the stranglehold of insurance companies. Under our present medical system, most physicians' incomes come primarily from insurance companies. Paperwork created by the insurance industry and licensing boards that is required of therapists, physicians, clinics and hospitals demands that each patient be given what is called an "ICD" (International Classification of Disease) code for their medical condition. This ICD code puts a name on your disease or condition. No one can fit in the cracks. You must have an ICD code to classify your illness. Despite the fact that it is absurd to assume that all patients will fit into a description found in some pre-designed code-book, everyone is required to have an ICD. If there is no ICD the financial medicine wheel quickly comes to a halt for that patient and for the doctor treating them. Records are incomplete without these codes and bills cannot be submitted to insurance companies without them. Consequently, physicians must identify the patient's diagnosis with an ICD code or the insurance companies will not pay them. As you might already have guessed, there is no ICD code for adrenal fatigue and the code for hypoadrenia is usually reserved for Addison's disease. Patients also depend on the insurance companies to pay for whatever therapy they receive, but an insurance company will only pay for certain therapies that are approved as appropriate for each ICD code (diagnosis). If the doctor does not use an approved therapy for his diagnostic (ICD) code, there will be no payment. Without insurance coverage of the costs, most patients as well as most doctors are unwilling to proceed with any medical treatment. As a result, adrenal fatigue rarely gets treated, even if the physician knows it exists.

The Lab Tests of Adrenal Function Do Not Diagnose Adrenal Fatigue

Hypoadrenia means Addison's disease to most doctors. Therefore the only tests they run to detect hypoadrenia are the tests for Addison's disease. This puts you in a "no-win" situation. If you present your symptoms to your doctor, he may think your symptoms do not justify running the tests since they are not severe enough to signify Addison's disease. If your doctor does run the lab tests, you probably will not test positive for Addison's disease and so you will be pronounced "healthy" and dismissed. If you suggest an alternative test, such as a saliva test for hormone levels that could pick up signs of non-Addison's hypoadrenia, chances are your doctor has never heard of hormone saliva tests. If he has, he may not know that they are as accurate and valid as blood tests, but more sensitive, or that they have been verified and written up in scientific papers and are accepted by many insurance plans. He will probably dismiss the test's usefulness even though it is a very valuable diagnostic tool for adrenal fatigue. Either way you lose. Unless you have an exceptional doctor, you may come away discouraged, doubting your own symptoms, humiliated for having taken any initiative concerning your health, and possibly with a prescription for tranquilizers or an appointment with a psychiatrist.

The Medical Establishment Dismisses Knowledge Provided By Alternative Medicine

The bond between medicine and the pharmaceutical and insurance industries has created a nearly unbreakable medical establishment that undermines the development of any other form of healthcare, including self-help. Until 1992, members of the American Medical Association (AMA) were even forbidden to associate in any way with practitioners of alternative medicine ("quacks," as the AMA called them). Even now most medical doctors continue to eschew alternative medicine as inferior to their professional standards. Information about such wide-ranging topics as therapeutic nutrition, oriental medicine and herbology is frequently suppressed or dismissed as unsubstantiated. This is unfortunate since these areas of learning have much useful knowledge about health and illness that does not fall within the narrow confines of acceptable "modern" medicine.

All of these factors negatively affect people suffering from adrenal fatigue. Despite the fact that every doctor's office frequently sees patients presenting with symptoms of low adrenal function, doctors do not check for it. If it has no ICD code, it simply does not exist. The vignette at the beginning of this chapter was a true incident, written by a woman recounting what she experienced when she consulted a doctor for adrenal fatigue. This did not take place in a small town located in some remote area, but occurred in a fashionable and supposedly progressive women's clinic in Malibu, California. It is an all too painful illustration that even when patients are well informed enough to request testing for mild hypoadrenia, it is probable that their doctors will only think in terms of

Addison's disease or nothing. It is even more rare for physicians to offer patients the available natural therapies for this condition.

Another good example of this is Karen, a medical writer. While writing an article about adrenal fatigue, she became aware that she had many of the symptoms of adrenal fatigue. She consulted her doctor about her suspicions and suggested she be tested for it. Instead of acknowledging that she presented clear symptoms of low adrenal function, he dismissed the notion and told her to, "Go home, get married and have a baby." If Karen had followed this advice instead of trusting her own intuition that something truly was wrong, she would have become even more severely depleted from the extra strain that marriage, pregnancy and motherhood would have put on her adrenals.

In short, from the doctors' point of view, this is just another health fad. Why should they worry about it, even if they do hear complaints about these same symptoms every day in their offices? If it does exist, the tests they use do not test for it and the treatments they use do not alleviate it.

The next chapter contains an adrenal fatigue questionnaire I have developed in conjunction with other health minded doctors over the last 20 plus years. It has proven its worth countless times and continues to be a valuable clinical tool. If you are reading this book because you suspect you, or someone you care about, suffers from adrenal fatigue, the questionnaire will reliably help you determine if you and/or your loved ones suffer from adrenal fatigue, and if so, how severe it is.

Part Two

Do I Have Adrenal Fatigue?

Chapter 8

Completing the Questionnaire

The following questionnaire is the most important tool in this book for determining if you have hypoadrenia (adrenal fatigue). In conjunction with other doctors over the past 2 decades, I have compiled the indications of adrenal fatigue covered by this questionnaire. Although it has not been standardized, I have found it to be extremely valuable clinically and it has consistently proved its worth time after time. It covers most of the signs and symptoms that are indicators of adrenal fatigue. Your answers to the questions will create a picture of how functional or dysfunctional your adrenal glands are and will help you to determine possible sources of this problem in your life.

Often adrenal fatigue becomes more extreme after a significant event such as an accident, surgery, illness or emotional trauma. Therefore, it is helpful when answering the questionnaire to think about the last time you felt well and the circumstances surrounding it. It is not critical that you have an exact date in mind, but a relative period after which your health began to deteriorate. If there is no particular time after which you noticed a change, do not worry about it. Adrenal fatigue frequently comes on gradually with no identifiable date of onset.

Instructions
The questionnaire is easy to take. Simply read each statement, decide its degree of severity, and then place the appropriate number beside each statement. Note that 0 stands for never or rarely, 1 is occasionally or slightly, 2 is moderate in frequency and intensity, and 3 is severe, constant and/or interferes with your daily living. There may be some statements you feel like putting a 5 beside. However, resist this temptation and only put 3 as the maximum value. Otherwise it confuses the final scoring. Try to be as objective as possible; mark a symptom how it really is rather than worse or better than it is. The more objective you can be about yourself, the more realistic will be your outcome. Do not labor over any one statement as the cumulative score is what is most important.

One column in the questionnaire is titled "Past" and one "Now." The past refers to your life before the date you entered under "The last time I felt well." If you cannot determine a specific date, then pick a relative time after which your symptoms seemed to noticeably worsen. Write this date at the top of the "Past" column so that you do not forget it. All your responses in the "Past" column will be about how you felt <u>before</u> that date. The "Now" column is not necessarily about today, but about how you feel generally now, in this present time frame or since the date you entered at the top of the "Past" column.

After you have completed the questionnaire, you will add the numbers in each column, as directed, to find your total scores. Then you will go on to the "Interpreting the Questionnaire" section to determine the state of your adrenal health.

You might find that you have some symptoms not mentioned in this questionnaire. It is not meant to be exhaustive but it adequately covers enough symptoms and signs to accurately determine the presence and the degree of adrenal fatigue. This questionnaire has proven itself extremely useful clinically over the past 20 years. Remember that this questionnaire is for your benefit. The more accurate and objective you can be, the more valuable will be your results. If you answer the questionnaire honestly, your answers will not only help you to determine your degree of adrenal fatigue, but will also give you useful information and insight into your present condition.

Adrenal Questionnaire

Today's Date: _12/11/07_

Instructions: Please enter the appropriate response number to each statement in the columns below.

0 = Never / Rarely
1 = Occasionally / Slightly
2 = Moderate in Intensity or Frequency
3 = Intense / Severe or Frequent

I have not felt well since _FEB_ when _2006_
                (date)   (describe event, if any)

Predisposing Factors
Past Now

1 _1½_ _1_ I have experienced long periods of stress that have affected my well being.
2 _2_ _2_ I have had one or more severely stressful events that have affected my well being.
3 _1_ _0_ I have driven myself to exhaustion.
4 _0_ _0_ I overwork with little play or relaxation for extended periods.
5 _0_ _0_ I have had extended, severe or recurring respiratory infections.
6 _0_ _0_ I have taken long term or intense steroid therapy (corticosteroids).
7 _1_ _1_ I tend to gain weight, especially around the middle (spare tire).
8 _0_ _0_ I have a history of alcoholism &/or drug abuse.
9 _0_ _0_ I have environmental sensitivities.
10 _0_ _0_ I have diabetes (type II, adult onset, NIDDM).
11 _0_ _0_ I suffer from post traumatic distress syndrome.
12 _0_ _0_ I suffer from anorexia.*
13 _2_ _2_ I have one or more other chronic illnesses or diseases.
   _1½_ _6_ **Total**

Key Signs & Symptoms

Past Now

	Past	Now	
1	2	2	My ability to handle stress and pressure has decreased.
2	3	3	I am less productive at work.
3	2	2	I seem to have decreased in cognitive ability. I don't think as clearly as I used to.
4	3	3	My thinking is confused when hurried or under pressure.
5	2	2	I tend to avoid emotional situations.
6	2	2	I tend to shake or am nervous when under pressure.
7	1	1	I suffer from nervous stomach indigestion when tense.
8	1	1	I have many unexplained fears / anxieties.
9	3	3	My sex drive is noticeably less than it used to be.
10	2	2	I get lightheaded or dizzy when rising rapidly from a sitting or lying position.
11	1	1	I have feelings of graying out or blacking out.
12	1	1	I am chronically fatigued; a tiredness that is not usually relieved by sleep.*
13	1/2	1 1/2	I feel unwell much of the time.
14	0	0	I notice that my ankles are sometimes swollen – the swelling is worse in the evening.
15	3	3	I usually need to lie down or rest after sessions of psychological or emotional pressure/stress.
16	3	3	My muscles sometimes feel weaker than they should.
17	0	0	My hands and legs get restless – experience meaningless body movements.
18	0	0	I have become allergic or have increased frequency/ severity of allergic reactions.
19	0	0	When I scratch my skin, a white line remains for a minute or more.
20			Small irregular dark brown spots have appeared on my forehead, face, neck and shoulders.
21	2	2	I sometimes feel weak all over.*
22	2	2	I have unexplained and frequent headaches.
23	2	2	I am frequently cold.
24	2	2	I have decreased tolerance for cold.*
25	2	2	I have low blood pressure.*
26	2	2	I often become hungry, confused, shaky or somewhat paralyzed under stress.

27 __0__ __0__ I have lost weight without reason while feeling very tired and listless.

28 __1__ __1__ I have feelings of hopelessness or despair.

29 __1__ __1__ I have decreased tolerance. People irritate me more.

30 _____ _____ The lymph nodes in my neck are frequently swollen (I get swollen glands on my neck).

31 __0__ __0__ I have times of nausea and vomiting for no apparent reason.*

__45__ __45__ **Total**

Energy Patterns

Past Now

1 __1__ __1__ I often have to force myself in order to keep going. Everything seems like a chore.

2 __1__ __3__ I am easily fatigued.

3 __2__ __2__ I have difficulty getting up in the morning (don't really wake up until about 10:00 AM).

4 __2__ __3__ I suddenly run out of energy.

5 __1__ __1__ I usually feel much better and fully awake after the noon meal.

6 __3__ __3__ I often have an afternoon low between 3:00-5:00 PM.

7 __2__ __2__ I get low energy, moody or foggy if I do not eat regularly.

8 __0__ __0__ I usually feel my best after 6:00 PM.

9 __1__ __1__ I am often tired at 9:00-10:00 PM, but resist going to bed.

10 __0__ __0__ I like to sleep late in the morning.

11 __0__ __0__ My best, most refreshing sleep often comes between 7:00-9:00 AM.

12 __0__ __0__ I often do my best work late at night (early in the morning).

13 __0__ __0__ If I don't go to bed by 11:00 PM, I get a second burst of energy around 11:00 PM, often lasting until 1:00-2:00 AM.

__13__ __14__ **Total**

Frequently Observed Events

    Past Now

1 _O_ _O_ I get coughs/colds that stay around for several weeks.

2 _O_ _O_ I have frequent or recurring bronchitis, pneumonia or other respiratory infections.

3 _O_ _O_ I get asthma, colds and other respiratory involvements two or more times per year.

4 _O_ _O_ I frequently get rashes, dermatitis, or other skin conditions.

5 _O_ _O_ I have rheumatoid arthritis.

6 _O_ _O_ I have allergies to several things in the environment.

7 _O_ _O_ I have multiple chemical sensitivities.

8 _O_ _O_ I have chronic fatigue syndrome.

9 _3_ _3_ I get pain in the muscles of my upper back and lower neck for no apparent reason.

10 _2_ _2_ I get pain in the muscles on the sides of my neck.

11 _O_ _2_ I have insomnia or difficulty sleeping.

12 _O_ _O_ I have fibromyalgia.

13 _O_ _O_ I suffer from asthma.

14 _O_ _O_ I suffer from hay fever.

15 _2_ _O_ I suffer from nervous breakdowns.

16 _O_ _O_ My allergies are becoming worse (more severe, frequent or diverse).

17 ____ ____ The fat pads on palms of my hands and/or tips of my fingers are often red.

18 _1_ _1_ I bruise more easily than I used to.

19 ____ ____ I have a tenderness in my back near my spine at the bottom of my rib cage when pressed.

20 ____ ____ I have swelling under my eyes upon rising that goes away after I have been up for a couple of hours.

    _9_ _9_

The next 2 questions are for women only

    Past Now

21 _____ _____ I have increasing symptoms of premenstrual syndrome (PMS) such as cramps, bloating, moodiness, irritability, emotional instability, headaches, tiredness, and/or intolerance before my period (only some of these need be present).

22 _____ _____ My periods are generally heavy but they often stop, or almost stop, on the fourth day, only to start up profusely on the 5th or 6th day.

    _____ _____ **Total**

Food Patterns

    Past Now

1 _2_ _1_ I need coffee or some other stimulant to get going in the morning.

2 _1_ _1_ I often crave food high in fat and feel better with high fat foods.

3 _0_ _0_ I use high fat foods to drive myself.

4 _2_ _0_ I often use high fat foods and caffeine containing drinks (coffee, colas, chocolate) to drive myself.

5 _2_ _2_ I often crave salt and/or foods high in salt. I like salty foods.

6 _____ _____ I feel worse if I eat high potassium foods (like bananas, figs, raw potatoes), especially if I eat them in the morning.

7 _2_ _1_ I crave high protein foods (meats, cheeses).

8 _3_ _1_ I crave sweet foods (pies, cakes, pastries, doughnuts, dried fruits, candies or desserts).

9 _3_ _3_ I feel worse if I miss or skip a meal.

    _15_ _9_ **Total**

Aggravating Factors

    Past Now

1 _1_ _1_ I have constant stress in my life or work.

2 __1__ __0__ My dietary habits tend to be sporadic and unplanned.
3 __0__ __0__ My relationships at work and/or home are unhappy.
4 __0__ __0__ I do not exercise regularly.
5 __0__ __0__ I eat lots of fruit.
6 __0__ __0__ My life contains insufficient enjoyable activities.
7 __0__ __0__ I have little control over how I spend my time.
8 __0__ __0__ I restrict my salt intake.
9 __0__ __0__ I have gum and/or tooth infections or abscesses.
10 __0__ __0__ I have meals at irregular times.
__1__ _____ **Total**

Relieving Factors

Past Now

1 __3__ __3__ I feel better almost right away once a stressful situation
is resolved.
2 __3__ __3__ Regular meals decrease the severity of my symptoms.
3 __2__ __1__ I often feel better after spending a night out with friends.
4 __3__ __3__ I often feel better if I lie down.
5 _____ _____ Other relieving factors _____
_____

__11__ __10__ **Total**

Scoring and Interpretation of the Questionnaire

A lot of information can be obtained from this questionnaire. Follow the instructions below carefully to score your questionnaire correctly. Then proceed to the interpretation section.

Total Number of Questions Answered

1. First count the total number of questions in each section that you answered with any number other than zero. Enter the "Past" and "Now" totals separately, entering each in the appropriate boxes for each section of the "Total number of questions answered" scoring chart on the next page. For example, if you answered a total of 21 questions in the "Past" column and 27 questions in the "Now" column of the "**Key Signs and Symptoms**" with a 1,2 or 3, your total number of questions answered score for the "Past" column in that section would be "21" and for the "Now" column would be "27." Note that there are no entries for the first section of the questionnaire entitled **"Predisposing Factors."** This section is dealt with separately and is not included in the summary below. Therefore, your first entry into the summary boxes will be for the "**Key Sign and Symptoms**" section.

2. After you have finished entering the number of questions answered in both columns for each section, sum all the numbers for each column and the total in the "Grand Total - Total Responses" boxes on the bottom row of the scoring chart.

3. All the boxes in the "**Total Number of Questions Answered**" chart should now be filled.

Then go on to the next part of the scoring.

Total Number of Questions Answered

Name of Section	Total Responses	
	Past	Now
Key Signs & Symptoms Number of questions -31	21	21
Energy Patterns Number of questions -13	8	8
Frequently Observed Events Number of questions - 20 for men 22 for women	4	4
Food Patterns Number of questions -9	7	6
Aggravating Factors Number of questions -10	3	1
Relieving Factors Number of questions - 4	4	4
Grand Total - Total Responses	47	44

Total Points:

This part of the scoring adds up the actual numbers (0,1,2 or 3) you put beside the questions when you were answering the questionnaire. Add these numbers for each column in each section and enter them into the appropriate boxes in the chart below. Then, sum each column to get the Total-Points-Past and Total-Points-Now scores. Enter these totals in the bottom 2 boxes to complete this part of the scoring.

Total Points

Name of Section	Total Points	
	Past	**Now**
Key Signs & Symptoms Total points possible -93	43	45
Energy Patterns Total points possible -39	13	14
Frequently Observed Events Total points possible – 60 for men 66 for women	9	9
Food Patterns Total points possible –27	15.	9
Aggravating Factors Total points possible -30	1	
Relieving Factors Total points possible -12	11.	10
Grand Total –Total Points		
Total Responses = Severity	94	37

Interpreting the Questionnaire

The questionnaire is a valuable tool for determining **if** you have adrenal fatigue and, if you do, the **severity** of your syndrome. Of course, the accuracy of its interpretation depends upon you completing every section as accurately and honestly as possible. Because there is such diversity in how individuals experience adrenal fatigue, a wide variety of signs and symptoms have been included. Some people have only the minimal number of symptoms, but the symptoms they do have are severe. Others experience a great number of symptoms, but most of their symptoms are relatively mild. That is why there are two kinds of scores to indicate adrenal fatigue.

Total Number of Questions Answered: This gives you a general "Yes or No" answer to the question, "Do I have adrenal fatigue?" Look at your "Grand Total – Total Responses" scores in the first scoring chart (Total Number of Questions Answered). The purpose of this score is to see the total number of signs and symptoms of adrenal fatigue you have. There are a total of 87 questions for men and 89 questions for women in the questionnaire. If you responded to more than **26** (men) or **32** (women) of the questions, (regardless of which severity response number you gave the question), you have some degree of adrenal fatigue. The greater the number of questions that you responded to, the greater your adrenal fatigue. If you responded affirmatively to less than 20 of the questions, it is unlikely adrenal fatigue is your problem. People who do not have adrenal fatigue may still experience a few of these indicators in their lives, but not many of them. If your symptoms do not include fatigue or decreased ability to handle stress, then you are probably not suffering from adrenal fatigue.

Total Points: The total points are used to determine the degree of severity of your adrenal fatigue. If you ranked every question as 3 (the worst) your total points would be 261 for men and 267 for women. If you scored under **40**, you either have only slight adrenal fatigue or none at all. If you scored between **44-87** for men or **45-88** for women, then overall you have a mild degree of adrenal fatigue. This does not mean that some individual symptoms are not severe, but overall your symptom picture reflects mildly fatigued adrenals. If you scored between **88-130** for men or **89-132** for women, your adrenal fatigue is moderate. If you scored above **130** for men or **132** for women, then consider yourself to be suffering from severe adrenal fatigue. Now compare the total points of the different sections with each other. This allows you to see if 1 or 2 sections stand out as having more signs and symptoms than the others. If you have a predominating group of symptoms, they will be the most useful ones for you to watch as indicators as you improve. Seeing which sections stand out will also be helpful in developing your own recovery program.

Severity Index: The Severity Index is calculated by simply dividing the total points by the total number of questions you answered in the affirmative. It gives an indication of how severely you experience the signs and symptoms, with **1.0 – 1.6** being mild, **1.7 – 2.3** being moderate, and **2.4** on up being severe. This number is especially useful for those who suffer from only a few of these signs and symptoms, but yet are considerably debilitated by them.

Past vs. Now: Now compare the total points in the "Past" column to the total points in the "Now" column. The difference indicates the direction your adrenal health is taking. If the number in the "Past" column is greater than the number in the "Now" column, then you are slowly healing from hypoadrenia. It is a good sign you are healing, but you will still want to read the following chapters to accelerate your improvement. If the number in the "Now" column is greater than the number in the "Past" column, your adrenal glands are on a downhill course and you need to take immediate action to prevent further decline and to recover. Now complete the section below before you finish reading the rest of the book.

Asterisk Total: Finally, add the actual numbers you put beside the questions marked by asterisks (*) for the "Now" column. If this total is more than **9**, you are likely suffering from a relatively severe form of adrenal fatigue. If this total is more than **12**, and you answer **yes** to more than **2** of the questions below, you have many of the indications of true Addison's disease and should consult a physician in addition to doing the things in this book. Be sure to read the section below, "Approaching Your Doctor," as well as other appropriate sections in this book before consulting a physician.

Answer the following questions only if you scored more than 12 on the questions marked with an asterisk (*).

Additional Symptoms (ones that are present now)
The areas on my body listed below have become bluish-black in color.
_____   Inside of lips, mouth
_____   Vagina
_____   Around nipples

_____ I have *frequent* unexplained diarrhea.

_____ I have increased darkening around the bony areas, at folds in my skin, scars and the creases in my joints.

_____ I have light colored patches on my skin where the skin has lost its usual color.

_____ I easily become dehydrated.

_____ I have fainting spells.

Interpretation of the "Predisposing Factors" Section: This section helps determine which factors led to the development of your adrenal fatigue. There may have been only one factor or there may have been several, but the number does not matter. One severely stressful incident can be all it takes for someone to develop adrenal fatigue, although typically it is more. This list is not exhaustive, but the items listed in this section are the most common factors that lead to adrenal fatigue. Use this section to better understand how your adrenal fatigue developed. Seeing how it started often makes clearer what actions you can take to successfully recover from it. This section also leads into a following section that explores in more depth how your adrenal fatigue developed.

Approaching Your Doctor

Now that you have decided that you have some form of adrenal fatigue, it is only natural for you to want to run and tell your doctor. Or you may want to have your doctor do further tests. If you skipped over the last chapter, a word of caution before you share your newfound revelations with him or her. First, your doctor may not believe that adrenal fatigue exists. Second, if he vaguely recognizes the term, he may want to run the test for Addison's disease. Since only 4 in a 100,000 have Addison's disease, chances are you will pass the test and he will conclude that there is nothing wrong with you. He may give you some tranquilizers, send you to a psychiatrist, tell you to quit reading the self-help books, or offer other unhelpful advice. Even many alternative physicians are not yet aware of the problems of adrenal fatigue. Believe it or not, the fact that adrenal fatigue is so common and so pervasive makes it more difficult to recognize. But regardless of what your doctor says, adrenal fatigue is real and the questionnaire in this book is a valuable tool in identifying its presence and severity. Although this book is written for people who have no medical background, it is based on a solid foundation of more than

2,400 scientific and clinical references relating to adrenal fatigue. However, the truly important questions are not how many studies relate to adrenal fatigue or whether or not your doctor recognizes it. The important questions are do you suffer from adrenal fatigue and if so, what can you do about it. To help you answer these questions, read on. The next chapter will help you determine how you came to have adrenal fatigue.

Chapter 9

How Did I Get This Way?

The purpose of this section is to develop a timeline or sequence of events that will reflect how your health may have changed with time, either improving or getting worse. This will help you see with more clarity what has affected your health and which associated events may have led to further problems that have gone unrecognized. Adrenal fatigue reflects the adrenals' inability to respond to stress, but remember that the sources of stress are additive and cumulative over time. Adrenal fatigue is usually preceded and aggravated by multiple events. It is very therapeutic to see how seemingly unrelated events combined to undermine your health.

Completing the "Health History Timeline" is like being a detective in a "who-done-it" mystery. In this case, the crime is the decline in your adrenal health and you are both the star detective and the victim (and sometimes the culprit as well). Your objective is to assemble as much information as possible regarding the events leading up to the crime. The timeline is a very useful tool for uncovering previously unrecognized sources of adrenal fatigue. Recording the events that preceded the onset of your fatigue and putting them in a meaningful, sequential order will help you recognize the contributing factors. The categories listed below are only guidelines for organizing this information. If you think there are other categories or incidents, list them as well. It will be easier to see the patterns of changes in your health with brief entries placed at their appropriate times, even if you want to write pages about an incident, be brief. You are now ready to complete the "Health History Timeline."

Health History Timeline
To complete the "Health History Timeline", review again the date you gave as the last time you felt well. Then start 2 years before this date and list the events as requested in the section below.

When completing this section, just recall the information to the best of your ability. Do not try to associate it with any signs or symptoms of the previous questionnaire. Simply enter it on the lines provided. If you need more space to complete any section, use a separate piece of paper. Remember, you are the most authoritative source of information about you, so now is your chance to be an expert on a subject of great interest and importance to you, **You!**

In the following section, list and date all the accidents, illnesses, emotional traumas, lifestyle changes, etc. that happened within the two years preceding the decline in your health. Even if you do not see any connection between these events and the symptoms you are experiencing now, write them down. There may also be long term, ongoing factors that have not changed. For example, you may have had a poor diet and little exercise for years before an illness or other specific event precipitated your adrenal fatigue. Write these down because, even though they did not begin within the two-year time frame, they were ongoing during that time. Poor dental work can also lead to hypoadrenia. If you have had root canals, amalgam fillings, gum infections, abscesses, teeth pulled or other dental work after which you noticed your health sliding (within 6-12 months), or if there were complications from dental work that seem to persist, it is important to list these. The mouth is an extremely important, but often unrecognized, factor in your overall health. In some cases it has been the pivotal key to health. The timeline can provide surprising information to help you recover. Like many things, the more you put into it, the more benefit you will receive.

Health History Timeline

Surgeries:
Date: _____ Incident: _____
Date: _____ Incident: _____
Date: _____ Incident: _____

Hospital visits:
Date: _____ Incident: _____
Date: _____ Incident: _____
Date: _____ Incident: _____

Sicknesses: severe colds, flu, bronchitis, pneumonia, severe sore throat, and other infectious diseases; accidents, injuries or incidences of severe pain; long term disorders (degenerative, chronic, or auto-immune)
Date: _____ Incident: _____
Date: _____ Incident: _____
Date: _____ Incident: _____

Dental work: root canals, implants, gum disease, extensive amalgam restorations (silver fillings)
Date: _____ Incident: _____
Date: _____ Incident:

_____
Date: _____ Incident: _____

Emotional events: lost job, moving, changing jobs, death of close friend or relative, separation, divorce, financial difficulties, shocks, traumas.
Date: _____ Incident: _____
Date: _____ Incident: _____
Date: _____ Incident: _____

Prescription or over the counter medication/recreational drugs: adverse reaction to, unpleasant side effects of, or chronic intake
Date: _____ Incident: _____
Date: _____ Incident: _____
Date: _____ Incident: _____

Other incidents:

Date: _____ Incident: _____

Date: _____ Incident: _____

Date: _____ Incident: _____

Now that you have completed the "Health History Timeline", review the entire list and number the events sequentially by date. For example, if your accident happened in June of 1996, your surgery in August of 1996, you lost your job in February of 1997, and had a root canal in April of 1997, number them 1-4 in the order in which they occurred. Then go back and circle any events that stick out in your mind. These would be events after which you seemed to feel particularly tired or required an extended period of time to recuperate. The first events after which these symptoms occurred are likely to be the onset of your adrenal fatigue. The events before it probably helped precipitate it and the events afterward helped intensify it. Having the knowledge of how your adrenal fatigue began is often valuable in your treatment plan and is psychologically very gratifying. It takes away the impression that you were walking along one day and adrenal fatigue fell out of the sky and hit you. Instead it allows you to see that your adrenal fatigue had an origin and that you can identify the probable source. This immediately places you in a more powerful position.

Adrenal fatigue often comes in stages and its onset can only really be seen when you review the series of seemingly unrelated events leading up to the fatigue. Look and see if there is a pattern to the events that preceded your adrenal fatigue. If so, recall in detail how you felt after each of the events and make a few notes concerning your recollection of the times after those events. If it was after an accident, injury, surgery, or chemical poisoning that your energy became especially low or you developed many of the symptoms of adrenal fatigue (see questionnaire), you may never have recovered completely from that experience. In that case you may need to do further healing related to that event to completely recover from your adrenal fatigue. If so, be sure to look at the chapter titled "Trouble-shooting."

The next chapter explains how to do several different types of self-tests you can do yourself to further determine if your adrenal glands are under-functioning.

Chapter 10

Tests for Adrenal Fatigue You Can Do at Home

Iris contraction

"When exploring the pupil area reflex, I found that in the iris of these cases [adrenal insufficiency], although reacting readily to light, the contraction [of the iris] was flabby, lazy, in a word asthenic. By making the patient look at the light we see that immediately after the initial miosis the pupil starts to dilate slowly as if it does not want to, seems to try to contract again but the dilation gains the upper hand and, after a fight between miosis and mydriasis lasting for about 40 seconds, the pupil remains dilated in spite of the persistence of the exciting agent [the light]. This sign is consistent and present in all cases of hypoadrenia in all of its clinical forms. In the normal individual, it does not appear as I have investigated. All patients presenting this sign, which I should like to call asthenocoria, have been benefited by suprarenal medication" (Arroyo, CF. Med. Jour. and Rac., Jan. 2, 1924. cxix, pg. 25.

The quote above describes Dr. Arroyo's discovery in 1924 of a very useful method for detecting adrenal fatigue. You can do this test at home yourself. The only equipment you need is a chair, a small flashlight or penlight, a mirror, a watch with a second hand and a dark room. Darken the room and sit in a chair in front of a mirror. (See illustration "Iris Contraction Test for Hypoadrenia"). Then shine a flashlight across one eye (not directly into it) from the side of your head. Keep the light shining steadily across one eye and watch in the mirror with the other.

IRIS CONTRACTION TEST FOR HYPOADRENIA

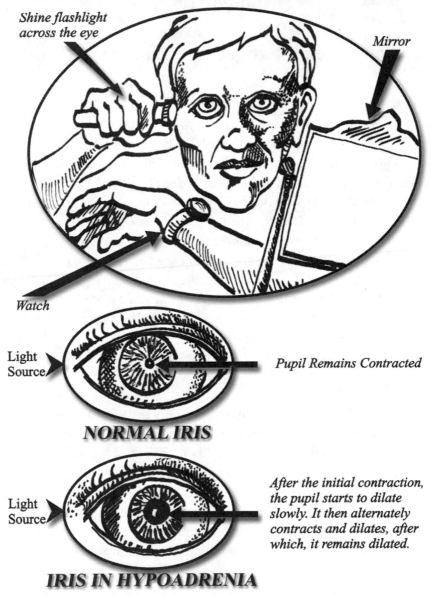

Shine flashlight across the eye

Mirror

Watch

Light Source → **NORMAL IRIS** → Pupil Remains Contracted

Light Source → **IRIS IN HYPOADRENIA** → *After the initial contraction, the pupil starts to dilate slowly. It then alternately contracts and dilates, after which, it remains dilated.*

You should see your pupil (the dark circle in the center of the eye) contract immediately as the light hits your eye. This occurs because the iris, a tiny circular muscle composed of small muscle fibers, contracts and dilates the pupil in response to light. Just like any muscle, after it has been exercised beyond normal capacity, it likes to have a rest.

The pupil normally remains contracted in the increased light. But if you have some form of hypoadrenia, the pupil will not be able to hold its contraction and will dilate despite the light shining on it. This dilation will take place within 2 minutes and will last for about 30-45 seconds before it recovers and contracts again. Time how long the dilation lasts with the second hand on the watch and record it along with the date. After you do this once, let the eye rest. If you have any difficulty doing this on yourself, do it with a friend. Have a friend shine the light across your eye while both of you watch the pupil size.

Retest monthly. If your eye indicates you are suffering from adrenal fatigue, this also serves as an indicator of recovery. As you recover from adrenal fatigue, the iris will hold its contraction and the pupil will remain small for longer. This diminished ability of the iris to remain contracted is present in moderate to severe adrenal fatigue, but may not be present in mild cases.

Low Blood Pressure and Postural Low Blood Pressure
"Hypoadrenia ordinarily spells hypotension" (Harrower, Henry R. Endocrine Diagnostic Charts. Harrower Laboratory, Inc. Glendale, California, 1929, pg. 79).

Blood pressure is an important indicator of adrenal function. Although there are other causes associated with low blood pressure, low adrenal function is probably the most common and the most neglected by doctors.

If your blood pressure drops when you stand up from a lying position, this almost always indicates low adrenals. This drop in blood pressure upon rising is called postural hypotension and can easily be measured at home. All you need is a blood pressure gauge (called a sphygmomanometer) from a local drug store, medical supply house, or on the internet. Get the type that takes your blood pressure for you without requiring a separate stethoscope. Some also have convenient printed readouts. After you know how to use your blood pressure measuring device, lie down quietly for about 10 minutes and then take your blood pressure while still lying down. (See illustration "Blood Pressure Test for Adrenal Fatigue"). Next, stand up and measure your blood pressure right after you stand. Normally blood pressure will rise 10-20mmHg

(mmHg = millimeters of mercury, the unit of measurement for blood pressure) just from standing up. If it drops when you stand up, you likely have some form of hypoadrenia or you may be dehydrated. If so, try it again on a day when you have had plenty of water. It will not work to just drink a glass of water and then try again right away because your tissues take a while to re-hydrate after drinking. If it still drops 10 mmHg or more when you are sure you are not dehydrated, you probably have some form of hypoadrenia. The more severe the drop is, the more severe is the hypoadrenia. An associated dizziness or lightheadedness may also be present when you stand, so do this test with someone beside you or have something you can grab on to in case you become dizzy or light headed.

BLOOD PRESSURE TEST FOR ADRENAL FATIGUE

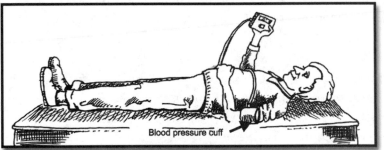

1. Lie down for 3 to 5 minutes rest. Take blood pressure while lying down.

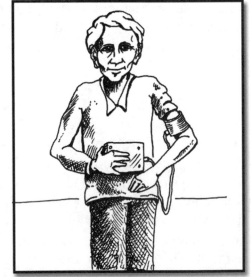

2. Stand and take blood pressure again. Blood pressure should rise 10 to 20mmHg or at least stay the same. In Adrenal Fatigue, the blood pressure will drop when standing from a lying position.

If you discover you are one of the many people with adrenal fatigue and low blood pressure, you should find your blood pressure increasing to normal as you follow the program in this book. Your lightheadedness and other related symptoms will also disappear as your adrenal health improves. Do not stop the program in the fear that it will get too high. Low blood pressure is no more desirable than high blood pressure. Just keep monitoring yourself and if your blood pressure starts to be consistently above 140/90 while lying down, then you will need to investigate the reasons for this abnormal elevation. Occasionally, someone can have high or normal blood pressure and still have hypoadrenia. This is usually due to the lack of elasticity in the arteries seen in atherosclerosis (hardening of the arteries). If your questionnaire indicates adrenal fatigue, but your blood pressure is elevated, consult an alternative doctor for the possibility of hardening of the arteries.* The recommended program in this book is safe for people who, for certain reasons, have high blood pressure despite having low adrenal function. This program does not produce high blood pressure. Rather it helps to normalize blood pressure by strengthening the adrenals. As your adrenals strengthen, your blood pressure will come back to normal so that when you stand up from a lying position it will actually rise 10-20 mmHg and you will no longer become lightheaded.

Note that if you are a complete vegetarian, your blood pressure may normally be around 95/65. If so, then your lower overall blood pressure does not necessarily mean you have hypoadrenia. However, a drop in blood pressure upon standing up from a lying position will still indicate hypoadrenia.

---

* The American College for the Advancement of Medicine (ACAM) specializes in training doctors to help atherosclerosis. You will find a list of doctors at their website at **www.acam.com**.

Sergent's White Line (present in about 40% of people with adrenal fatigue)

This test was first described in 1917 by a French physician named Emile Sergent, as a simple test for low adrenal function that is still useful today. To do this test, simply take the dull end of a ballpoint pen and lightly stroke the skin of your abdomen, making a mark about 6" long. Within a few seconds a line will appear. In a normal reaction, the mark made by the pen is initially white but reddens within a few seconds. If you have hypoadrenia, the line will stay white for about two minutes and will also widen. This test, although not always positive in people with hypoadrenia (about 40% of cases), is a slam dunk confirmation of the presence of hypoadrenia.

It is best to do all three tests: the iris contraction, blood pressure lying and standing, and Sergent's white line test. The first two are reliable indicators found in nearly every moderate to severe case of adrenal fatigue, but often not in mild cases. Sergent's white line is only present in moderate to severe hypoadrenia and, in borderline cases, may only be present when the adrenals are at a low ebb. Again, the questionnaire can be your guide, especially in mild cases because symptoms of adrenal fatigue usually precede signs.

In addition to these self-tests, there is a relatively new laboratory test that can be extremely useful for diagnosing and monitoring adrenal fatigue, if used properly. The next chapter will give you the information you need to have this lab test done correctly.

Chapter 11

Laboratory Tests for Adrenal Fatigue

None of the standard laboratory tests typically used by most doctors are designed to detect adrenal fatigue in its varying degrees of severity. (For more on this topic see the section below on "Problems in the Interpretation of Laboratory Tests.") Although it is possible to use several standard blood and urine tests to look for indications of hypoadrenia, their interpretation is inexact. The "normal" range for adrenal function on standard blood and urine tests includes everything but the most severe cases of adrenal malfunction, such as Addison's disease (extreme low) and Cushing's Syndrome (extreme high). So unless your hypoadrenia is this severe, your doctor will interpret your test results as indicating your adrenal function to be within the normal range.

However, there is a relatively new lab test that accurately measures several hormones, and is especially useful for measuring several of the adrenal hormones. It is called saliva hormone testing.

Saliva Hormone Testing

Saliva hormone testing measures the amounts of various hormones in your saliva instead of in your blood or urine. It is the best single lab test available for detecting adrenal fatigue and has several advantages over other lab tests in determining adrenal hormone levels. Saliva hormone levels are more indicative of the amount of hormone inside the cells where hormone reactions take place. Blood, on the other hand, measures hormones circulating outside the cells, and urine measures the spill over of hormones out of the blood and into the urine. Although blood and urine hormone tests have their uses, neither of them correlates with the hormone levels inside the cells. The level of a hormone circulating in the blood or excreted in the urine does not necessarily reveal how much of that hormone is getting into the cells. However, saliva testing for hormone levels is simple, accurate and reliable, and many studies have confirmed its accuracy as an indicator of the hormone levels within cells.

Besides providing this nice little peek at hormone levels inside the cells, saliva tests are easy to perform. All you have to do is spit into a small vial. The tests are non-invasive (no needles) and you do not even have to go to a laboratory to complete them. This means that they are an extremely useful way to monitor your degree of hypoadrenia and your progress over time because they can be repeated as often as needed. Saliva tests are also less expensive than blood tests for hypoadrenia. They can be done by many health practitioners, other than medical doctors, such as chiropractors and naturopaths, who may not have laboratory privileges in your state, but who perhaps know much more about adrenal fatigue than your family doctor or specialist. Some labs will run this test for you without a physician's signature, so it is possible to order the kit and do the test yourself. You can even obtain a saliva kit by mail and then send it back to the lab from anywhere in the United States. However, unless you know how to interpret a hormone test, it is far better to have a health practitioner familiar with saliva tests and adrenal fatigue do the interpretation for you. The health practitioner's experience and understanding of how particular test results relate to your whole health pattern is something that is difficult to provide yourself. In this case it is important to find a practitioner who has experience with adrenal hormone testing and interpretation, which is unfortunately not a procedure widely known to mainstream doctors.

The best way to determine your particular adrenal hormone (cortisol) levels is to use the saliva test that measures your cortisol levels several times per day. Typically, laboratories testing hormonal content of saliva have test kits that take samples four or more times per day. You merely carry around a few small tubes and, at designated times of the day, you spit into one of the tubes and recap it. The samples usually do not need to be refrigerated and can be sent by mail to the laboratory. For a list of laboratories that do accurate and reliable saliva testing, as well as a list of doctors familiar with this test, see our website at **www.adrenalfatigue.org**. By measuring your saliva hormone levels at least four times per day, you will be able to see for yourself where your cortisol levels are compared to the norms. After you receive your report, you can see whether low cortisol levels are responsible for the feelings of fatigue that you experience during particular times of day. Because saliva hormone levels correlate well with the amount of hormone inside the cells (tissue levels) and samples can be taken as needed without inconvenience or adverse side effects, saliva testing is often more useful than blood or urine testing of hormone levels.

How I Use the Saliva Hormone Tests

I use the saliva hormone test to confirm other signs and symptoms of adrenal fatigue. I start with a saliva cortisol screening test that measures cortisol levels at four different times during the day: between 6:00-8:00 AM (within 1 hour after waking) when cortisol levels are highest; between 11:00-12:00AM; between 4:00-6:00 PM; and between 10:00-12:00 PM. This shows how your cortisol levels vary during the day (something else you cannot easily do with blood or urine tests).

In addition, if I have a patient whose main symptom is fatigue and their questionnaire is inconclusive, or if someone has intermittent symptoms, I use the saliva test to determine if their symptoms are related to low adrenal function. Sometimes I have patients carry around some test vials with them so they can take saliva samples while they are experiencing a low period or other symptoms, at any time during the day. On each saliva sample they write the date and time. They also record, along with the date and time, information on a separate sheet of paper and send the vials off to the lab. When I get their test results back, I compare their saliva cortisol levels with the laboratory standards for the time they are experiencing symptoms. If the cortisol levels are low at those times, we know that low adrenal function is involved in the symptom picture. This gives me a way to assess adrenal activity at the time they were experiencing a symptom.

Another way I like to use the saliva test, when possible, is to compare samples taken when a patient is experiencing an energy high or low with samples taken during a regular day, when the patient is feeling relatively normal (baseline samples). After we have a baseline, these patients carry around some spare vials to take saliva samples at times when they are feeling especially good or especially bad. Again, they record the symptom(s) they were experiencing as well as the date and time (on a separate sheet of paper). They also record the date and time on each vial and send them off to the lab. This is an excellent way to determine whether the lows and highs you experience correspond to relatively low and high cortisol levels. To my knowledge, no other physician uses this method, but it is quite a handy method of determining cortisol levels in relation to symptoms.

I also usually measure DHEA-S levels with the saliva test as well because the adrenals are the primary source of DHEA-S (but not necessarily DHEA). Adrenal fatigue syndrome often involves decreased DHEA-S. The DHEA-S level is a direct indicator of the functioning of the area within the adrenal glands that produces sex hormones (the zona reticularis). Saliva tests for testosterone, the estrogens, progesterone and other hormones can also be done, if needed, and may be of value in working with adrenal fatigue. Testosterone and DHEA-S levels are two of the most reliable indicators of biological age. Testosterone and DHEA-S levels below the reference range for the person's age may be indicators of increased aging. If the cortisol levels are also decreased, the 3 tests together further indicate chronically-decreased adrenal function.

The Effect of Transdermal Hormone Replacement on Lab Results

When using transdermal replacement hormones (hormones applied through the skin, such as progesterone cream), the saliva values for those particular hormones frequently rise out of the testing range. These hormone levels will remain abnormally high on saliva tests until a few months after you stop applying them. Blood tests, on the other hand, will not reflect tissue levels of the transdermally applied hormone creams because the hormones from the creams are transported through the lymph to the cells rather than through the blood. The blood levels will not change even though more hormone is getting into the cells. So if you are using transdermal hormones, neither blood nor saliva test results are accurate indicators of your tissue levels. In this case, your symptoms (or lack of) rather than lab tests are better indicators of your own hormonal output. Symptoms are very closely related to tissue hormone levels of most hormones.

Similarly, if you use topical cortisone or related preparations, it is best to have a period of non-use of 1 week or more to get accurate indicators of tissue cortisol levels from saliva tests. Like progesterone, cortisol and its synthetic analogs used in topical creams can falsely elevate saliva levels.

Problems with the Interpretation of Standard Laboratory Tests in Adrenal Fatigue

If a doctor does not use the saliva hormone tests, piecing together a correct diagnosis of adrenal fatigue from other laboratory tests is more difficult. Most laboratory tests are designed to look for "disease" states in the human body and adrenal fatigue is not a disease per se. In addition, there has never been a reliable urine or blood test that checks for, and can definitively diagnose, mild forms of hypoadrenia. Currently available laboratory tests can be useful in the diagnosis of adrenal fatigue, but they require special training in their interpretation. In fact, common tests done as part of a routine blood work-up can be very useful in the detection of signs of adrenal fatigue if physicians know what to look for. However, standard laboratory tests have certain limitations of which you should be aware.

Laboratory tests are usually based on a population of so-called "healthy" people. But the fundamental flaw in using these tests to diagnose adrenal fatigue is that these "healthy" people were never screened for mild to moderate hypoadrenia themselves. They were only screened for severe hypoadrenia, i.e. Addison's disease. Thus the very standards to which laboratory tests compare patients are faulty from the outset because the population used to standardize the tests may include many people with some level of adrenal fatigue.

Another problem is that laboratory tests are defined and standardized according to statistical norms instead of physiologically optimal norms. That is, test scores are based on math rather than on signs and symptoms. When the adrenal function of a population is tested, all the individual scores are taken and averaged together. The resulting group average, called the "mean," is then used to calculate what is called a probability distribution. In this case the probability distribution is a statistical prediction of how often each score will occur when the adrenal function of a group of people is tested. When all the scores are lumped together, this probability distribution looks like a bell (See illustration "The Normal Bell Curve"). The most frequent scores occur close to the mean, thus forming the dome of the bell. Less frequent scores occur further from the mean and so form the slope and skirt of the bell. Only the highest and lowest 2.5% of the scores are considered to be outside the "normal range" and therefore indicators of actual disease. As a result, this statistical model only catches extreme adrenal dysfunction and misses all the rest.

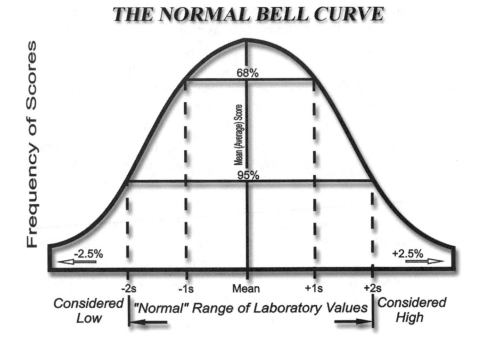

THE NORMAL BELL CURVE

In adrenal function the extreme low is Addison's disease and the extreme high is Cushing's disease. The other 95% represents an enormous variation in levels of adrenal function that is usually disregarded by lab computers and overlooked by doctors because the scores in this range do not fall into either of the two extreme, or "diseased" categories. By default, any scores falling within this wide range (95%) are considered "normal" (See illustration "So-called normal laboratory values for cortisol include all but the most extreme value"). The end result of basing laboratory test scores on statistics rather than on signs and symptoms is that many people who have mild to moderately severe adrenal fatigue are never accurately diagnosed; they look "normal" on the tests. To make matters worse, standards can vary from lab to lab and therefore it is not always possible to even compare the results of one lab with another.

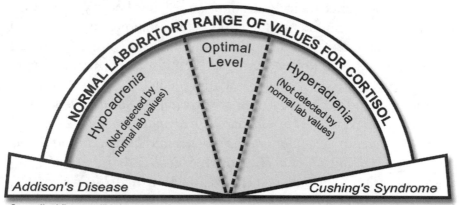

So called "normal" lab values for cortisol include all but the most extreme values

Additionally, standard laboratory tests also do not take into account the important factor of individual biochemical variation. One person's test results can vary significantly from another person's, with both test results being normal (See illustration "Variation in 'Normal' Values Between Individuals").

VARIATION IN "NORMAL" VALUES BETWEEN INDIVIDUALS

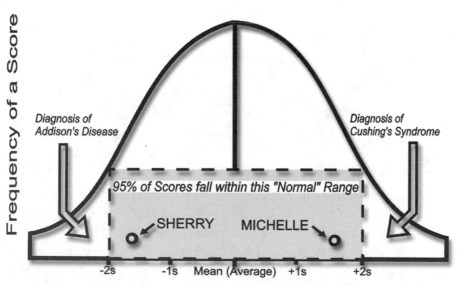

Both test results shown would be considered to have Normal Cortisol Values

This individual variation is not considered when scoring lab tests; you are either inside or outside the normal range. That means that your test score could even drop to ½ its normal value and still fall within the normal range. When your hormones drop to half their normal value, there are definite biochemical changes going on in your body, yet this may never show up as unusual on standard lab tests interpreted in the usual way (See illustration "Individual Variation of Blood Cortisol Values.") This concern has been voiced in one of the most authoritative texts in medicine, <u>Harrison's Principles of Internal Medicine</u>. *"Most hormones have such a broad range of plasma levels within a normal population. As a consequence, the level of a hormone in an individual may be halved or doubled (and thus be abnormal for that person) but still be within the so-called normal range." (Fauci, Anthony S. et al. (Ed). <u>Harrison's Principles of Internal Medicine</u> 14th ed. Vol. 1. McGraw-Hill, NY, p1970, 1998.)*

INDIVIDUAL VARIATION OF BLOOD CORTISOL LEVELS

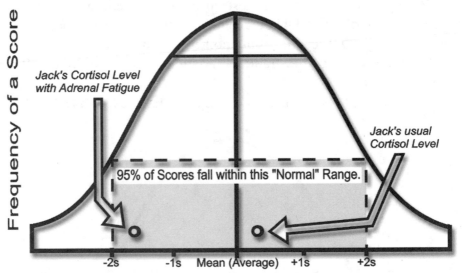

Cortisol Level has dropped dramatically but is still considered Normal.

Ideally, doctors would have baseline scores for each patient that had been obtained when the patient was feeling well and functioning at a healthy level. This way, when the patient becomes symptomatic and is functioning at a lower level, the test could be repeated and the resulting scores compared to the original scores. The difference would be quantifiable and the doctor could make an accurate judgment as to whether or not adrenal function in this patient is below his or her own normal. Perhaps future physicians truly interested in their patients' health will do this.

There is also a significant problem associated with the way laboratory results are reported. Scores are sharply demarcated as falling either within the normal range or outside the normal range. There is no gray area. Most doctors have taught themselves to look only at those scores outside the normal range. These are clearly indicated on laboratory test printouts. Therefore, if Marsha received a score of 2.0 on a lab test where the normal range was 2.0-5.0, she would be considered normal. But if she scored 1.9, her test score would be considered abnormally low and would be flagged as such by the computer printing her test results. In the first case, the doctor would consider her normal, tell her as much, and ignore the actual score. If, on the other hand, her score was 1.9, the doctor would surmise that there is something wrong with Marsha because she got an abnormal score on the test and act accordingly. In the doctor's mind at 2.0 she "didn't have it" and at 1.9 she "did have it." On most tests, laboratory error could account for more than the small difference between the 2 scores. It is important to realize that laboratory results are only indicators and that the actual scores, even when they fall within the normal range, may contain more useful information than "abnormal/normal." I encourage you to obtain copies of all your lab tests so you can see for yourself the actual test values that indicate what is going on inside your body.

Further complicating the problem of proper interpretation of laboratory data in adrenal fatigue is the fact that steroid hormones occur in more than one form in your body but most lab tests measure only one. Cortisol, for example, takes on three forms in your blood: 1) unattached to any other substance (free), 2) loosely bound and 3) tightly bound to blood proteins. The most common measurement for hormones is the amount of hormone not attached to anything, called the free circulating hormone. However, this usually represents a meager 1% of the total amount of hormone available. It does not measure the bound hormones, which act as reserves and become free hormones if needed. This reserve can be critical to proper physiological function. For example, very low circulating cortisol levels can be brought to within normal range by the administration of a synthetic cortisol. But people taking synthetic cortisol cannot withstand stress as well as people with naturally normal cortisol levels, even though blood tests for both show normal free circulating cortisol levels. Part of the reason for this is that although their free circulating cortisol level is increased by taking the synthetic cortisol, there is still a lack of the reserve cortisol bound to different tissues in the blood that is made available in cases of emergency. Blood tests can often be deceptive because they do not typically give you the whole picture. Therefore, even though both healthy people and people taking cortisol might show normal free cortisol levels, their response to stress will probably differ considerably. The test results would give a very deceptive picture of "normal" in the case of the person receiving the drug, as it tests only the most superficial layer of cortisol availability.

Yet another problem with most laboratory tests is that many steroid hormones, such as cortisol, have notable hormonal fluctuations throughout any given day. Cortisol levels at noon are normally quite different than cortisol levels at 8:00 AM. However, many labs disregard the time of day samples are taken and compare them all to values standardized for 8 AM. Often I have had doctors send their patients back to a lab to have a cortisol test redone at 8:00 AM because no one had told the patient to have the blood test at 8:00 AM. Most hormonal tests, but especially adrenal tests, are standardized for 8:00 AM testing. So, unless otherwise indicated, always have hormone blood tests done at 8:00 AM.

Stress is another factor that significantly affects adrenal hormone levels. Your cortisol level tested after a quiet, relaxing morning will be very different from your cortisol level tested when you are under stress before you arrive at the lab. To obtain a typical value, have your test on a typical morning.

This is not to say that current laboratory tests are not useful for diagnosing adrenal fatigue but simply that it is important for you and the physician interpreting them to understand their limitations and appropriate uses. Listed below are some of the standard laboratory tests typically used to detect Addison's disease that can also be useful for detecting milder forms of hypoadrenia if you know what to look for.

Useful Methods of Interpreting Standard Laboratory Tests in Adrenal Fatigue

The 24-Hour Urinary Cortisol Test: An analysis known as the 24-Hour Urinary Cortisol Test measures the hormones excreted in your urine over a 24 hour period. This lab test can be helpful as an indicator of the output of several adrenal steroid hormones including corticosteroids, aldosterone and the sex hormones. Although the laboratory range of what are considered normal hormone levels is too broad to be of much value in diagnosing all but the most severe cases of hypoadrenia, if your hormonal output is in the bottom 1/3 of the "normal" range you can suspect hypoadrenia. When this result concurs with your responses to the questionnaire, the diagnosis is relatively certain.

The interpretive value of this test is limited because all the urine for a 24-hour period is pooled in one container. Consequently, it excludes the valuable information about surges or drops in hormone levels at specific times in the day which many people with adrenal fatigue experience. At one time of day cortisol levels may be normal or even high, and during another time of day they may drop to dramatically below normal. But because all the urine samples of the day are pooled in this test, the highs and lows often cancel each other out making the results look deceptively "normal." To obtain specific information about your cortisol levels at particular times of day, do a saliva test.

Blood Tests: There are blood tests to measure circulating levels of the adrenal hormones aldosterone and cortisol, and others to measure the sex hormones related to adrenal function. But, by their very nature, blood tests divulge only the levels of the hormones circulating in the blood and do not reveal those inside the tissues, or potentially available to the tissues. However, when blood tests and urine tests are interpreted together by a trained practitioner who knows what to look for, a picture of your adrenal function can be pieced together, especially when the information is used in conjunction with your clinical presentation and medical history.

ACTH Challenge Tests: There is another kind of blood test, called an ACTH Challenge Test, which helps evaluate adrenal reserves and responsiveness and thus can help detect adrenal fatigue. In this test, baseline levels of circulating cortisol are first measured. Then a substance like Adrenal Corticotrophic Hormone (ACTH) that stimulates the adrenal output of hormones is injected. After the challenge substance is given, the circulating cortisol is re-measured to see how well the adrenals were able to respond to the stimulation. A normal response is for the blood cortisol levels to at least double. When cortisol levels do not double or rise only slightly, adrenal fatigue can be suspected. Although this test is usually done only if the blood cortisol levels are found to be low by some other indicator, I have known of instances in which the blood cortisol was well within the "normal" range, but failed to rise in response to the ACTH challenge. The ACTH Challenge Test has some value, even if cortisol levels are within the "normal" range, but it is important for the physician to realize that it is the reserve capacity of the adrenals and not their moment by moment response to stress that is being tested.

An alternative and more useful way of using the ACTH Challenge Test to detect adrenal fatigue is to combine it with the 24-Hour Urinary Cortisol Test. In this protocol, a 24-Hour Urinary Cortisol Test is given both before and immediately after the ACTH challenge. The results of the two 24-Hour Urinary Cortisol Tests are then compared. If the cortisol level of the second test is not at least double first, adrenal fatigue is present. This test can be a valuable indicator even if the first 24-hour test has cortisol values within the normal range.

There are several other blood and urine tests that can be of some use as indicators of hypoadrenia when used by physicians with special training. However, their value is limited and their interpretation is complex and beyond the scope of this book.

Although there are a few medical doctors who know how interpret these tests for adrenal fatigue, most do not. Even if they are willing to do the tests, most physicians will only pay attention to lab results that fall outside of the accepted norm, thus missing all but Addison's disease or one of the even rarer diseases that cause severe hypoadrenia. Since your test scores will probably not be out of the accepted normal range, your doctor will tell you there is nothing wrong with your adrenals. What would be more accurate would be to say that your adrenals are not in failure or near failure. That is all that conventional interpretation of most urine and blood tests can determine. Single lab tests are merely separate pieces of a puzzle that must be assembled carefully before the hidden picture is accurately revealed. This is another reason why I prefer the saliva test; it gives clearer and more direct indications of hormone levels at the actual site where they are utilized – inside the cell. None of the blood or urine tests typically give you as much useful information about your adrenal fatigue as you will get from the combined use of the questionnaire, clinical self-tests described in this book, and saliva hormone tests.

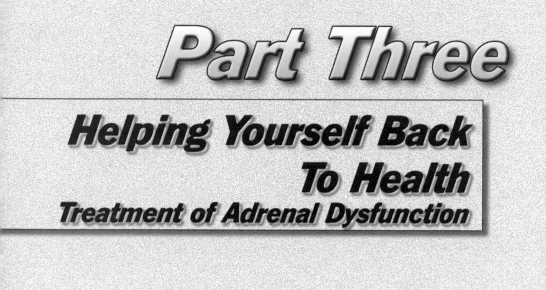

Part Three

Helping Yourself Back To Health
Treatment of Adrenal Dysfunction

The Good News

One of the few good things about adrenal fatigue is that you can do most of what is necessary to recover and regain your adrenal health, yourself. You do not have to give your power to someone else in the hope that they know what they are doing because they have a license to practice and to prescribe magic pills to make you well. There are no magic pills for adrenal fatigue but there are certainly key lifestyle changes and nutritional supplements that will greatly facilitate your recovery.

Healing from adrenal fatigue requires a combination of things; first and foremost, your recovery depends upon your **lifestyle**. How you spend your energy, how you conserve your energy, and how you create energy are all extremely important. Your recovery is also contingent on **what you eat and drink**, as well as on **the thoughts you feed your mind** and **the beliefs you base your life on**. A great thing about the program described in this book is that it gives you almost total control over your recovery process. You can design it, implement it, monitor it, adjust it and receive the many benefits from it. This is a wonderful opportunity because, in our society, there is the tendency to give this power away to someone else.

However, this power comes with its own challenges. At this writing, there is not a lot of direct support for people recovering from adrenal fatigue. I hope there will soon be facilities and support groups across the US and the rest of the world but, at this time, you are mostly on your own. The irony is that we have a nation rampant with people suffering from various stages of adrenal fatigue being served by doctors who are unaware of its existence, even though they see it nearly every day in their offices.

For this condition, most of you will have to become your own physician. Ask for help when you need it from friends, from public services, or any available source, but remain in charge of your recovery. The authority to design and implement your own program is a very powerful position. This book will tell you what to do. A complete recovery program is contained in these pages for most of you, but you must do what it says to do and keep following your own recovery. Being in charge is important for adrenal health; researchers have found from earlier experiments that rendering an animal helpless is one of the most rapid ways to deplete its adrenals. Putting yourself in charge does not mean doing it all yourself. As mentioned earlier, you should solicit the help of anyone or anything that will lead to your healthy recovery, as long as it does not compromise their health or well being.

The first, and arguably the most important, part of your recovery program will be concerned with lifestyle. It is the first chapter on recovery and should be first in your priorities. I promise you that the happiness and greater health you will experience when you institute the lifestyle changes in this book will be more than worth the effort it takes to make the needed changes.

The chapter titled "Food" contains certain foods and beverages that feed your adrenals and facilitate recovery. This section also includes a chapter on tracking down hidden food allergies because people with adrenal fatigue often have **food allergies or sensitivities**. This is followed by chapters on particular nutrients and **nutritional supplements**, as well as **herbs** and other substances that can strengthen the adrenals and facilitate recovery. **A sample daily program for adrenal recovery** is provided, along with chapters on **trouble-shooting** problem areas and commonly asked **questions and answers**. Now turn to the first chapter – "Lifestyle" – and begin your journey back to health and happiness.

Chapter 12

Lifestyle

Lifestyle is extremely important in your program for recovery from adrenal fatigue. As early as 1919, physicians pointed out that the influence of lifestyle was paramount in both the creation of and the ultimate recovery from adrenal fatigue (Harrower, 1919). These early writings reported that unless patients changed their lifestyles to reduce the sources of adrenal strain and developed new lifestyles to allow their adrenals to recover, complete healing was seldom seen. I have found the same with the patients in my practice. Elements of lifestyle are frequently the cause and the aggravating factors of adrenal fatigue that stand in the way of healing. When you understand these factors in your own lifestyle, you have the power to recover by making the necessary changes.

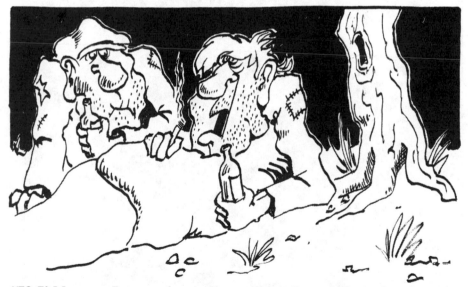

"If I'd known I was going to live so long, I would've taken better care of myself."

One of the first principles in healing is to remove the cause and the aggravating factors of the illness. For example, a wound must be cleaned and disinfected before applying the dressing otherwise the remaining debris and germs will aggravate it and prevent complete healing. The same is true in healing from adrenal fatigue. In most instances, there are lifestyle components that either caused or contributed to the adrenal fatigue and that often continue as aggravating factors. The illustration "Health Drain" shows some of the common components of our lives that make our health go down the drain. Therefore, it is essential to remove the health limiting factors if the adrenals are to recover and heal properly.

HEALTH DRAIN

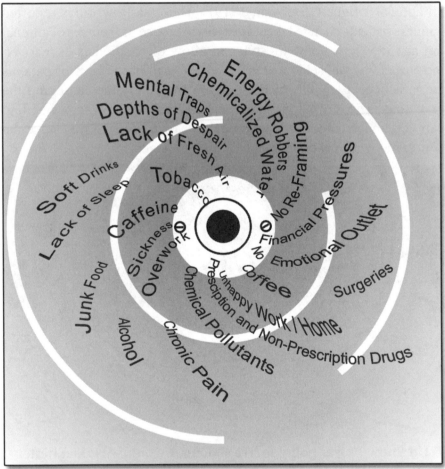

For more than seventy-five years we have known that the adrenal glands cannot heal from fatigue unless they have the opportunity to rest. Long periods of bed rest are not feasible for most people, nor are they usually necessary. The particular kind of rest you need when you have adrenal fatigue comes not so much from lying down, but from standing up for yourself, and from removing or minimizing the harmful stresses in your life.

Discovering how you can do this carries a double benefit because a sense of powerlessness or helplessness is the most debilitating and stress-inducing emotion there is. Any situation, no matter how bad, is more tolerable and less stressful when you feel you can do something about it; even when doing something about it means changing yourself rather than the situation. It is important that you take yourself seriously and find out what you need to make yourself well. Use this book as a tool to help you decide what and how to change in order to de-stress your body and improve your life.

The following sections explore many of the lifestyle factors that can cause or perpetuate adrenal fatigue and ways that you can eliminate them from your life. Find out what aspects of your life are draining you but then, most importantly, take an active hand in helping yourself back to health by doing what needs to be done to shift the advantage in your direction.

Separating the Good from the Bad and the Ugly
It is important to be able to distinguish which things in your life are contributing to your health and which things are detracting from it. So the first step in helping yourself obtain a lifestyle you love is to make a complete and thorough list of all the things that are beneficial to your life and health, and all the detrimental things in your life.

To help you get clear on this I use the following very simple but informative exercise. Take a piece of paper, date it and draw a vertical line down the center. At the top of the left column put "good for me" and at the top of the right column put a "bad for me." In the "good" column list all the things that you feel contribute to your health and well being. These can be physical or leisure activities, eating patterns, exercises, relationships, work, family, emotional patterns, attitudes, beliefs, dietary supplements, and any other things that make you feel good and contribute to your sense of well being.

Do not list things that "should" be good for you, or which you do not really find pleasurable or beneficial. Do not idealize and put what ought to be good for you. Reach into your heart and health and find what makes you feel good and what you love in life. List all things that bring you pleasure and add to your life, even if you haven't done them for a while.

In the "bad" column, list <u>everything</u> that seems detrimental to your health and well being. Again, they can be physical, emotional, attitudinal; they may be work or family related situations, relationships, eating and drinking patterns, or anything you are doing or are involved with that is not good for you.

If some aspects of a situation are good and some bad, separate them out. For example, you may have a job that you love, but the grueling hours and the fast pace are exhausting. In this case you put your job in the "good" column and the excess hours and high pressure demands in the "bad" column.

Use as many sheets of paper as you need. Take as much time as necessary. You may have to do this in 2 or 3 sessions, but really look to see what is working and what is taking away from your life, until you have a complete inventory of the good and the bad. There is no maximum or minimum number of items to put in either column. This is not a test. There is no pass or fail, no right or wrong answers. The more forthcoming you can be with information, the more you can help yourself. The following is an example of a Good For Me/Bad For Me chart.

Good For Me *(makes me more alive, healthy, happy)*	Bad For Me *(drains me, takes away my energy and health)*
Friendship with Sarah	Smoking
Bike riding	Being a couch potato – makes me sluggish and grumpy
Quiet reading	Resentment of John for leaving me
Eating regular meals	Not eating regularly – makes my head thick, lower energy.
Saturday night jazz	Working more than 1 night/week
Breathing fresh air all day	Being a perfectionist
Learning speed reading	Being around Martin
Being around friends	Not telling people how I really feel
	Staying up too late

Review each column and then circle the five most significant entries in each column. Rank each of those five from 1 to 5, with 1 being the most important and 5 being the least. Now go back to the top 5 in the "bad" column. Identify exactly what about these items is so hard on you. Look at them under a microscope until you have a clear picture of the main things in your life that are negatively affecting your health.

Select the worst one from the "Bad" column (the one you ranked number 1). See clearly how much it is detracting from your life. Commit to eliminating this item from your life. Devise a plan for accomplishing this and the date by which it will be done. Write down your resolve and put it in some private place you will see often. If it is too personal or you do not want it seen by others, make a symbol to remind you of your commitment and place the symbol on your mirror or somewhere you see several times a day. Be reasonable, but be committed to your happiness.

After you have eliminated its negative influence on you, go to #2 on your "Bad" list and do the same. Continue until the first five have been eliminated or rendered powerless in your life. If you get stuck, you might want to read the section "Three Things You Can Do."

Now go to the "Good" column. Note the five things you have circled. Review your life to see how you can do more of the five things you have circled or things like them. The idea is to have more and more good things in your life as you eliminate or render powerless the negative ones, tipping the balance in favor of a life you love to live. Write these ideas and your action plans down in detail because you will be referring back to them later in the "Three Things You Can Do" section.

Locating the Energy Robbers

The major symptom that is most disturbing for anyone suffering from adrenal fatigue is indeed fatigue. In most cases of adrenal fatigue, there are life situations that are draining, such as being around a certain person or group, in a particular building or environment, at work or at home or in some other specific situation that leaves you feeling excessively tired or stressed. Therefore, finding out what drains you and tires you out will help uncover the external factors using up your adrenal resources.

These external factors are what I call the *energy robbers*. Imagine your energy being like water in a barrel. If the barrel has holes in it, then more water has to be continually poured into it in order to keep the barrel full. The more holes or the larger the holes, the more difficult it is to keep the barrel full. Energy robbers are like holes in the barrel preventing you from being full of energy. It would seem silly to keep demanding more and more energy from your body instead of just plugging as many of the holes as possible. Every time you eliminate or minimize one of these energy robbers in your life, it is like plugging one of the holes in the barrel, allowing your energy reserves to begin to rebuild. As you become aware of what is robbing you of your energy and make the necessary changes, you will see significant differences in your energy levels. Freeing yourself from the energy robbers in your life is much easier once you have identified them. Over my twenty-two years of practice I have found the following simple procedure to be one of the most useful methods of helping my patients gain insight into the energy robbers and fatigue producing factors in their lives.

On a fresh sheet of paper make a heading **"Energy Robbers"** and list everything and everyone in your daily life that takes away your energy. Many of these will be the same as the items you listed in the "bad" column of the "Separating the Good from the Bad and the Ugly" exercise, but in this one look at your life in terms of what makes you feel more tired or worn out. What or whom do you feel drained around? It can be anything from a food to a perfume, an activity, a nagging memory, a co-worker or a spouse. It may be a building, a room or a situation. There may be many heads to this dragon but it is worth the effort. The following are areas where I often find energy robbers in a patient's life.

Energy Robbing People: As you go about your day, notice if there are certain people in your life that seem to make you feel more tired, listless, helpless, frustrated, angry or fatigued when you are around them. It may be a casual acquaintance, a social friend, or even a relative, spouse or parent. People you feel drained by or feel worse after coming into contact with are energy suckers (robbers) in some way. These people usually do not intentionally drain your energy. In fact, they are seldom aware that they are having that effect. It is not necessary at the moment to explore the reasons why they deplete you but just to become aware of who drains your energy. Some people can be energy suckers at one time, and not at others. Try to be sensitive to when this is occurring. There are some people you have to test the water with each time you come into contact with them. Sometimes you feel okay in their presence, other times you are drained by them.

Being aware of the energy suckers in your life will allow you to change how you interact with them. Changing your social contacts is sometimes the key to tipping the scales in your favor for recovery. No matter how many right things you put into your body and your lifestyle, their positive effects can be undermined by too much contact with people who are energy suckers. Therefore, if you look at your life and you find that energy suckers are a factor, it is important to do something about it. If they are people you know casually or have little contact with, you should consider eliminating them altogether from your life. If you find that someone is robbing you of your energy during a particular interaction, end your contact as quickly as possible at that time.

It is more difficult when the energy robbers are people you are very involved with. If it is a spouse you can comfortably talk to, tell him that there are certain times he takes away your energy and that during those times you need to minimize your contact with him. You might work out a signal to let him know when he is robbing you of your energy so he can stop. Or if it is someone you cannot easily communicate with, which is in itself a sign of a probable energy sucking situation, you must do what you can on your own. If this is pervasive throughout your relationship, you should rethink this relationship. Patients often tell me that they feel guilty for minimizing their contact with friends or family members even when that person is robbing them of their energy. But it is important for you to realize that nobody has a right to your energy. Your energy is your energy to use to stay alive and healthy. The same is true for every other person.

For example, I had a patient who was suffering from severe adrenal fatigue and was finding it difficult to recover. After doing the "Energy Robbers" exercise, she discovered that she had several energy suckers in her life. She felt guilty if she did not have regular contact with these people and continued to listen to their long stories of woe and hardship on the telephone. Unfortunately, the calls occurred daily so she was continually drained by her contact with these people, including her mother. For this woman, part of her prescription was to eliminate contact with these energy suckers, at least for the time being, and to absolutely minimize contact with her mother. In order to facilitate this, she monitored her calls and picked up only those that were necessary and did not answer or respond to calls from the energy suckers. She notified them that, as part of her doctor's orders, she had to limit her social contacts and phone calls but that, if it was all right with her doctor, she would contact them at a later date. With her mother she no longer took direct calls, but communicated with her briefly on the telephone, only when necessary. As part of my instructions to her, she was not to talk to her mother for more than three minutes at a time and only twice per week. If her mother started to drain her during those telephone conversations, she was to say that the conversation was making her feel bad and that she needed to go. In addition, this woman worked on ridding herself of her own sense of shame and guilt so that she would no longer be vulnerable to emotional manipulation and would, in the future, choose friends she felt good around. Although these energy suckers were not the major factors causing her adrenal fatigue, until they were removed, she was not able to recover.

Energy Robbing Work and Home: If you feel weakened or de-energized by home or work conditions, it is usually specific aspects of these that are the energy robbers, not the entire situation. Particular duties, tasks, hours, environmental factors or people may zap your energy. You might feel great while working with clients but exhausted while preparing reports, or full of energy outdoors but tired soon after you get to work.

Sometimes the solution needs to be rather unconventional. For example, I know of one company president who was overwhelmed with work. He identified phone calls as being one of the chief energy robbers in his life. It was not so much that each phone call was draining him, but that the calls so frequently interrupted his other tasks that it was hard to get things done. His solution, though radical, was to not answer the phone at all. Instead, he let the answering machine take all of his messages. He set aside two prescribed times during the day to return phone calls, and re-turned them as briefly as possible. Whenever possible, he delegated the return phone call to someone else in his office to further minimize the negative impact of the task that drained him.

Energy Robbing Environment and Food: You might think of the environment as the great outdoors but the environment that concerns us in this book is what is all around you. It includes things like the lighting in your home and workplace, cooling and heating, air quality, the fabrics, fragrances and cosmetic preparations you wear, and the many other details of your daily surroundings. These factors and the particular foods you eat can be serious energy robbers that drain your adrenal resources. If you feel groggy or tired in particular locations or clothing, or after eating certain foods, or around some odors and fragrances, then examine which foods and environmental factors are energy robbers for you. Removing or changing the offending items can do a lot to alleviate these body burdens and free up your energy.

Three Things You Can Do

Now that you are more aware of what and who is taking your energy, we can talk about some ways to deal with them. The most valuable thing I learned in Psychology 101 is that there are three things that you can do when you are in a difficult situation.

> **(1)   You can change the situation.**
>
> **(2)   You can change yourself to fit (adapt to) the situation.**
>
> **(3)   You can leave the situation.**

Three Things You Can Do In Any Undesireable Situation

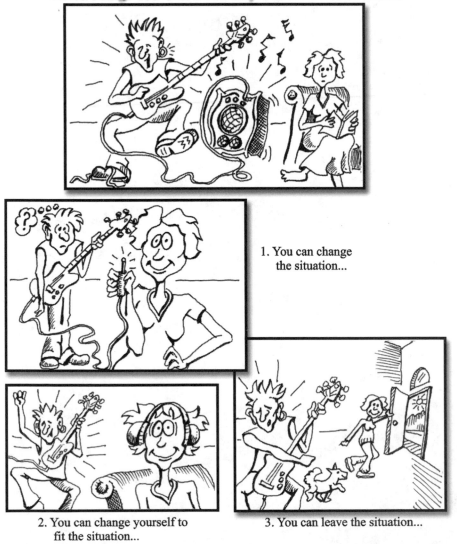

1. You can change the situation...

2. You can change yourself to fit the situation...

3. You can leave the situation...

An important preliminary step to healing your adrenals is to take a close look at your life with the purpose of identifying what is draining you and to pinpoint which factors worsen the problem and which relieve it. You have already done this with the help of the exercises from the previous chapters: the questionnaire, the health history timeline, separating the good from the bad and the ugly, and locating energy robbers.

The next step is to use this information to decide whether you can (1) leave the situation(s), (2) adapt yourself to the situation(s), or (3) adapt the situation(s) to you in order to actively change this negative to a neutral or a positive. Leaving is often not possible or appropriate and is a decision that only you can make, but this book may help you to see what is possible and appropriate to eliminate from your life so that you can move forward to regain your health. Most of the following sections in this chapter are devoted to showing you the many possible ways you can effectively use the second and third options to recover from, and prevent further, adrenal fatigue. You can use the help of friends and family or any resource you can think of to make the necessary changes, but decide <u>now, as you go through this book,</u> what you are going to do about it. I cannot emphasize enough how important your decision to act is.

Remember that stresses are additive and cumulative. Removing or neutralizing your largest source of stress will make a very significant difference to your adrenal glands and to your health and well being. Most of the time, if you take care of the big ones, the smaller ones will take care of themselves. Your body has a natural ability to handle stress and remain healthy. In fact, a certain amount of stress is beneficial. It is only when the stresses are overwhelming in quantity, duration or intensity that the systems in your body start to break down.

Let me illustrate how taking action to change the energy robbers in your life works with a couple of examples from my own practice. Both involve abusive relationships as major contributors to their adrenal fatigue, but each had a different solution.

Stephanie was a patient who came to me for a myriad of complaints, including most of the symptoms of adrenal fatigue. She was in a difficult relationship. Her husband frequently abused her and she blamed herself, believing that her own inadequacies were the reason for his abusiveness. After completing the energy robbers exercise, she saw that self-blame and worrying about her husband's reactions were taking up most of her energy. She realized then that even though she was not perfect, she did not deserve to be so badly treated. This insight allowed her to recognize that although she loved her husband, his abusiveness was destroying her. Stephanie had no idea where else she could go with her two children but her new understanding gave her the courage to search for alternatives. She found that the local police help find shelters for and protect women and children in her situation. She first tried asking her husband to quit his physical abuse but found no cooperation there. So one day while he was at work, she and the children went to a secret safe house where they were protected. She took part in re-education and self-esteem courses, changed jobs and, with the help of therapy, saw how she had picked this abusive relationship to confirm her own sense of inadequacy and guilt. Working through this, she became a happier and much less stressed woman. She was able to establish a new, non-abusive life in which she felt healthier physically as well as emotionally and psychologically. Stephanie successfully employed all three options for change: she left, she changed her situation and she changed herself once she empowered herself to act. As a result her life improved and her adrenal fatigue lessened greatly.

Another patient in a similar situation had quite a different response. *Jeannie was a petite woman. She and her husband were pig farmers, but both of them also held other jobs. Jeannie would occasionally come into the office with marks on her face and body. Once when I asked her about this she confided in me that financial stress and her husband's abusiveness were causing her adrenal fatigue. Whenever the stress became too much for him, he would get drunk and then take out his frustrations on her physically. He was never violent when he was sober, so I asked Jeannie if she would have a serious talk with him about his abusiveness. He must understand that the abuse had to end, she would not tolerate it any longer. When I saw her a few months later she was feeling much more energetic and less tired. Her face was bright and sparkly and I knew that something had happened to improve her health.*

When I asked her what had changed, she innocently said, "Doctor, the last time I was here, I heard what you said about getting Tom's attention and making him know that I was serious. One night after he came home from drinking and chased me around the table a couple times, he went in and fell asleep on the bed. It was then that I remembered your words. I knew that I had to get his attention and he had to know that I was serious or things would never change. Even though he was drunk, I knew it had to be tonight or I might never have the courage to do anything again. So I went to the bed where he was passed out on his back, and I hit him square in the face with a cast iron frying pan. He woke up with his eyes as big as saucers and I said, 'Tom, do I have your attention?' He nodded his head yes. I said, 'Tom, you can't keep on doing this to me. Do you understand?' He nodded his head yes with big ups and downs. Then I said 'I hope so, because Tom if you ever do this to me again I don't know what I'm going to do next time, do you hear me?' Again, he nodded his head up and down and then I walked back into the kitchen. I felt a lot better. We never mentioned it again and I don't know what he told his workers the next day when he went in with his face all black and blue, but Tom's been a different man ever since."

Now I would never have advised anyone to do what she did and it was certainly far from what I had imagined her doing. However, in her own way, Jeannie changed herself through regaining a sense of power in her life and changed her situation by taking effective action. What she did helped her to reverse her debilitating adrenal fatigue. She loved her husband but was being brutalized by him. She was being physically and emotionally drained by her sense of helplessness and powerlessness in her situation. What is important is that she empowered herself and took action. Hopefully, some other less violent action would have been equally as effective.

Changing the Stress Inside

Let us look at some stress reducing ways to adapt to a situation that cannot currently be changed. There are a number of popular techniques made available in books, audio programs and seminars for deflecting the negative influences around you. Many of these involve using your imagination and sense of humor. Neurolinguistic Programming (NLP) offers many effective exercises for altering your perception, and thus your feelings, about a person or situation. For example, you might picture an intimidating person dressed in a diaper instead of a suit, distort his face in your mind, or make his nose lengthen, eyes widen and ears grow while singing very softly to yourself "M-i-c-k-e-y M-o-u-s-e". This is especially useful with an unpleasant boss. Or you might put up an imaginary shield between you and the other person so that his energy bounces away from you and back towards him, making him feel bad instead of you. Often when you change the way you relate to a person or situation, you undergo a process called *reframing*. Although the term "reframing" was coined by NLP, the technique has been used since humans developed imagination.

Reframing

Leslie was a bright, energetic physician who had just completed ten years of research on a new treatment for TB, when she had her "day in hell." On her way to Dallas to meet with a group of investors about funding her TB project, her car broke down and she had to hitchhike to the airport. Just after the plane took off she realized she had left her presentation in the stranger's car and, as a result, she lost her bid with the investors. To top it off, when she returned home that night she discovered her car had been stolen from the roadside.

The next morning she could barely crawl out of bed. She thought she must be sick, but in the following weeks her energy continued to be so low she had to drag herself through each day. She could not seem to concentrate or focus on her work, she had trouble sleeping even though she was so tired she was ready to fall into bed by 8 PM, and she started putting on weight. Everything seemed like a chore and she felt so discouraged about her project, she considered quitting.

Then one sleepless night as she sat in a tired stupor in front of her TV, she heard a man talking about a "near death experience" he had had after being struck by lightning. What got Leslie's attention was how enthusiastic and grateful for his life this guy was, despite some overwhelming health problems resulting from his accident. He said that the most important thing he had learned from his experience is that each person's life, and how he or she lives it, matters. This really struck home with Leslie. Over the next few days she began looking at her difficulties differently, as information about where she was off-track in her life rather than as an overwhelming force knocking her down. What if she said "Yes!" to whatever life threw her way instead of only to the things that went her way? Using this new attitude she saw that she had too much ego wrapped up in her project and that her work obsession had alienated her from other people and activities she enjoyed. She had become impatient, demanding, inflexible and unrealistic in her expectations of herself.

Using these insights and some others, Leslie changed her approach to her work and her personal life. She began to regain her energy, focus, and enthusiasm as she started taking better care of herself and reconnecting with coworkers and friends. She rewrote the prospectus for her project, with the thought in mind that she would consider every opportunity that came up rather than pushing for just one big venture. This eventually resulted in a very satisfactory partnership with a group of investors who shared her interest in improving healthcare in developing countries.

Several years later Leslie thought back on her "day in hell" and with amazement realized it had been one of the luckiest days in her life. She would never forget how much better she started to feel in every way once she learned to look for the opportunities in even the worst difficulties.

Have you ever looked at one of those pictures containing a hidden image? At first you look and look from every angle, but all you can see is the regular picture. Then suddenly your focus shifts, the hidden image appears and you see it so differently that it becomes impossible not to see it that way. *Reframing* is a similar process of changing focus in which new information and/or a new point of view alters the way you see something. When you change how you see something you also change how your body responds to it. That is why one of the most effective ways to lessen the stressful effects of an unavoidable, difficult situation is to *reframe* or refocus your perception of the situation. This often allows you to adapt yourself to the situation in a more positive way or gives you a key to changing the situation for the better. In the story above Leslie reframed several traumatic events that had stressed her beyond her capacity and exhausted her adrenals. This worked so well for her that she was able to completely recover from her adrenal fatigue. Leslie's story demonstrates that it is possible to look at something that seems completely negative as something positive and have your body respond accordingly. It takes some imagination and effort but reframing can literally be a lifesaver.

Sometimes, the way circumstances unfold allows us to reframe miserable experiences into beneficial ones (like finding out that a negative lab test result was an error, giving you a new lease on life). However, it is usually up to us to "turn lemons into lemonade" by consciously altering how we see our difficulties in order to experience them as something better (just as Leslie did by using the mistakes she made as keys to unlocking the good things in her life). If we wait around hoping life will present us with a series of happy endings we will probably be disappointed. However when we choose to use reframing techniques to shift our perceptions about situations that have been wearing us out with stress, we empower ourselves to stay healthy. We change how our bodies actually experience and respond to these situations. The psychological changes produce physiological changes that directly affect our health.

Many times, changing the impact of a situation is not as difficult as you imagine it will be. If you look at a situation from a different angle or allow your attitudes or beliefs about it to change, quite often the stress and tension that the situation provokes will begin to diminish. For example, if you go to work every day and think your boss hates you, or you dread going because of the unpleasant people you work with, you are really seeing yourself as the victim in this situation. Instead, you could decide that this is really a master's training course on how to handle difficult people that you are taking while looking for another job. This way you can benefit from studying these people and your reactions to them.

Changing your responses puts you back in control of the situation. You can then pick one reaction each week that you want to change, or somehow diffuse, and continually work at mastering yourself so you are no longer a victim. In other words, you turn it into an opportunity for getting something you want or need instead of allowing it to be an obstacle to what you want or need. Each time you lose your temper or get uptight, instead of blaming or criticizing yourself, realize that you need more practice in deflecting other people's negativity and maintaining a positive emphasis on your own perceptions and goals.

The positive changes you make will give you more confidence that you can actually find a work situation that you would enjoy; something you might have thought was impossible a few months before. Remember we are not required to sell our souls in order to work. That is a belief that some of us hold and, as a result, we find ourselves working for companies that demand it.

It surprises many people to discover that not only is it possible to change a belief about something but that changing the belief often changes the situation. If, for example, you believe you must exhaust yourself at work in order to get ahead, then you are in a real bind. The only way you can win is to lose. If you win at your job, you lose with your health and if you are not exhausted, you must not be doing your job.

A belief is like an ***internal equation*** you live by. In this example if you can replace your equation that *job success = exhaustion* with an equation like *job success = focus with relaxation*, then new possibilities can arise for you. In the first equation you have a sense of powerlessness and your job controls you; in the second equation you are empowered to have much more control over yourself and your job experience. What you believe (your equation) about success in this case governs your freedom to choose work attitudes and behavior that either lead to health or to debilitation and possibly to actual success or failure. For example, if you have to work late some evenings, you can set a limit on how much is reasonable for you to finish and how many extra hours you are willing to put in to meet your job goals. Then while doing the work you can use techniques like deep breathing to stay focused and relaxed. In a relaxed state, you will usually work more effectively than you do when you put yourself under the gun, so you might even get the job done faster. The important result for your health is that you can do whatever you have to do with less stress.

Reframing Exercise I: Turning Lemons into Lemonade

Here is a simple set of exercises to help you decrease your internal stress load by reframing.

1) Write down negative self-talk: For two days pay attention to your self-talk (the things you say to yourself but do not speak out loud). Notice, in particular, the negative messages you give to your self and the things you tell yourself when you are upset. Jot these things down in a single column on a piece of paper. It is easier to keep track if you carry a little notebook with you. For example, Jane ate three doughnuts for breakfast and then thought of herself as fat and ugly with no willpower, so she wrote down:

> *fat*
> *ugly*
> *no will power*

2) Scoring: After the two days, sit down with your list and add up how many negative messages you gave yourself. This will give you an idea of how much energy you are putting into making yourself feel bad. Anything over 2 or 3 a day is wearing a negative groove in your mind. Then count how many times you gave yourself a particular message (for example, Jane told herself she is fat 10 times) and mark that total beside each message. Using those totals, rank your messages from most frequent to least frequent. This will give you a clearer idea of what you feel the most stressed about. In our example, Jane was in a difficult relationship with food and her self-image.

3) Discovering what you want: Across from the negative message, write it's opposite in positive terms. For example, Jane wrote slim next to fat, beautiful next to ugly and strong will power next to no will power. Now look at the top 5 messages in your positive list and think about what would be different about your life if all, or most, of the things in this positive list were true. This will help you to understand what it is that you want in your life that you currently do not feel you have. For example, when Jane thought about being slim, beautiful and having lots of will power, she realized it would make her feel more in control of her own life (more powerful), respected by other people and more lovable. What she really wanted was empowerment, respect and love but she had been focusing instead on her appearance and eating habits. In a way this gave her some sense of control in her life because these were more tangible things to deal with. Now write down what your lists reveal that you really want in your life that you currently do not have.

4) Reframing: The next step is to look at how you can reframe the troublesome areas of your life so that they can start giving you what you want, instead of what you do not want. For example, after writing down what she wanted, Jane decided that the best place to start was to find a way to get respect and love through her relationship with food. This was the most difficult and frustrating area of her life at the moment. She began to see that her body was like a child depending on her care, rather than an out of control tyrant. When she felt cravings for fattening, unhealthy foods she recognized that her body was sending her a signal that she should listen to, just as she would respond to a child crying.

5) Act according to your reframed perception: Once you have reframed that difficult situation, begin interpreting everything that happens in that situation according to your new positive framework and then act accordingly. In the example of Jane, instead of trying to either suppress or give in to her cravings, she used cravings as opportunities to discover what she needed at that moment so she could take the appropriate action. She may have needed food, or she may have needed exercise, or rest, or a deep breath, or to speak her mind at home or work. By using food cravings as an aid rather than an obstacle to getting what she wanted, Jane found her relationship with food improved tremendously. She began by reframing her perception of her body from tyrant to dependent child. This transformed her eating habits into an opportunity to learn how to give herself what she really wanted rather than a reason for not getting what she wanted. By treating her body with love and respect she ended up empowered to find the things she wanted in other areas of her life as well. Reframing shifts your focus from the wall to the doorway.

Reframing Exercise II: Act As If

This is a much shorter exercise and should be done in the spirit of play. It will help you to loosen up your perceptions about your life. Imagine that you have a magic wand that can change one, and only one, thing about any situation. For example, when you go in to work tomorrow, you will think of yourself as a millionaire who does not have to work but chooses to; or the next time you find yourself getting enraged behind a slow driver during rush hour, you will transform her in your mind into your beloved aunt who told you wonderful stories when you were little. Sometimes even the most outrageous and ridiculous images can help begin to dissolve the negative associations you have with problem areas in your life. Have fun with this exercise and do it every day.

Reframing Exercise III: Up in Smoke

The purpose of this exercise is to help you let go of whatever it is you are holding on to too tightly so that a new perspective has a chance to emerge. You will need a pencil, three small pieces of paper, a candle and/or matches and a small fire proof container or surface.

Light the candle if you have it. On the first piece of paper write down in a few words one source of unhappiness, a problem or a regret that you have in your life right now. Take a moment to just hold that thought in your mind and become aware of all the feelings you have about it. Then hold the end of the paper in the candle or match flame and drop it into the container. Watch and make sure it burns up completely. Then take a deep inhalation and as you exhale slowly, exhale that problem out of your body, let it go.

On the next piece of paper write down in a few words one change that you believe has to happen before you can be happy right now. Take a moment to just hold that thought in your mind and become aware of all the feelings you have about making the change and where your belief about it comes from. Then hold the end of the paper in the candle or match flame and drop it into the container. Watch and make sure it burns up completely. Then take a deep inhalation and as you exhale slowly, exhale that belief out of your body, let it go.

On the third piece of paper write down in a few words one thing that would be different about your life if you were happy. Take a moment to just hold that thought in your mind and become aware of how you feel about it. Then hold the end of the paper in the candle or match flame and drop it into the container. Watch and make sure it burns up completely. Then take a deep inhalation and as you exhale slowly, exhale that expectation out of your body, let it go. Just spend a few moments quietly listening to your breath and enjoying the peace. You may find that you will see things differently after this exercise.

The following exercises open the door for you to make use of another very important aid to healing from adrenal fatigue, relaxation.

Relaxation
The Relaxation Response: Learning to relax is another way to adapt yourself to difficult situations with less stress and debilitation. People tend to think of leisure activities as relaxation. However, physiological relaxation is a set of specific internal changes that occur when your mind and body are calm. It is not the same as sleep, rest or having fun. Physiological relaxation is the one internal state that can protect your body from the harmful effects of too much stress. Without a doubt it is extremely important to your health. Although it can occur in a wide variety of circumstances (ranging from athletic competitions to meditation), it rarely occurs spontaneously in modern life.

In the late 1960's a Harvard cardiologist named Herbert Benson, MD began a series of studies investigating the physiological changes that take place in meditators while they are meditating. He called these changes collectively *the relaxation response*. From these studies he discovered that no matter how the relaxation response is elicited, the resultant internal changes are quite consistent. The body shifts from sympathetic to parasympathetic nervous system dominance; breathing, heart rate, and oxygen consumption slow down; muscles relax; the brain predominantly generates the slower alpha waves; and blood pressure may drop. These changes occur within a few minutes of beginning an activity that produces the relaxation response, whereas they happen very gradually over hours while sleeping and often not at all while engaging in a leisure activity.

Of particular relevance to adrenal fatigue recovery is that during the relaxation response, stimulation of your adrenal glands diminishes so they can rest and, in addition, all the tissues in your body become less sensitive to stress hormones secreted by your adrenal glands. This means that every part of your body has a chance to return to normal and recuperate instead of being constantly on red alert.

Methods for producing the relaxation response are described in detail in many widely available books and courses. Effective techniques include most forms of meditation, yoga, ta'i chi, qi gong, guided imagery, biofeedback and deep breathing, among others. I suggest you find a class nearby because nothing can replace a good teacher. However the following simple exercises are known to reliably elicit the relaxation response with practice and will get you started. All of them are centered on your own breathing for two reasons: you always have your breathing available to focus on, and slow, deep breathing turns off the alarm signal that drives your adrenal glands to overwork. The more you practice these exercises, the quicker and easier it will be to experience physiological relaxation with all its mental and physical benefits. If you are suffering from adrenal fatigue it is essential that you learn at least one of these methods and incorporate it into your life.

Relaxation Response Exercises
1) Belly-breathing: This is the most natural kind of breathing, although it may feel unfamiliar initially. If you have ever watched a baby or an animal breathing you have seen belly-breathing; the belly rather than the chest expands and contracts. This allows the air to reach the lower part of your lungs where there is a rich blood supply and it triggers the relaxation response within a few minutes. It is just about impossible to be tense and belly-breathe at the same time.

Take 10 minutes when you will not be interrupted. Either lie or sit on a comfortable surface that fully supports your body. Place your hand palms down on your abdomen, just below your navel. Close your eyes and, at first, just pay attention to your breathing without trying to change it; listen to the sound of it, feel it moving in and out of your nose and throat, notice how far down into your body it seems to go. Then imagine that you have a balloon inside your lower belly, under where your hands are. As you inhale, try to inflate that balloon; as you exhale, let the balloon deflate. Do not expand your chest as you inhale, just your belly. It is best to breathe through your nose for this exercise but if for some reason you cannot, then it is okay to breathe through your mouth. Continue inflating and deflating the balloon for at least 5 minutes. Belly-breathing may feel awkward or forced the first few times you try it but pretty soon it will feel quite natural. After all, this is the way you used to breathe when you were little.

2) Slowing down your breath: This is a very simple method that you can use even when you are in the midst of doing something else. Whenever you notice you are feeling tense and uptight, check and see how you are breathing. Most people under stress either alternate holding their breath with taking barely perceptible short breaths, or take rapid shallow breaths. After you become aware of your own breathing, consciously relax your belly and slow down your breathing. It works best if you focus on slowing down your exhalation rather than your inhalation. With each exhalation you can say to yourself, "slow down." That is all there is to it – simple but surprisingly effective!

3) Counting your exhalations: This is a variation on slowing down your breath that should be done when you can set aside 10 minutes of time to focus on it. Get comfortable in a relatively quiet place and begin belly-breathing. This time count slowly from 5 down to 1 with each exhalation. Your mind will probably wander many times, but each time you catch your attention drifting, just calmly bring it back to counting from 5 to 1 during each exhalation. Do this for at least 5 minutes. When you can keep your attention on your breathing for 5 minutes, you can move on to deeper meditation methods.

4) Repeating a mantra or affirmation: Spiritual disciplines have traditionally used repeated phrases or sounds for prayer and meditation. Gregorian chants and the rosary are examples from the western tradition. The mantra, a specially chosen sound/phrase used in meditation, is an example from the eastern tradition that has become popular in the west through Transcendental Meditation (TM). It seems that the repetition of particular kinds of sounds, words or phrases is a very effective way to clear your mind and trigger the relaxation response when practiced daily. You can get many of the benefits of physical and mental relaxation from this method yourself, even just using a sound, word or phrase you choose yourself.

First you need to choose a word, phrase or sound that is calming to you. Some examples that other people have chosen are, "relax," "peace," "I am still," "I release the past," "I open my heart," "Om," and so on. Take 15-20 minutes in a quiet place where you will not be disturbed. Sit or lie down with your back straight and close your eyes. Focus your attention either between your eyebrows (mind center) or in the middle of your chest (heart center). Allow your breathing to slow down and deepen. When you feel settled, begin repeating your word/phrase/sound out loud or silently. You can repeat it on each inhalation and on each exhalation. Your mind will wander many times, but each time it does just gently bring it back to your phrase. You may find yourself frequently falling asleep at first, but keep coming back to the exercise. Do this for at least 15 minutes once or twice a day and you will be amazed at the change in how you feel.

5) Progressive relaxation: This is a particularly good exercise for you if you have a lot of stress related aches and pains or if you think you cannot relax. With practice it trains your body to release tension and relax more easily.

This exercise takes about 10-20 minutes and is best done lying down. Some people use it to help themselves fall asleep. Take a few slow breaths to get settled and then, starting with your toes, first tighten the muscles in your toes as tight as you can, hold for about 10 seconds and then relax your toes. Next tighten up the muscles in your feet, hold for 10 seconds, and then relax. Continue repeating this procedure all the way up your body until one by one every part of your body has been tensed and then relaxed: calves, knees, thighs, buttocks, hips, abdomen, back, chest, hands, arms, shoulders, upper back, neck, face, scalp. After you have completed this, imagine a wave of relaxation rolling up your body each time you inhale and imagine this wave washing all tension out of your body each time you exhale. Do this for a few minutes and then just rest, breathing slowly. You will find that the relaxation you experience with this exercise will get deeper with practice.

6) The Quiet Pond: Have you ever stood beside a quiet pond away from buildings and people. If you have, you know how spending some time by the pond, letting everything else fade as you take in the full experience of the pond, just seems to cause all your cares and burdens to slide down off your shoulders and slip away. It is amazing how refreshing a few minutes beside a pond can be. If you have not had that experience, maybe you have had one of your own; a place you can go that is so peaceful, comforting and renewing, it is hard to leave.

I believe everyone has the capacity to carry their own peaceful pond around inside them and, with practice, access it at will. If you have such a place, take time to recall it in your mind daily. Find your quiet pond every day, even if it is for only a few minutes or even for a few breaths. Take time for relaxation every day. When you associate the feelings you have about your quiet place and bring those feelings of quiet peacefulness into your consciousness, you are doing more than feeling good. You are helping establish balance in your nervous system. You are activating the part of the nervous system called the parasympathetic nervous system that is responsible for healing and repair. Calling forth those images and feelings, even briefly, helps offset the stress building up inside.

If you are able to do this at a specific time each day, your body will soon know when it is time and will begin to bring forth the image and the feelings without any conscious effort on your part. I used to meditate at one time during the day but then switched to another time. It took my body a few days to switch, but during the transition time I could feel it preparing to meditate a few minutes before the old time was near. If you can return to your quiet inner pond at approximately the same time every day, you will soon receive help in relaxing from your unconscious. Find your quiet pond deep inside where you can refresh yourself daily regardless of where you are, what you are doing or what is going on around you.

Unstructured Time

In addition to learning to produce the relaxation response, it is important to schedule some unstructured time into every week (every day if you can). The idea of resting one day a week has long been part of our Western culture, but in modern life it seldom happens. What I mean by unstructured time is a period of a few hours or more during which you do not have any planned activities or goals to accomplish. You can spend this time doing whatever you feel like without worrying about being productive or about what other people think. You can putter around the house, take a leisurely stroll or do anything that you enjoy, although it is best not to spend it watching TV or sleeping. This unstructured time gives you an emotional and mental break from the constant striving and measuring of productivity that is driving your adrenals to exhaustion.

Vacations

Taking some time off every year to rest, renew and enjoy yourself pays big dividends to your health and well-being, if not to your finances. Vacationing one to two weeks twice a year and traveling to somewhere new at least once a year can refresh your body as well as your mind and spirit.

Relaxation leads to improvement of another important element in the healing process, adequate deep sleep.

Sleep

Sleep is very important to full adrenal recovery but the twist is that sleeplessness is sometimes one of the signs of adrenal fatigue. In any case, how and when you sleep will affect your level of adrenal fatigue or replenishment.

When to Sleep

For people with adrenal fatigue (most people), it is important to be in bed and asleep before your second wind hits at about 11:00 PM. Riding your second wind and staying up until 1:00 or 2:00 in the morning will further exhaust your adrenals, even though you may feel more energetic during that time than you have felt all day. In order to avoid this pitfall, make sure that you are in bed and on your way to sleep before 10:30 PM, so that your adrenal glands do not have a chance to kick into overdrive for that second wind.

Although most people's schedules do not allow it, it also helps to sleep in until 8:30 or 9:00 in the morning. There is something magical about the restorative power of sleep between 7:00-9:00 in the morning for people with adrenal fatigue. Even when your night has been restless or your sleep fitfull, catching those couple of hours of sleep between 7:00-9:00 AM can be remarkably refreshing.

The reason for this is that while you are sleeping during those morning hours your adrenals have a chance to rest, allowing your cortisol levels to rise. Normally cortisol levels rise rapidly from 6:00 AM to approximately 8:00 AM, but quite often in adrenal fatigue these levels do not rise as high and/or drop faster than normal. Also when your cortisol levels are lower, as in adrenal fatigue, it takes longer to feel fully awake in the morning. Sleeping in, therefore, is not only restorative for your adrenals but also helps you feel much better when you wake up and during the rest of the day. Some of my patients have told me that they can even get up between 2:00 and 4:00 AM, do some work, return to bed, and still feel fine during the day as long as they go back to sleep before 7:00 in the morning and remain asleep until 9:00 AM. I do not recommend doing this, but it does illustrate the important fact that <u>when</u> you sleep is significant as well as how long you sleep. Unfortunately many of us cannot sleep in during the weekdays so if this is the case for you, sleep in on the weekends if at all possible. It is not self indulgent, it is essential. Knowing when to sleep can make all the difference to how you feel.

What If I Can't Sleep?

There can be several reasons for sleeplessness with adrenal fatigue. If you are waking between 1:00 and 3:00 AM, your liver may be lacking the glycogen reserves needed for conversion by the adrenals to keep the blood glucose levels high enough during the night. Blood sugar is normally low during the early morning hours but, if you are hypoadrenic, your blood glucose levels may sometimes fall so low that hypoglycemic (low blood sugar) symptoms wake you during the night. This is often the case if you have panic or anxiety attacks, nightmares, or sleep fitfully between 1:00 and 4:00 AM. To help counteract this have one or two bites of a snack that contains protein, unrefined carbohydrate, and high quality fat before going to bed, such as half a slice of whole grain toast with peanut butter or a slice of cheese on a whole grain cracker. See the "Food" chapter in this book for more suggestions and specific information.

Both too high and too low nighttime cortisol levels can cause sleep disturbances. To determine if this is a problem for you, simply do a saliva cortisol test at night and compare your night sample levels with your own daytime levels and with the test standards for those times. To do the night test, take a saliva sample at bedtime, another if you wake up during the night and a third when you wake up in the morning. Write the time each sample was taken on the vial and in your notebook on a separate sheet of paper. If cortisol is the culprit, your cortisol levels will be significantly higher or lower than normal for those times. If your night time cortisol levels are too low, you may sleep better when you exercise in the evening, before going to bed because exercise tends to raise cortisol levels. If your nighttime cortisol levels are too high, try doing one of the relaxation or meditation exercises to calm you down before going to bed. The specific yoga posture called the alternate leg pull can be quite helpful in getting to sleep or returning to sleep. This is a basic yoga posture that almost any yoga book or video will describe but an instructor is preferable because there is some subtlety to doing this posture.

Here is a list of some additional things you can do to improve your sleep.

1) Above all, go to bed before 10:30 PM and stay in bed until 9:00 AM as often as possible, even if it is just on the weekends. It is amazing how restorative sleeping until 9:00 AM is for the adrenals.

2) Be sure to get enough physical exercise during the day. Try varying the kinds of exercise you do, their intensity or when you exercise. Many people have told me swimming at night helps them sleep.

3) Certain postures in yoga, ta'i chi and qi gong can also be helpful. Check with a teacher of these disciplines to find out which postures or exercises would specifically help you.

4) Avoid coffee, caffeine containing beverages and chocolate because they act as stimulants. These can interrupt sleep patterns and increase morning lows. Even if they are consumed early in the day, they can disrupt sleep and make the next morning harder to negotiate.

5) Some people are photosensitive and watching television or looking at a computer screen keeps their melatonin from rising and inducing sleep. If you are having difficulty going to sleep and usually are staring at a TV or computer screen late at night, try having an 8:00 PM limit on these visual stimuli.

6) If your cortisol levels are low late at night, try exercising in the evening,

as exercise raises cortisol levels and may afford you a sound night's sleep.

7) There are particular nutritional supplements that can be beneficial. Often **melatonin** (0.3 - 1.3 mg.) taken 30 minutes before bedtime helps establish normal sleep patterns. **Calcium citrate** (500 mg.) taken with 50 mg. of **5-hydroxytryptophan (5HTP)** at night before retiring is also relaxing and helps many people sleep through the night. **Trace mineral tablets** taken at the evening meal also help relax the body. **Adrenal extracts** taken ½ hour before bedtime often help those with adrenal fatigue fall asleep and remain asleep. If your adrenal fatigue is moderate or severe, try this one first.

8) The hypothalamus is very important in regulating sleep. Although accurately testing hypothalamic function is complicated, a simple test you can do yourself is to try taking 1-4 tablets of **hypothalamus extract** and 10-40 mg. of **manganese** before bedtime and see if your sleep improves. Sometimes the hypothalamus tablets need to be combined with the adrenal extracts to normalize sleep

9) There are also several herbs commonly used to promote better sleep such as hops (whole plant), catnip (leaves), valerian (root) and licorice (root). Although not known as a sedative, the herb ashwagandha can help indirectly through its ability to normalize cortisol and sex hormones, both of which can produce sleep disturbances.

If none of these help and your life is being deleteriously affected by lack of or interrupted sleep, check your local area or the website for the location of the nearest sleep center. Several cities around the country have these centers that specialize in helping individuals determine the cause of their sleep disturbances.

Take Short Horizontal Rests During the Day

During the day, you will probably notice that you have particular times when you feel more lethargic, cloudy headed, tired or have other symptoms of adrenal fatigue. Try to schedule your breaks so that when these occur, you can physically lie down for 15-30 minutes. Lying down is much more restorative than sitting, for the person with adrenal fatigue.

Laughter

You have heard it said, "Laughter is the best medicine." Nothing could be truer for the adrenal glands. When you laugh, stress decreases and all the mechanisms in your body relax. When the body is relatively free of stress, even during those brief moments of levity, the adrenals are much freer to recover and rebuild.

In the book <u>Anatomy of an Illness</u>, Norman Cousins describes his struggle with ankylosis spondylitis, a disease that causes eventual fusing of the bones of the spine. Unwilling to believe his doctors' prognosis that he would be immobilized for life, frozen into either a sitting or standing position, he did some research on his own. What he discovered was that the anti-inflammatory properties of cortisol, secreted by the adrenal glands, are extremely important in overcoming the deleterious effects of ankylosising spondylitis. Through his own investigations, he found two important keys to helping rebuild the adrenals: laughter and vitamin C. After unearthing this information, Cousins prescribed laughter for himself daily, in addition to taking vitamin C. He did everything possible to make himself laugh, including watching funny movies, reading humorous books, cartoons, jokes, comic strips, and anything else that would cause him to laugh. As a matter of fact, he laughed so much he was disruptive to the rest of the patients in the hospital ward and had to be moved to a private room where he could laugh his way back to health. His therapy was successful. He made a full recovery based only on his prescription of daily laughter and humor, vitamin C, and a change of lifestyle that included rest, away from his hectic life.

Each one of these elements is important, but never underestimate the tremendous value of laughter and enjoyment as a recuperative tool. So prescribe laughter for your life. Do not take yourself and others so seriously and look on the lighter side. Make it a point to laugh several times every single day, especially when you don't feel well. Laughter not only makes your day better, but it is good therapy.

There is a simple but effective eastern meditation practice that relates to this. It consists of arranging your face in a half-smile while you are alone. You do not have to feel like smiling or even think of anything that makes you smile; the facial expression itself is enough to allow you to feel more peaceful inside and less stressed.

Physical Exercise

Exercise is probably the last thing you feel like doing if you are hypoadrenic. But before you skip this section, listen to all the good things it will do for you. And remember that dancing and making love are exercise too!

Benefits of exercise: Rapid breathing expels volatile gases out of your body that become harmful if they build up. The increased blood flow helps keep plaque from building up in your arteries while stimulating your liver to perform its 3,000+ functions more efficiently. Cell function improves with the accompanying acceleration of carbon dioxide, oxygen and nutrient exchange. Exercise normalizes levels of cortisol, insulin, blood glucose, growth hormone, thyroid, and several other hormones and puts more oxygen into your brain. These are only some of the benefits of exercise. One of the greatest advantages of exercise is how much better it makes you feel in every way!

Exercise also decreases depression. An acquaintance of mine used to run a residential psychiatric institution in Jackson County, Illinois. The two most significant changes that Jay made when he took over its directorship were to eliminate sugar, which composed up to 70% of some of the inmates diets, and to have a daily exercise program for all residents. He found that these two things alone decreased depression dramatically among the patients at the mental hospital. Depression is a common finding in adrenal fatigue. There are studies that show that exercise can be as effective in treating depression as are some pharmaceutical agents. It is empowering as well as rejuvenating.

Lee was an ambitious 25-year-old undergraduate student in psychology, who also owned part interest in a nightclub. Managing the nightclub from 6:00PM to 3:00AM and attending classes from 7:00AM to noon was a challenge but he enjoyed both. Eventually, Lee worked out a schedule that enabled him to work, attend classes and complete his studies. The only thing he had to leave out was sleep. With his new schedule, he slept only on Sundays and Wednesdays, except for occasional catnaps. He kept himself going with a combination of coffee, Coca-Cola and alcohol. This lasted for a little more than a semester. Although he consistently fell asleep in classes, he was able to finish his undergraduate degree and graduate, and even made the honor roll. After graduation all he seemed to want to do was rest. Of course for him, just running the nightclub without having to attend school was as good as a rest.

However about the time he was starting to get his old energy back, his girlfriend wrote to him from Colorado and asked him to move out there so that they could be together. In eager anticipation of getting married, he sold his nightclub and drove to Colorado. Unfortunately, within a week of arriving in Colorado, his fiancé ended their engagement. Emotionally devastated and now running low on money, he got a job working construction. The physical activity was good for his body and over the next few months he felt better working outside in the open air and having virtually no responsibilities other than to show up in the morning at work. When he was ready he left Colorado and went on to new endeavors and relationships with his vitality restored.

Lee is an example of someone who had adrenal fatigue, but who adjusted his lifestyle in a way that allowed him to recover, even though he remained very active. He rested emotionally and mentally while engaging in vigorous physical exercise. Although Lee obviously had relatively strong adrenal glands and good energy reserves, his story reflects the healing power of physical exercise.

What kind of exercise is best? Exercise that is beneficial for adrenal fatigue recovery should be enjoyable. It should not be highly competitive, grueling or debilitating. What you need is something that increases lung capacity, muscle tone and flexibility while having fun. (See illustration "Exercises – combine aerobics, anaerobics and flexibility").

Yoga with breathing exercises, ta'i chi, kick boxing, swimming, fast walking, dancing, and any number of team sports and exercise programs are all good ways to get your body moving. Pick something that is enjoyable to you. Remember you are not working out to run a marathon or set new records, but to bring your body back to life and take pleasure

EXERCISES - COMBINE AEROBICS, ANAEROBICS AND FLEXIBILITY

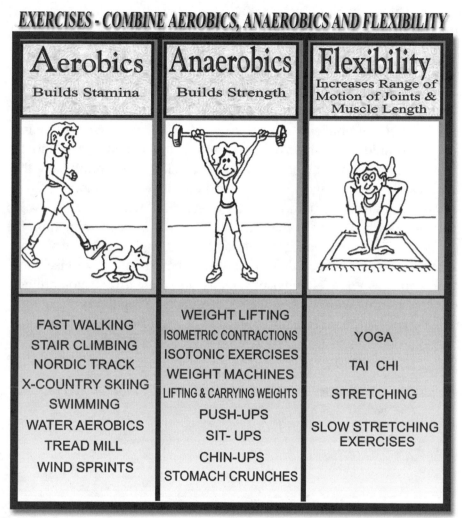

Aerobics	Anaerobics	Flexibility
Builds Stamina	**Builds Strength**	**Increases Range of Motion of Joints & Muscle Length**
FAST WALKING STAIR CLIMBING NORDIC TRACK X-COUNTRY SKIING SWIMMING WATER AEROBICS TREAD MILL WIND SPRINTS	WEIGHT LIFTING ISOMETRIC CONTRACTIONS ISOTONIC EXERCISES WEIGHT MACHINES LIFTING & CARRYING WEIGHTS PUSH-UPS SIT-UPS CHIN-UPS STOMACH CRUNCHES	YOGA TAI CHI STRETCHING SLOW STRETCHING EXERCISES

in it again. There will be days, especially when you first begin exercising, that you do not feel like doing anything physical. When this happens, instead of forcing yourself to exercise, start slow and gently work into it. In other words, do not let the exercise become another stressor in your life. When part of you resists, simply treat that part with kind understanding, acknowledge its resistance, but do not let it undermine your commitment to your health. People with adrenal fatigue often feel too tired to exercise. However, if you set a routine time to exercise, no matter how you feel, you will soon experience the rewards of your self-discipline.

How do I know if I am exercising correctly? Exercise at your own pace and not the pace of the person next to you or your friends. If you get tired, rest or quit for a while or for the day. If you are tired the next morning, take it easier the next time. As your stamina increases, gradually increase your exercise. The purpose of exercising in this program is not necessarily to become stronger, but to increase your body's tone, flexibility and aerobic capacity. Two weeks after you start exercising daily you should notice that you are beginning to feel better. You should feel good after a workout and should only be slightly or mildly sore the day after. If you feel worse after a workout or the next morning, you probably exercised too hard and need to step it down a notch. Type A personalities who are out of shape are particularly prone to doing this. In their minds, they are in much better condition than they actually are and so make more demands on their bodies than they should. Exercise done properly makes you feel better physically and mentally. If you are not experiencing this within a few weeks of starting a regular program, either cut back a little or try a different kind of exercise. The most important requirement is that exercise becomes enjoyable for you.

Chapter 13

Food

You probably agree that even in the best of times you need food to survive and be healthy. Adrenal fatigue is definitely not the best of times and so the food choices you make become even more important to your survival and health. The old computer saying, ***"garbage in = garbage out"*** applies here as well; if you make inadequate food choices (garbage in), your body will make inadequate responses (garbage out) to the demands placed on it (stress). When your adrenals respond to stress the metabolism of your cells speeds up, burning many times the number of nutrients normally needed. By the time you are in a state of adrenal fatigue, your cells have used up much of your body's stored nutrients and are in desperate need of new supplies just to continue to function, let alone heal. Good quality food is the best source of these nutrients; there is no substitute. The nutritional supplements described in Chapter 15 can increase your ability to heal and speed your recovery, but without a foundation of nutritious food intake, you will not make much progress.

"We cannot over emphasize the importance of a proper diet" Dr. John Tintera – The Hypoadrenia Cortical State and its Management. New York State Journal of Medicine, Vol. 55 #13, July 1, 1955, p.11.

It is crucial for you to read this chapter so you will understand which foods help your healing process and which foods are detrimental. If you think you already know a lot about food and nutrition, I still ask you to read this chapter because anyone with adrenal fatigue syndrome is missing something in their food intake. They are lacking the essential nutrients they need to meet the increased demands their cells experience under stress. In many cases of adrenal fatigue, poor diet is one of its main causes but in <u>all</u> cases of recovery from adrenal fatigue, a nutritious diet is a major factor.

The Connection between Adrenal Fatigue and Low Blood Sugar

The adrenal hormone cortisol helps keep blood sugar at adequate levels to meet your body's demands for energy. However, when your adrenal glands are fatigued, cortisol levels drop lower than normal. This makes it more difficult for your body to maintain normal blood sugar levels. As a result, people with adrenal fatigue (hypoadrenia) tend to also have low blood sugar (hypoglycemia).

If you have adrenal fatigue, when you eat is almost as important as what you eat. Low blood sugar is in itself a stressful situation that further drains your adrenals. Therefore avoiding letting your blood sugar levels drop too low by eating natural, high quality food at frequent, regular intervals will make a difference to your adrenal health as well as to your energy level. Many people suffering from mild hypoadrenia push themselves, often going for long stretches without a proper meal. This further taxes the adrenals because the lower the blood sugar levels, the more cortisol it takes to normalize them. If you have adrenal fatigue you should not follow the eating pattern that some popular books present as the perfect adrenal diet. This supposed 'adrenal diet' consists of yogurt for breakfast; fruit, a green salad and a slice of whole grain toast four hours later, for lunch; and a light supper, six hours after that. This eating pattern is appropriate only for the person with very strong or over-functioning adrenals. The lack of adequate protein, essential fatty acids, and good quality carbohydrates, as well as the long time between meals in this program, will worsen the symptoms of adrenal fatigue.

People suffering from adrenal fatigue who were used to having lots of energy before they became hypoadrenic tend to choose foods and drinks that energize them at the expense of the adrenal glands, such as coffee, colas and fast foods. They soon learn that fats provide more sustained energy than sweets, so they drive themselves with high-fat fast foods. The problem is that the fat found in processed and fast foods is the wrong kind of fat, the carbohydrates are the wrong kind of carbohydrates because they are refined and have little or no food value, the protein is of inferior quality, and the meals generally offer very little actual nutrition. The caffeine in the coffee and colas temporarily drives the adrenal glands, which further depletes adrenal reserves and causes a roller coaster blood sugar effect. At the end of a day of this, these people often feel pretty wrecked. Add those days up into years and you get the idea. As they continually kick their adrenals with over consumption of fast food and caffeine and deprive their bodies of certain restorative nutrients, their adrenal glands become more and more fatigued and difficult to stimulate*.

Weight Gain and Cortisol Levels

As if this is not bad enough already, people in this predicament usually overeat in their attempt to bolster their lagging energy and then end up gaining weight. The temporary increase in cortisol levels produced by driving the adrenals with too much fast food and caffeine causes people with chronically low cortisol to put on weight because even a temporary excess of cortisol causes fat to be deposited around the middle (the spare tire or swallowed-a-beach-ball look). The added weight adds to their lethargy, making them eat more and more of the wrong food to get through the day. If only they knew when and how to eat, they would be able to keep their energy steady without resorting to this destructive pattern. The solution to this vicious cycle is covered in the sections below.

When to Eat

One of the major dietary mistakes made by people with low adrenal output is not eating soon enough after waking. It is extremely important if you have hypoadrenia that you **eat** <u>**before**</u> **10:00 AM.** You need to replenish your waning glycogen (stored blood sugar) supply after the previous night's energy requirements. Even a small, nutritious snack is better than having nothing at all. However there are two factors that tend to diminish your appetite during the early morning hours. Between 6:00 and 8:00 AM, cortisol levels typically rise rapidly, peaking at around 8:00 AM, and while your cortisol levels are higher, you may not feel like eating. In addition, the low liver function that often accompanies low adrenal function also suppresses early morning hunger. If your liver is very congested, you may sometimes even feel an aversion to food in the morning. Nevertheless, this does not change your need for energy intake and so you must eat some nutritious food before 10:00 AM to keep your body from having to play catch-up during the rest of the day. See the section on "What to Eat" for some suggestions about ways around this.

---

* An overview of the physiology of adrenal fatigue, cortisol levels and hypoglycemia (low blood sugar) is given in Chapter 22 in the section entitled "The Interaction of Low Cortisol, Adrenal Fatigue and Hypoglycemia".

An early **lunch, before noon,** is also better than a later lunch because your body quickly uses up the morning nourishment and needs the next installment; **11:00 – 11:30** is usually the best time for lunch. You should also eat **a nutritious snack sometime between 2:00 and 3:00 PM** to sustain you through the dip in cortisol levels that typically occurs between 3:00 and 4:00 PM in most hypoadrenics. When cortisol levels drop, you do not as readily manufacture or mobilize stored energy from proteins and fats as you do when your cortisol levels are normal. Therefore, taking in food between 2:00 and 3:00 PM allows you to coast through this low energy time much more smoothly. Your **evening meal should be eaten around 5:00 or 6:00 PM**. If you are like most people suffering from adrenal fatigue, you will feel your best after your evening meal. If you do not feel your best after the evening meal, you may be eating the wrong foods for supper.

Later in the evening, **before bed, just a couple of bites of a high quality snack** is often the key to successfully getting through the night without panic attacks, sleep disturbances, anxiety reactions, or feeling wrecked in the morning. The section on what to eat or drink will give you guidelines about these snacks.

If you feel too hungry or if you feel the symptoms of hypoglycemia creeping up on you during the day, then you have waited too long to eat and you should eat something nutritious (not sweet) right away. However, it is much less taxing on your body to eat before you get to the point of being over-hungry or have signs and symptoms of hypoglycemia, especially when your adrenals are weak. The quantity can be small as long as the food provides good quality protein, fat and complex carbohydrates. Make as many refueling stops as you need on your daily flight. Remember that a good fuel supply keeps you from crashing.

What to Eat and Drink
Energy From Food: If you suffer from adrenal fatigue you will do best combining fat, protein and starchy carbohydrates (such as whole grains) at every meal and at every snack. Your body converts fats, proteins, and starch or carbohydrates into a blood sugar called glucose. Despite the fact that your body uses glucose for fuel, eating sugar or sugary foods and fruit juices is hard on your body. It makes blood sugar rise too high, too fast, and subsequently fall too low, leaving your body starving for

fuel again. You can read more about this in the chapter on anatomy and physiology, but for now, remember that foods that are converted too quickly into energy will quickly let you down. Fats, proteins, and starchy carbohydrates eaten together provide a steady source of energy over a longer period of time because they are converted into glucose at different rates. The starchy carbohydrates are converted fairly quickly, the protein takes longer and the fats take the longest to be converted into energy. Combining these three as energy sources puts less strain on every part of your body, including your adrenals.

To Salt or Not to Salt – There is No Question: Salt craving is a common symptom in all stages of adrenal fatigue. The physiological reasons for this are explained in Chapter 22 on physiology and anatomy. But suffice it to say that this is your body's way of crying out for something that it needs. Our salt-phobic society has deprived millions of people struggling with adrenal fatigue of something that would decrease their symptoms and speed their recovery. They have taught their bodies to ignore the urge for salt because it is politically incorrect to salt food. Most of this fear of salt is due to the myth that it causes high blood pressure.

However, the majority of people with adrenal fatigue have low blood pressure, not high. For over seventy years it has been known that people with Addison's disease benefit from the addition of sodium (salt) to their diet. In fact, Loeb, a prominent physician and researcher, was even able to maintain Addison's patients (before the advent of corticosteroids) by the use of large quantities of sodium in their diet. Salt is a welcome addition to the diet in adrenal fatigue because it not only helps increase blood pressure, but also helps restore some of the other functions related to sodium loss within the cells. So if you have cravings for salt, get out the saltshaker and use it.

If you are concerned about your blood pressure, simply buy a sphygmo-manometer (blood pressure cuff) from a drugstore, the internet or medical supply store, and monitor your blood pressure yourself. Although it is true that a small percentage of people are sensitive to sodium and develop high blood pressure as a result of its intake, the majority of people with normal blood pressure do not experience a rise in blood pressure with moderate salt intake. Those with low blood pressure may experience a temporary increase toward normal when they add sodium to their diet. However this does not lead to high blood pressure. If your blood pressure rises to over 140/90, then cut back on salt.

In most cases of adrenal fatigue, salt intake benefits those who add it to their diet. So unless you are one of the rare people with adrenal fatigue and high blood pressure, salt your food. In fact, some of the symptoms of adrenal fatigue are caused by your body's needs for salt.

Sea salt is a good source of salt. It contains more trace minerals than regular table salt but note that it often does not contain iodine. Some of the most nutrient rich sources of salt are kelp and a preparation of salt and sesame seeds called gomasio. To improve the nutrient content of sea salt it is a good idea to mix it half-and-half with kelp. This combination will be especially beneficial for those suffering from severe adrenal fatigue.

This does not mean that excessive salt intake is good for the person not suffering from adrenal fatigue. Excessive salt can be detrimental, especially when combined with a diet high in refined carbohydrates and fat or for the person with mildly elevated adrenal function. As your adrenal glands get stronger, you will usually lose your taste for salt. If you are concerned that you are taking in too much salt, decrease the amount and watch yourself closely. If your symptoms increase or you do not feel as good, then you probably still need a little extra help from salt.

Conversely, foods high in potassium such as fruit (especially bananas and dried figs) make adrenal fatigue worse. This is another reason you should avoid fruit and fruit juices in the morning. Not only do they contain a significant amount of fructose (fruit sugar), they also contain high amounts of potassium. This results in a dangerous duo for people with hypoadrenia. A nice "healthy" fruit and yogurt breakfast will put a lot of hypoadrenic people on the floor. In fact, one sign of hypoadrenia is increased fatigue or shakiness after a high fruit breakfast.

Nutrients From Food
As mentioned above, what you eat is a fundamental aspect of your adrenal recovery program. For this reason it is important for you to under-

stand the different components of foods and how they affect your adrenal health.

Scientists divide food into the components of energy, nutrients, and fiber. The energy portion provides fuel that is converted by your body into energy (usually glucose) and includes fats, proteins and carbohydrates. Nutrients are the vitamins, minerals and other substances in food that nourish your body. Fiber, the indigestible plant cell wall portion of food, also serves important functions in keeping your body healthy. The following sections describe how various foods and nutrients affect adrenal health.

Proteins

Good quality protein available from meat, fish, fowl, eggs, dairy and various plant sources is essential to adrenal recovery. Avoid processed proteins such as lunchmeats, processed cheese and TVP (texturized vegetable protein). Proteins have more food value and are easier to digest when eaten lightly cooked or raw. The amino acids are delivered intact (and therefore more usable) in uncooked or lightly cooked food rather than in the denatured (irreversibly changed) form produced by high heat or long cooking. However, it is always necessary to fully cook poultry and pork to avoid potential microbial danger and to make sure that raw fish, shellfish and beef are free from contamination. If you can be sure of the safety of the source, then sushi, sashimi and ceviche are excellent sources of protein, as is steak tartare and similar preparations from fresh organically raised beef. Raw or lightly cooked eggs and goat milk or goat cheese also provide protein that is exceptionally easy for your body to assimilate.

Many people with adrenal fatigue also have lowered levels of the hydrochloric acid (HCL) necessary to properly break down protein foods in the stomach. If you have this problem you may experience gas, bloating and heaviness in your stomach after eating a meal containing protein foods. Because of these unpleasant after effects, people with low hydrochloric acid often choose to eat less protein and more carbohydrate foods. This only compounds the problem, by aggravating adrenal fatigue with too much carbohydrate and too little protein consumption. The solution is to take a digestive aid with meals that provides supplementary HCL along with other factors such as pepsin, trypsin, papain and/or digestive enzymes that help your body to properly break down protein.

Proteins from vegetable sources are also fine if they are combined correctly to provide all the amino acids you need. Legumes (beans) must be eaten with whole grains, seeds or nuts to make a complete protein. However, it is my experience that vegetarians suffering moderate to severe adrenal fatigue have tremendous difficulty recovering on a strictly vegan (no foods from animal sources) diet. If you are a vegetarian and you have adrenal fatigue, you will do much better if you modify your diet to include eggs, miso (Japanese bean pasta), sea vegetables, yogurt, as well as combining your grains with beans, seeds and nuts at every meal.

Dairy foods (milk, cheese, yogurt, kefir) are excellent sources of protein for some, but many people are unable to digest certain fractions of dairy food either because of an allergy to milk protein (casein) or an absence of the enzyme needed to break down milk sugar (lactose). If you know that you are sensitive to dairy foods, then of course do not include them as a source of protein. If you are not certain, refer to the chapter titled "Food Allergies and Sensitivities." to find out how to determine if you are sensitive to dairy or other foods.

Carbohydrates
Carbohydrates are prevalent in a very broad class of foods that includes grains, vegetables and fruits, but not all carbohydrates are alike. A simple way to divide carbohydrates into three useful categories is as 1) sweet or sugary, 2) starchy, and 3) non-starchy. These categories generally correspond to fruits, grains, and vegetables, respectively.

The sweet or sugary carbohydrates predominate in foods that taste sweet (honey, sugar, syrups, dried or fresh fruits, fruit juices, milk, soft drinks, desserts such as pies, cakes, pastries, and anything that is made with sugar). They provide a quick source of energy that at first rapidly drives the blood sugar up only to let it drop to a low about an hour later. These foods are the most detrimental early in the day. After coffee and a doughnut for breakfast you may feel great for a while, but it may take you the rest of the day to recover from the inevitable low that follows. A whole day of skimpy eating spiked with sugary snacks can leave you feeling exhausted and even hung-over the next morning. The "roller coaster" energy this kind of food provides is especially detrimental for people with low adrenal function. You will therefore do better to greatly limit sweet and sugary foods. The best choices in this category are fruits and fruit drinks sprinkled with some salt. Avoid the white flour and sugar combinations such as pies, cakes, cookies, doughnuts, etc. If you do eat any of these fast energy foods, do not have them by themselves but rather combine them with protein and fats.

Starchy carbohydrates are found mainly in grains and certain root vegetables. The grains can be divided into two subgroups: refined and unrefined, which reflect the amount of processing they have been subjected to. Unrefined grains (whole grains) are minimally processed and still contain their nutrient portions as well as their starchy portion. Your body metabolizes energy from them more slowly, which means that you get more sustained energy as well as nutrients from them. They are also rich sources of the vitamins and minerals needed to metabolize them into energy. Good sources of unrefined carbohydrates are brown rice, whole wheat, buckwheat, unpearled barley, whole oats, unhulled millet, quinoa, and amaranth. Cook and eat them pretty much the way they come from nature, simply washed and steamed in a covered pot with a little salt and the appropriate amount of water (usually twice as much water as grain). Whole grains take anywhere from 15 minutes to an hour to cook, depending on the grain. One note of caution – most people with adrenal fatigue do not do well having cereal grains (even those made from whole grains) in the morning. Check your own reactions, but be careful of grains and breakfast cereals as your first food of the day. An occasional bowl of oatmeal (not instant) seems to be all right.

In contrast, refined grains (refined carbohydrates) have had everything removed in the refining process but the white, starchy portion on the inside of the grain. The nutrients (vitamins and minerals) necessary to metabolize the energy (inner starchy) portion are contained in the outer portion of the grain that is milled away when the grain is refined. Since the nutrient portion of the grain is now missing, your body has to either rob nutrients from itself or get them from a different food source in order to metabolize energy from the refined grain. Over time this leads to the nutritional bankruptcy we experience as poor health, sickness, chronic illnesses, and many subtle deteriorations in health (garbage out).

Unfortunately, many of the favorite menu items of our culture such as pasta, white rice, bread, pastry, and all baked goods made from white flour are made from these refined grains. A similar problem occurs with sugar cane, beets and corn when they are refined into sugar or corn syrup. Approximately three feet of sugar cane makes one tablespoon of white sugar. That means that three feet of nutrients and fiber are lost to produce one tablespoon of naked calories. Continually consuming these naked (energy without nutrients) calories leads to nutrient deficiencies. Nutrient deficiencies lead to impaired physiological function. Impaired physiological function leads to the structural and pathological changes we know as chronic illnesses. Because the purpose of food consumption is to provide your body with the energy AND the nutrients you need, avoid foods that are energy only (i.e. sweets, white flour products, and refined naked calories). Make them an occasional exception rather than the daily rule. Use the Dietary Wheel given later in this chapter to help you plan and eat your way to health.

Choose whole foods over refined foods. But if you are going to choose refined foods, choose pasta over white sugar products. Pastas sustain blood sugar for about three times as long as white sugar products. Both, however, cause a net loss of nutrients since they both have had the vitamins, fiber, minerals and other food values stripped from them in processing. This net loss negatively affects your health with time. If these foods compose a significant part of your diet, you will end up with one form or another of nutritional bankruptcy.

The Glycemic Index
The glycemic index has been brought to the public's attention through the recent popularity of low carbohydrate diets. It assigns a value to how much each food raises blood sugar and was originally intended for use by diabetics. This index only considers the extent to which a food elevates your blood sugar and is not concerned with a food's nutrient value, or the sustainability of the energy a food provides.

For this reason the glycemic index should not be used as the sole guide for making food choices. A good example of the misconceptions that arise when food value is based only on glycemic value appeared in a recent brochure from a diabetic association. It showed a chocolate brownie on one side of the brochure and a potato on the other and asked, "Which raises your blood sugar more?" The answer, that both raise it the same, is essentially true (actually the potato raises your blood sugar slightly more than a brownie). However their inference that eating brownies is okay because it has the same effect as eating potatoes is quite false. Although both of these foods should be used with caution by people who have blood sugar problems, each of them is metabolized differently. The potato has many nutrients in its skin (which should always be eaten with the potato), whereas the brownie is composed mainly of white flour and sugar that robs your body of nutrients while it is being metabolized into blood glucose. Use the glycemic index chart to help maintain steady blood sugar levels, but recognize that it does not provide information about nutrients contained in the food, nor the sustainable energy of a food. Always pick whole foods when you have a choice. A copy of the glycemic index is included in Appendix A and on the website.

Vegetables

Every day you should include 6-8 servings of a wide variety of vegetables in your meals, especially the vegetables that are naturally highly colored (bright green, red, orange, yellow, purple). In addition to carbohydrates and proteins, vegetables provide vitamins, minerals, antioxidants, and a high amount of fiber. They also provide important constituents such as proanthrocyanadins, anthrocyanadins and other elements essential for health but not considered in the typical energy or nutrient categories. Make sure you have at least three highly colored vegetables with each of your noon and evening meals. You will not gain weight with these vegetables but, by including them, you will give your body many of the factors it needs to improve your overall health with time.

Vegetables can be steamed, sautéed, stir-fried, deep-fried, baked, boiled, grilled, blanched or eaten raw. It is actually better to use a variety of techniques to prepare vegetables because different nutrients are made available through different cooking methods. For example, nutrients like vitamin C and folic acid are vulnerable to heat and do not survive cooking. However, other vitamins such as the carotenoids (vitamin A related substances) and some of the minerals become more available if the vegetables are cooked before being eaten. Therefore, if you combine a variety of preparation techniques with a wide variety of vegetables, you will increase your chances of getting the most complete range of available nutrients from the vegetables.

One class of vegetables eaten by most coastal cultures is seaweed. There are many kinds, but nearly all are rich in trace minerals, good quality vegetable protein, and are easily digested. Most oriental stores and some health food stores carry a variety of these nutritious foods and can tell you how to prepare them. Seaweeds are some of the most nutritious vegetables you can eat.

Sprouts are another source of exceptionally high quality concentrated nutrients. Almost any bean or seed can be sprouted. Sprouts are easy to grow, inexpensive and contain nutrients often deficient or missing in diets. They can be used in salads, soups, vegetable dishes, and eaten with any vegetable, grain or meat. Any person in a health food store or co-op should be able to tell you how to grow sprouts. If not, there are several books and booklets available that contain simple instructions. Ounce-for-ounce, sprouts rank at the top as a source of nutrients. People who have an abundance of sea vegetables and sprouts in their diet usually enjoy good health. Note: Obtain your seeds for sprouting from a health food store or other food outlet. Seeds sold to be planted often contain pesticides and other chemicals that can be harmful if swallowed. Check with a knowledgeable person in the store if you have any doubts about whether the seeds can be used for sprouting.

A list of vegetables is located in Appendix B. Use this list to widen your usual choice and find new and interesting flavors.

Vegetables high in sodium and thus helpful in supporting adrenal recovery include the following (given in descending order of sodium content):

<u>Highest sodium content</u>
Kelp
Green Olives
Dulse
Ripe (black) olives

<u>High sodium content</u>
Hot red peppers

New Zealand spinach
Swiss chard
Beet greens
Celery (leaves and root)
Zucchini

A vegetable soup recipe that has proved helpful in restoring adrenal function during the active, chronic, and recovery phases of infectious disease is given below. This high-energy soup called "Taz" comes from Dolores S. Downey's "Balancing body chemistry with nutrition seminars," Cannonburg, MI 49317, page 158.

Adrenal Recovery Soup
16oz. green beans
1 cup chopped celery
1 zucchini, sliced
1 medium onion, chopped
1 cup tomato juice
1 cup spring water
2 tbsp. raw honey
1 tsp. Paprika
1 cup chicken broth
pepper to taste
Combine ingredients and simmer for one hour until vegetables are tender.

Fruit
People with adrenal fatigue and blood sugar problems should go lightly on fruits, especially in the morning. But if you exercise early in the day, it may be possible for you to handle a small amount of fruit for breakfast. Exercise elevates cortisol and aldosterone levels, which in turn raise sodium levels in your blood, allowing for greater tolerance to the effects of fruit. However, be very careful of fruit consumption and if you notice that you become more tired, thick headed or start to experience other symptoms of either low blood sugar or low adrenals, then eliminate fruit in the morning.

Any fruit that you do eat should be organically grown. Many people who suffer from adrenal fatigue are sensitive to chemicals in foods. Several sprays are used on commercially grown fruits and, although they are considered safe by government standards, they still adversely affect a significant portion of people with adrenal fatigue. Buy your fruit from organic farmers, if possible, or health food stores and grocery stores who carry unsprayed or certified organic fruits and vegetables. If you cannot find organic or unsprayed fruit and vegetables, soak the produce in 3 quarts of water with 1 teaspoon of bleach added for 15 minutes, rinse well and dry, or use one of the vegetable washes that are now available in many grocery and health food stores. This will help remove most of the chemicals on the skins of the fruits and vegetables.

Below is a short list of fruits people with adrenal fatigue do better with and those they should avoid. A complete list of fruits is available in Appendix C. Remember that quantity, quality and time of day are all important in your fruit intake. As a general rule do not have fruit in the morning, eat only organic fruit that has not been sprayed with chemicals that could keep you tired for days, and eat only modest amounts at any one time. If the fruit has been sprayed with chemicals while growing (i.e. not organic) do not eat the skin. The extra nutrients are not worth the chemical poisons you eat with the outer surface. Nutritional deficiencies are much more easily rectified than chemical toxicities. Buy organically grown fruit whenever possible. Always wash fruit before eating.

Fruit Guide For People With Adrenal Fatigue	
Preferred fruits	**Fruits to avoid**
papaya	Bananas
mango	Raisins
plums	Dates
pears	Figs
kiwi,	Oranges
apples	Grapefruit
grapes (only a few)	
cherries	

Fats & Oils

Fats and oils have gotten a bad rap in North America over the past few years. Although it is true that most North Americans consume too much fat in their daily diet (40-55% of daily calories), it is also true that a disproportionate number of North Americans suffer from hypoadrenia. People with adrenal fatigue often crave fats and oils, partly because foods high in fats make them feel better for longer than low fat or sweet foods. Some fats also contain cholesterol needed by the adrenal glands to make the steroid hormones essential for adrenal activity throughout your body. Ideally, fats should not make up more than 20-25% of your total daily calories but it is very important that they are the right kind of fats.

Despite this huge over-consumption of fat, most North Americans are sadly lacking in the essential fatty acids that promote good skin quality, reduce inflammation and slow down the aging of body tissues. The type and quality of fats in your diet is critical because they become a major part of your cell walls, nerves and the membranes of your body. So do not simply decrease your fat intake but look closely at what kinds of oils and fats you eat to make sure you are choosing ones high in essential fatty acids that nourish your body. An excellent book on the subject of the essential fats is Udo Erasmus' book "Fats that Heal, Fats that Kill." Below are a few things you should know about fats and oils.

Saturated and Unsaturated Fats: Fats and oils are composed of 3 fatty acids stuck to a glycerol molecule. The fatty acids are chains of carbons that vary in length from 4 to 24 carbons, with an acid stuck on the end. Each carbon is connected to the next by either a single bond or a double bond. If all the carbons in the fatty acid chain are connected by only one bond between them, it is called a *saturated fat* (like butter, coconut oil and lard). When there is one double bond in the whole fatty acid chain, it is called a *monounsaturated fat* (like olive oil). If there is more than one double bond in the chain, it is called a *polyunsaturated fat* (like canola, peanut and safflower oil).

The common belief is that saturated fats are bad, polyunsaturates are good, monosaturates are best. The truth is that each has its uses. The oils least damaged by heating include: coconut, palm, palm kernel, cocoa butter, butter, refined peanut, refined avocado, high oleic sunflower, high oleic safflower, sesame oil and olive oil, in that order. Saturated fats withstand heat the best, and so do not become rancid or toxic as easily as other fats when heated. Use saturated fats for cooking (baking, broiling, sautéing, frying), but use the minimum amount needed to do the job and do not reuse them. You can recognize saturated fats by their ability to remain solid at room temperature. Butter, animal fat, palm and palm kernel oil, and coconut butter are common sources of saturated fats.

Monounsaturated fats can be used for low heat cooking, but should not be used for high heat or lengthy cooking. You can recognize monounsaturated fats by their property of being liquid at room temperature but solid when refrigerated. Olive oil contains a high amount of monounsaturates. Rapid stir frying, sautéing, and similar methods are acceptable ways of using these oils. When sautéing or stir-frying, put a little water in the pan before the oil to keep the oil from getting too hot, add garlic, onions or scallions to help decrease the rancidity caused by heating the oil, and use only small amounts of oil. Although these are the safest fats to cook with, none of these oils contain appreciable amounts of essential fatty acids. They are simply "less bad for you" because they do not break down as easily with heat.

Avoid deep fried foods. If you have cancer or any chronic degenerative disease, do not eat fried foods at all. If you have adrenal fatigue, only eat fried foods once a month or less, the cost to your health is just too high a price to pay for the sake of convenience or habit.

Polyunsaturated fatty acids are relatively fragile, even at room temperature and go rancid much more quickly than the other fats. Their average shelf life is only a few weeks after opening. The more heat and light they are exposed to, the more quickly they go rancid. Unstable as they are, we need certain polyunsaturates in our diet to be healthy. So although they should not be used for cooking, they should be added to food after it has been cooked, or used in salad dressings.

Essential Fatty Acids: Polyunsaturated fatty acids come in 2 categories, non-essential and essential. Non- essential fatty acids are those the body can make by itself from other fats and oils. Essential fatty acids are the fatty acids we need to get from food because we cannot make them ourselves. Luckily, there are some plants and animals that do make them. We can get our essential fatty acids by eating them and the oils made from them. Essential fatty acids are very important for us to consume in adequate amounts in order to maintain good health. Lack of intake or imbalances in the essential fatty acids has been shown to lead to a myriad of health problems.

There are 2 types of essential fatty acids, alpha-linolenic and linoleic. Alpha-linolenic acid belongs to the Omega 3 group of fatty acids and linoleic acid belongs to the Omega 6 group. Omega 3 fatty acids have more double bonds (3 to 6) and come from colder, more northern climates. Examples of foods high in omega 3 fatty acids are salmon, sardines, soybeans, walnuts, flax seeds, and in smaller amounts, dark green plants. Omega 6 fatty acids have fewer double bonds (2-4) and come from more southern plants such as sesame, sunflower, safflower, and corn. Both groups of essential fatty acids are extremely important to your health. An improper balance of essential fatty acids fosters the development of many conditions such as heart and circulatory disorders, arthritis and cancer, and the adrenals inevitably become involved in these diseases.

Because these oils contain a high number of double bonds, they are relatively unstable, so buy them in small quantities and keep them in the freezer. They stay liquid even in the freezer. Be selective; buy oils that are unrefined and pressed in cool temperatures (under 100 degrees F) from raw, organically grown seeds, and packaged in light-proof (dark, non-transparent) containers. You can find these oils in specialty stores, health food stores and on the internet. A good way to check for freshness and quality is the sniff test. Remove the cap when you get it home and smell the oil. It should have a pleasant smell, reminding you of the seed it was made from. If it smells fishy, bitter, like varnish or has another off-smell, return it because it is rancid and has probably been over-refined, over-heated, or had solvents used in its extraction.

The right balance of essential fatty acid intake contributes significantly to adrenal recovery, as well as to your general health. For optimum health the best balance of essential fatty acids is a 4:1 ratio of omega 6's to omega 3's. One easy way to get the right amount of essential fatty acids in this ratio is to mix 1 tablespoon of flax seed oil with 1 tablespoon of sunflower or safflower oil daily. Add this mixture, <u>uncooked</u>, to food just before you eat it (as salad dressing, mixed in with vegetables, sauces or grain, added to smoothies, etc.). My favorite way to add these oils is to mix a little soy sauce into them and use it in place of butter or margarine. It is very pleasant tasting when used as a condiment in this way.

Another great way to make certain your essential fatty acid intake is adequate is to follow these simple rules.

Getting the Essential Fatty Acids You Need

- Mix flax seed oil with safflower or sunflower seed oils in a 1:1 ratio
- Consume 1-2 tablespoon (uncooked) per day, sprinkled on meats, vegetables, grains, etc.
- Use only fresh, raw, cold pressed, unrefined oils
- Buy only organically grown oils stored in lightproof containers
- Keep all oils in the refrigerator or freezer
- Squeeze one capsule of 400 IU vitamin E (mixed tocopherols) into every ¼ cup oil
- Eat cold water ocean fish (except tuna, mackerel and swordfish.*) as a source of omega 3 oils
- Eat fresh seeds and nuts (except peanuts) as a source of omega 6 oils
- Avoid all hydrogenated or partially hydrogenated oils (read labels on food)
- Use lower temperature cooking methods (see cooking tips above)
- Eat fried foods only occasionally
- Avoid all deep fried foods
- Avoid restaurant foods cooked with oils

* These fish are too high in mercury.

But even if you do eat the right quantity of essential fatty acids in the right ratio, their value can be negated if you also consume poor quality or hydrogenated oils. The problems created by hydrogenated, partially hydrogenated and poor quality fats will be covered in detail in the section below on "Foods to Avoid." Read labels, do not buy any foods containing them and avoid fried foods in restaurants. If you continue to eat them, even though you are eating the right essential fatty acids as well, you will lose the very valuable, health enhancing aspects of essential oils, and promote body processes that spawn cancer, heart disease, arthritis, obesity and other chronic ailments. Needless to say, you will also make it more difficult for your adrenals to recover.

Seeds and Nuts as a Source of Essential Fatty Acids
Choosing the right seeds and nuts - Seeds and nuts are an important source of essential fatty acids that your body converts into a number of different substances it needs. For example, if there is not enough cholesterol in your diet, your adrenal glands will manufacture the cholesterol needed to produce all the adrenal steroid hormones. This cholesterol is made from fatty acids derived from the oils you eat. As mentioned above, other substances manufactured from these oils become an integral part of the structure of your cell walls, nerves and membranes. Obviously, the better the quality of the oils and fats you eat, the easier it is for your body to produce good quality cell structures and hormones.

The following seeds and nuts are good sources of essential fatty acids, as long as they are purchased fresh and stored properly. Listed to the right side of most seeds and nuts, there are brief descriptions of what these seeds and nuts look like when they are fresh. You must make sure of their freshness when buying seeds, nuts, fish, and the oils from them. Rancid oils make the symptoms of adrenal fatigue worse and should absolutely be avoided. In parenthesis are the signs of rancidity for that particular seed or nut.

Seeds (raw only)
- Sesame Seeds, unhulled, – tan or black (shiny, bitter tasting or stale smelling seeds are rancid)
- Pumpkin Seeds – green (shiny seeds are rancid)
- Sunflower Seeds - mouse gray (brownish or shiny seeds are rancid)
- Flax Seeds - reddish brown (slightly fishy smelling seeds are rancid)

Nuts (raw only)
- Filberts – brown skin, creamy meat (shriveled nuts or nuts with dark spots on meat are rancid)
- Cashews – light beige, no skin (darkish brown or shiny cashews are rancid)
- Almonds - light brown skin, pale creamy meat (shriveled nuts or nuts with dark spots on meat are rancid)

- Brazil Nuts – dark brown skin, pale creamy meat (brown streaks on meat indicate rancidity)
- Macadamias – very pale cream color (shiny nuts or brown spots indicates rancidity)
- Coconuts, fresh – heavy, plenty of liquid, hard unbroken shell, white sweet smelling meat   (fermented odor, brownish or shriveled meat indicates rancidity)
- Pecans – smooth shell, brown and cream meat (shiny, oily or shriveled nuts are rancid)
- Walnuts - smooth shell, brown and tan meat (shiny, oily or shriveled nuts are rancid)
- Peanuts – reddish skin, cream to light tan meat (shriveled, darkened or hard nuts are rancid; organically grown nuts, stored cold, are less likely to be contaminated by aflatoxin)
- Chestnuts – dark brown, plump, smooth shell with cream colored meat (shriveled, hard or dark meat indicates rancidity; nuts may also have bluish mold on the inside)

All seeds and nuts should be purchased raw and stored in the freezer to avoid rancidity. Although it is preferable to eat them raw, if you want roasted nuts, you can easily dry roast them. Simply heat them in a cast iron skillet on medium-low heat, stirring frequently, for about ten minutes, or bake them on a cookie sheet in an oven preheated to 200°F for approximately 20 minutes. Another way to make a great adrenal-friendly snack is to sprinkle soy sauce made from organically grown soybeans and free of MSG over nuts and seeds, just before or just after you roast them. Do not use oil for roasting nuts. After dry roasting, the nuts should be again stored in the freezer and be ready for instant use. Either raw or dry roasted nuts are great as a snack, incorporated into meals, blended into nut drinks, sprinkled onto salads, and used in many other ways. Avoid all nuts and seeds that have been commercially roasted or deep-fried. The high heat and poor quality oils used in this process usually make them go rancid quickly. Rancid oils are poisons and need to be avoided. They interrupt the normal metabolism of oils in the body and contribute to free radical damage in the cell walls. It is worth paying a little more for higher quality raw nuts and getting the benefits of their fresh oils than it is to submit your body to the destructive effects of rancid oils.

Rancid nuts and oils can especially play havoc with mental processes in subtle ways that are sometimes difficult to detect, but that interfere with daily life. Many more people are sensitive to rancid oils than realize it. Read the chapter "Food Allergies and Sensitivities" to learn how to find out if you are one of these people. I have known of several instances in which skeptical patients were surprised to see many positive changes in their mental functioning as well as in their health once they switched to eating raw seeds and nuts, stored in the freezer, and started using only organically grown, cold-pressed oils. A couple of interesting and dramatic examples are included in the section "Food sensitivities that are not allergies" in the chapter titled "Food Allergies and Sensitivities." Whenever you have an adverse, allergic or sensitivity reaction to a food such as rancid oil, your adrenals have to once again draw on their resources to compensate for the stress and to rebalance your body chemistry.

Tips on Cooking with Oil – Even though it is important to consume the essential oils above, you do not want to cook with them. Fats and oils containing essential fatty acids break down easily with heat to form harmful free radicals, thus it is best to cook with oils low in essential fatty acids. Use the following chart to select your cooking oils. Note that none of the oils given in the table contain many essential fatty acids. Therefore, relying on these oils alone for your fat intake will result in essential fatty acid deficiencies. If you cook with oils, use one kind for cooking and add the oils high in essential fatty acids to your food just before serving. The oils listed below are more resistant to the toxic, free radical and rancid effects created by the heating of oils. Even these still break down if heated excessively though, so to protect yourself do the following:
- Avoid all deep-frying and browning
- Put a little water into the pan first before you add the food to be cooked
- Add the food before the oil
- Use only a small amount of oil (less than a tablespoon)

Oils for Cooking (in order of preference)*
Coconut
Palm Kernel
Cocoa Butter
Butter
Refined Peanut & Avocado
High Oleic Sunflower & Safflower
Sesame
Olive

(from Erasmus, Udo. Fats That Kill, Fats That Heal, p 129)

Summary of What to Eat
1) The Dietary Intake Wheel for adrenal fatigue, shown on the next page, summarizes what you should eat if you have adrenal fatigue. Here are 9 easy rules to follow.
2) Eat a wide variety of whole, natural foods.
3) Combine a fat, protein and carbohydrate source with every meal.
4) Eat lots of vegetables, especially the brightly colored ones.
5) Salt your food to a pleasant taste.
6) Eat mainly whole grains as starchy carbohydrate sources.
7) Combine grains with beans, seeds or nuts to form a complete protein.
8) Avoid fruit in the morning.
9) Mix 1-2 tablespoons of essential oils into grains, vegetables and meats daily.
10) Eat high quality food; it becomes you.
11) By following these simple guidelines, your food intake will help you recover from adrenal fatigue.

If you have moderate to severe adrenal fatigue, you will probably do better by increasing your protein intake and decreasing the starchy (whole grains) and sweet (fruit) carbohydrate content of your diet. Of course, sugar and white flour products should be eliminated altogether (see below). As you improve, you should gradually be able to handle the starchy carbohydrates (grains) and eventually the fruits in greater proportion. Re-read the section on proteins to become familiar with the most valuable ones for recovery.

Now that you know what to eat, it is important for you to also learn what foods to avoid. These are foods that can wreck your biochemistry, hormone balance, and eventually your health. Read the next section to find out how to protect your health by knowing which foods work behind the scenes to sabotage your health.

DIETARY INTAKE WHEEL FOR ADRENAL FATIGUE

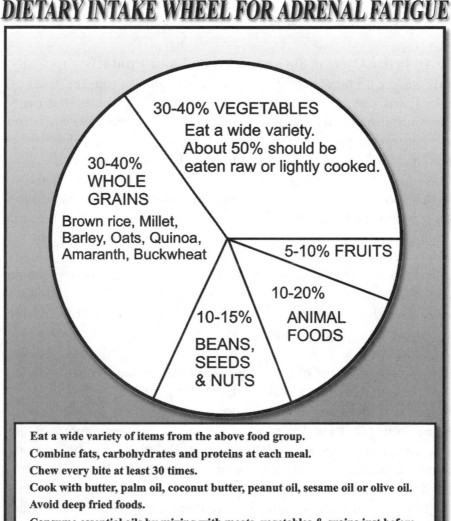

30-40% VEGETABLES
Eat a wide variety.
About 50% should be
eaten raw or lightly cooked.

30-40% WHOLE GRAINS
Brown rice, Millet,
Barley, Oats, Quinoa,
Amaranth, Buckwheat

5-10% FRUITS

10-20% ANIMAL FOODS

10-15% BEANS, SEEDS & NUTS

Eat a wide variety of items from the above food group.

Combine fats, carbohydrates and proteins at each meal.

Chew every bite at least 30 times.

Cook with butter, palm oil, coconut butter, peanut oil, sesame oil or olive oil.

Avoid deep fried foods.

Consume essential oils by mixing with meats, vegetables & grains just before serving.

Avoid the following foods: cakes, pies, doughnuts, cookies and other foods containing white flour, sugar and chocolate.

Avoid the following drinks: coffee, colas, alcohol, black tea and hot chocolate.

What Not to Eat

It is hard to say which is more important when you have adrenal fatigue - what to eat or what not to eat! Eating the wrong foods or combination of foods can throw you off for hours and even days, so do not even try to sneak something by; it is just not worth the price you have to pay. Pick the foods that are recommended and stick with them. The further you deviate from them, the more problems you are likely to have and the more difficult it will be to balance your body chemistry.

The Addictive Cycle of Sugar and White Flour Products: Ironically, foods made with these ingredients such as doughnuts, rolls, pies, cakes, cookies, crackers, candy bars, and soft drinks are the ones that many people suffering from adrenal fatigue crave. This is because when you have adrenal fatigue you also usually have hypoglycemia (low blood sugar) and foods made from refined flour and/or sugar quickly raise your blood sugar. Unfortunately, they raise your blood sugar so high and so fast that too much insulin is released in response. This excess insulin then causes your blood sugar levels to crash, leading to hypoglycemic symptoms and more cravings. Furthermore, sugar and white flour are entirely naked calories, the metabolism of which drains an already depleted body of the vitamins and minerals it needs to heal or to maintain itself. Furthermore, because of their disruptive effects on your body's metabolism, these substances can also produce cravings and compulsive behavior, and become addictive.

Millions upon millions of people in industrialized nations are addicted to white flour and sugar products. Look at the typical coffee break. It happens at 10:00 in the morning, approximately two hours after break-fast, and consists of a coffee and doughnut or some other combination of refined white flour and sugar. This temporarily drives your blood sugar up and the insulin soon follows. As mentioned above, the excess secretion of insulin causes a rapid drop in your blood sugar. Normally, when your blood sugar starts to fall, the circulating cortisol triggers certain proteins and fats to be converted into blood sugar to compensate for this drop. But when your adrenals are fatigued, the amount of cortisol in circulation is low and cannot keep up with the demand to create new blood sugar. Consequently, your blood sugar continues to drop unchecked to even lower levels. As luck would have it, this happens about 11:30 to 12:00 when you can usually stem the plunge with lunch.

But again, people often polish off lunch with a cup of coffee, a soda, or a dessert, which drives blood sugar artificially high once more. They know that if they do not end the meal this way they will become sleepy at around 2:00 PM. However, the reason they get sleepy after a meal is that their repeated consumption of refined carbohydrates has, over time, reduced their ability to secrete enough digestive juices to totally digest the food. Then, of course, around 3:00 PM, there is another crash typical of low adrenal function. To avoid this, many people take another coffee break at 2:00 PM at which they consume more refined carbohydrates to get the blood sugar up and going. Or they may continually drink coffee or soft drinks all afternoon. By the end of the day, if you follow this typical pattern, you probably feel like a wreck because you have consumed the kinds of foods and beverages that have taken your blood sugar on a roller coaster ride. If you replace the items made with white flour like pies, cakes, cookies, crackers, most desserts, commercial breads and pastas, and all caffeine containing or sweet drinks like sodas with foods that contain nutrients and not just energy, you will quit robbing your body of what it needs. More than that, you will be able to get off the perpetual hypoglycemic roller coaster ride that leaves you fatigued, inefficient, and aging more quickly inside.

The Hidden Message in Chocolate Cravings: Yep, we finally got to it. You thought we were going to gloss right over chocolate and not mention it. If you have a piece of chocolate once or twice a year, you can probably skip this section. However, if you crave chocolate, would almost be willing to kill for chocolate, or if chocolate is a coveted part of your diet, then you need to read this.

A craving for chocolate can sometimes actually be your body's craving for magnesium, since chocolate contains large amounts of magnesium. This is especially true in women who crave chocolate before they menstruate or who have PMS. Magnesium helps mediate the symptoms of PMS because it is intimately involved in the manufacture of progesterone. A lack of magnesium can lead to inadequate progesterone levels, producing the PMS symptoms. In the body's wisdom, it craves chocolate because chocolate is rich in magnesium. The unfortunate aspect, however, is that chocolate is also high in caffeine and a caffeine-like substance, theobromine, that over stimulate the adrenals leading to further adrenal fatigue. Much of the fine balancing of the sex hormones is accomplished by the adrenals, and the increase in adrenal fatigue leads to increased PMS. So chocolate ends up increasing PMS even though it contains magnesium.

Therefore it is much better to use your craving for chocolate as a reminder to get your magnesium from some other source. The easiest solution is to supplement your diet with 400 mg. of magnesium per day. Presently, the best form of magnesium for the cost is magnesium citrate. It is readily available, easily absorbed and effective. For severe cases of PMS, take magnesium all month long. For mild cases, take it from the time of ovulation (12th to 14th day from the first day of your cycle) until the next cycle starts. That physical craving for chocolate should decrease rapidly, often within one to two weeks after beginning the magnesium supplement, and should disappear or remain negligible as long as the amount of magnesium intake remains adequate. Foods high in magnesium such as kelp, almonds, cashews and other nuts, sesame seeds (brown), whole wheat, peas, and beans should also be increased.

The Evils of Hydrogenated and Partially Hydrogenated Oils: Hydrogenated and partially hydrogenated fats are oils that have been altered chemically to have certain properties (like remaining solid at room temperature) that have nothing to do with your health. Three common examples are vegetable shortening, margarine and the oil in commercial peanut butters. These adulterated fats are used in almost all commercially prepared food items found in grocery stores and in many restaurant foods. So even in our fat-phobic society, we still consume a tremendous amount of the wrong kinds of fats and oils. A great deal of these bad fats and oils are eaten in the pre-prepared products mentioned earlier.

You learned in the section about seeds and oils just how valuable and important the right kinds of fats and oils are to your health. The good fats are those that the body can use to build tissue, such as nerve and cell wall membranes, and the bad fats are the ones that block this from happening. When you eat foods containing hydrogenated and partially hydrogenated fats they disrupt normal fatty acid metabolism in your body. **They use up the enzymes that normally would be utilized by the good oils, and prevent your body from creating quality cell membranes and nerve sheaths**. As a result, your body cannot transform essential fatty acids into the materials it needs to make various cell wall components and other structures.

A recent clinical study in Canada demonstrated that the metabolism of good oils into substances needed by the body was completely blocked when the people in the study were given hydrogenated or partially hydrogenated oils. This means that the margarine you have been eating instead of butter is probably doing you more harm than good.

Therefore, read the labels on everything that you buy. You may be surprised to see just how many of the foods you eat contain hydrogenated or partially hydrogenated oils or fats. Any time you see hydrogenated or partially hydrogenated oils or fats, put that food back on the shelf and **do not buy it**. Alternatives are available in health food stores and in the grocery store, if you look carefully.

Even though you may crave these familiar foods, eating them seriously interferes with your ability to heal. What you are really craving are the essential fatty acids. Go back and re-read the sections "Getting the essential fatty acids you need" and "Seeds and nuts as a source of essential fatty acids" to know how to truly satisfy your body's craving.

Avoid Deep Fried Foods: Most deep fried foods are fried in hydrogenated or partially hydrogenated fats. These fats are kept at high temperatures and are often reused. As the oil is heated above a certain temperature or reheated, it breaks down, forming toxic free radicals and becoming rancid. This means that eating deep fried food causes not only the same problems as hydrogenated fats but also the additional problems created by toxic free radicals. Because free radicals are produced when oils break down with heat, you should also avoid food fried in oils high in essential fatty acids (cold pressed sunflower, flax, peanut, safflower, etc.) or any foods fried at a high temperature or for long periods of time.

Avoid "Fast" Foods and Junk Foods: There are numerous problems with typical fast food and junk food. They all contain white flour, sugar, hydrogenated fats, or all three. Often their ingredients are poor quality (cheap) with little nutrient value, and artificial colors, flavors and preservatives are used to make up for this. What nutrients they do have are frequently lost while they are kept hot or stored for long periods of time. It is questionable whether some junk foods are even food at all. You do not need these "foods," they only create havoc with your biochemistry, make you fat, and leave you feeling wrecked after the insulin rush is over.

Avoid Foods You Are Allergic or Sensitive To: It is important to completely eliminate all foods and food substances that you are allergic or sensitive to. Unless there is an anaphylactic reaction (cannot breathe) or hives, most people are not aware that their symptoms may be a reaction to a food they are sensitive too. Chapter 14, "Food Allergies and Sensitivities" will explain the role food allergies and sensitivities play in adrenal fatigue. It describes in detail how you can find out what foods you may be allergic or sensitive to, if any, and what you can do to help yourself if this is a factor in your adrenal fatigue.

Avoid Foods You Are Addicted To: Foods you crave are often foods that contain substances you are addicted to for reasons that may involve food sensitivities and/or hypoglycemia. Eating these foods places more stress on your adrenals and so you should avoid them. Refer to the section on food addiction in the next chapter for more information.

How to Eat
The Act of Eating - How you eat can have as much affect on your adrenal glands as what you eat. Before you start a meal, it is important to prepare your body so it can begin the complicated process of digestion, absorption, and utilization of energy and nutrients. If you have any control over your eating environment, choose a peaceful spot with pleasant surroundings. If you do not, think of pleasant surroundings and use things like headphones or photos to change your environment. Play music or other relaxing sounds through your headphones and visualize or look at things in your environment that are relaxing or beautiful. Think of enjoyable things. Eating with friends is also a good idea. Congenial conversation and good company promotes relaxation and digestion. Rushing through meals while focusing on work or problems, and eating with people or in situations that make you tense are bad for your health.

Eat your food sitting down, not standing up at a counter, not running from one place to another, not driving nor lying down but actually sitting in one place peacefully. Before you start to eat, take a moment to calm yourself.

Take a deep breath and let it out after you are seated and ready to eat. Take a second deep breath, hold it for a few seconds, and then let it out. Take a third breath, breathing in deeply from the abdomen, hold it for a longer time, and then let it out. The idea is not to see if you can turn blue while holding your breath, but to help your body relax. When you are relaxed the part of your nervous system that is responsible for digestion and absorption is free to function properly. Holding your breath for ten to twenty seconds is a good way for your body to begin to relax.

Next, take a moment to be grateful because just by the fact that you are alive, you have many blessings. Bringing your body and mind together with your breathing and gratitude settles your body and prepares it to eat. If at all possible, eat your meal peacefully and slowly. Eating peacefully and slowly also helps you digest your food more completely, allowing you to get the most value out of your food and experience fewer digestive problems. It also is more refreshing.

Chew your food well because chewing properly makes a surprisingly significant difference to good digestion. The instructions for chewing are very simple; chew, chew, chew. (See Illustration "When you eat, think of trains…"). Chew 30 times per mouthful if at all possible. If you have digestive upsets or difficulty digesting food, chew 60 times per mouthful. With diabetic patients and patients with digestive problems, I always have them chew 100 times per mouthful because the more thorough the chewing, the more completely the food particles are mixed with saliva which contains enzymes for digestion. In addition, the act of chewing is a relaxing one.

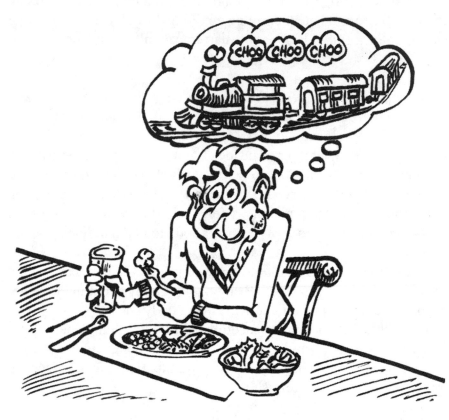

When you eat, think of trains....choo...choo...chew!

Avoid rushed and hectic meals and gulping down your food because that is exactly the opposite of what your body needs to recover from adrenal fatigue. The combination of sitting down to eat, taking time to breathe, experiencing gratitude before eating, eating peacefully and slowly, and chewing well is a very relaxing and restorative process that aids the entire body. Eating and the act of eating then become therapeutic in themselves.

If you have hypoglycemia, which is very common in people with adrenal fatigue, having several small meals during the day may be better than one or two large ones. Many people with blood sugar irregularities find that more frequent small meals work better for them than one or two large meals. Even in the smaller meals, it is important to chew very well, at least 30 times per mouthful.

Even when you eat and drink the right things, in the right way, hidden food sensitivities may be bringing down your adrenals. The next chapter will tell you all about hidden food allergies and sensitivities. If you have times when you feel bad for no reason, read on because this and other symptoms such as brain fog, sporadic poor coordination, and many other symptoms related to adrenal fatigue can be caused by your reactions to food.

Beverages

Drink Me – People with adrenal fatigue often crave caffeine or cola beverages because of the stimulatory effect of the caffeine. The difficulty with this is that caffeine also over-stimulates the adrenals, which leads to further fatiguing when the caffeine wears off. Therefore, many people with adrenal fatigue get through the day by kicking their adrenals with several cups of coffee and beverages containing caffeine or by combining caffeine, sweets, and chocolate (which contains caffeine and a caffeine-like substance). Although this makes them feel better temporarily, this regimen will eventually exhaust the adrenals even more, leading them into further difficulties. Therefore, avoid caffeine containing foods and beverages.

Below is a list of beverages that work better for people with adrenal fatigue. Those that need preparation have an asterisk beside them and there will be instructions for how to prepare them listed on the following pages. Several of the drinks listed are accompanied by necessary explanations.

Green Tea – Green tea is better for your adrenals than regular (black) tea or coffee. Even though it has a small amount of caffeine, it contains high amounts of antioxidants and other nutrients. Green tea has been noted for its anti-cancer or cancer protection qualities. It is pleasant tasting, refreshing, easy to make, and can be taken hot, cold, or at room temperature. If the green tea you buy tastes very strong or bitter, it is poor quality, so try another brand. It is readily available in some of the larger grocery stores, as well as in high quality health food stores and oriental markets.

Barley Tea – Barley tea is tea made from roasted barley. Available in tea bags at most oriental markets and some health food stores, it can be drunk hot or cold. I use it in the summer in place of regular ice tea, keeping a gallon jar of it in the refrigerator. It is pleasant, with a light, roasted taste. You can also easily make your own barley tea by roasting unhulled barley on a cookie sheet in a 200 degree oven until it turns brown and has a roasted fragrance. After it cools, store it in plastic bags to keep it fresh.

Twig Tea or Kukicha Tea – Twig or Kukicha tea is made from the small twigs of the tea plant. It is prepared by boiling some of these twigs in water and can be taken hot or cold. One of the advantages of twig tea is that it has a nice roasted taste. It also has the same viscosity as coffee, although it does not taste like coffee. I found that some people miss the consistency of coffee as much as the stimulation and so twig tea provides a good substitute with that consistency. It is available in some oriental stores, health food stores, and from all microbiotic outlets.

Bancha Tea – Bancha tea is another tea available from oriental markets. There are many different kinds of bancha teas, some have small tea leaves, some have twigs, and some are combined with roasted rice. Any of them are all right to consume and each has its own unique flavor. Again, the bancha tea can be taken hot or cold and is versatile in its uses.

Herbal Tea – Over the last twenty years a tremendous variety of herbal teas have come on the market and are now produced by large commercial companies. Because there is such a variety of teas, it is difficult to comment on each of them. As a general rule, it is important that the herbal teas contain only herbal teas and are not mixed with black teas. Herbal teas can be taken hot or cold, can be mixed with nut milks, and are very refreshing.

Water - You might think that the topic of water would be very straightforward. However, water is actually quite a complicated issue. The difficulty is twofold: 1) the poor water quality in most city water supplies contains toxic substances especially detrimental for people suffering from adrenal fatigue, and 2) people with low adrenals have specific problems with their internal water balance.

City water supplies include one or more of the following health hazards: high pH, increased particulate matter, toxic metals, and toxic chemicals including excessive chlorine or fluoride. Bacterial, viral and even parasitic contaminants are also problems. As a result, unless you have done adequate research on your own water supply and determined it to be safe, you may be risking short or long term health problems by drinking your local water. Even some bottled waters are known to contain contaminants. The recommended solution for this is to have a water purification system installed at the tap or in your house. The system you purchase should filter for chemicals (chlorine, toxic industrial chemicals such as PCBs & TCE, toxic metals, pesticides, herbacides, fungacides, microorganisms, rust and particulate matter) but leave the minerals in the solution. It is also important not to drink softened water because it softens your bones and teeth.

To check the quality of your water, try these simple tests. 1) Use a chlorine indicator (from a swimming pool supply company) to determine its chlorine concentration. No chlorine is best, but the lower the better. 2) With a simple pH meter (from a local electronic supply or hardware store) measure the water's pH. If the pH is much over 7.6, then the water is too hard and probably has too much particulate matter. 3) Get a bottle of colloidal silver, 15 parts per million (from a health food store or the internet), and drop a capful (1 tsp) into an 8oz glass of water. If the water becomes cloudy, then the water is probably contaminated with microorganisms. To do a control test, drop the same amount of colloidal silver into 8oz of distilled water. It should remain clear. The cloudier the water, the more microorganisms are in the water.

Water poses a specific problem for people with adrenal fatigue because they tend toward dehydration but can easily over dilute the circulating electrolytes (sodium, potassium, magnesium and chlorine) in their blood by drinking too much water. The balance of sodium and potassium significantly affects the symptoms experienced by people with adrenal fatigue and drinking plain water alters this balance (see "Anatomy and Physiology" in chapter 22 for explanation). Therefore although they are often thirsty, drinking water may make them feel worse. To help balance the ratio of water to sodium and avoid this problem try adding ¼ to ½ teaspoon salt (sodium chloride) to every glass of drinking water. You will probably find that the lightly salted water actually tastes better than regular water if your adrenals are low because the salted water is more beneficial to your body. Certainly you will feel much better because your body needs both the salt as well as the water. If you are feeling especially draggy or fatigued, add more salt to the water. If you have an aversion to salted water, then you probably need less or no salt in the water Too much salt in the water will make you nauseated so adjust according to taste.

Drinking salted water just after you wake up can help you to function better in the early morning. Having another glass with a snack at around 2:00 PM can also lessen or sometimes prevent the lows typi- cally experienced in adrenal fatigue between 3:00 to 4:00 PM. My patients have demonstrated over and over again how important salted water is to coping with and recovering from the symptoms of adrenal fatigue. Some have been able to assess the level of their adrenal function simply by their desire for salt.

A Caution with Fruit Juices - Fruit juices and fruit drinks are not good beverages to have in any quantity if you are hypoadrenic and/or hypoglycemic. Once in a while they can be tolerated, diluted or in small quantities. Add a pinch of salt to help balance the high potassium content of fruit juice. You may find that it tastes better to you with the salt as well. Do not drink fruit juices early in the morning or anytime you are experiencing major symptoms of adrenal fatigue. If you start experiencing increased low adrenal symptoms within 90 minutes of drinking fruit juice, then the fruit juice is probably at fault and you should avoid it in the future. Orange juice seems to be especially detrimental to people with adrenal fatigue. It might be the concentrated fruit sugar, the pesticides in the rind (most orange juice is made by grinding the entire orange rind and all oranges are heavily sprayed). Avoid orange juice especially before noon if you suffer from adrenal fatigue. So the take home message from fruit juices is do not drink them in the morning, do not have them by themselves, and only drink them in small quantities.

Vegetable Juices - Fresh vegetable juices contain many nutrients that are excellent for the body. Almost any vegetable can be juiced, and the flavor is sometimes a touch of heaven. Combinations like carrot/celery/

beet or carrot/parsley are rich in color, high in vitamins and phytonutrients, and help stimulate the liver. However, too much juice at one time can drive blood sugar up too high in some people, causing them to crash between 3/4 and 1-1/2 hours later. Adding a pinch of salt and eating food with the juice helps minimize this reaction but it is always best to drink these juices in small quantities (4-6oz) at intervals rather than drinking a large amount all at once. It is also best to drink them fresh from the juicer. You can buy juicers from many health food stores. Juicers of lesser quality, but adequate, can also be found in department stores and specialty shops.

Canned tomato or vegetable blend juices are becoming more popular for work breaks, with snacks and as an alternative to cola or alcoholic beverages at social gatherings. Put a celery stick or lemon a slice in a Virgin Mary (a Bloody Mary without the vodka) and you can avoid social commentaries about not consuming alcohol at parties. The only downside to this is that you have to endure the drunks when they think they are so funny. But it is a small price to pay for feeling good the next day and not taxing your health. Always read the ingredients on commercial vegetable juices; many of them contain sugar, corn syrup or fruit juice. These ones should be left on the shelf.

Milk
Cow's Milk - Milk can be both the perfect whole food and the source of many problems. My experience is that people suffering from adrenal fatigue do not do well with cow's milk. There are several reasons for this. One is that cow's milk contains a high amount of lactose (milk sugar). We know that approximately 50% of Whites, 90% of Blacks, and nearly all Orientals are lactose intolerant. When you drink a glass of milk, you are drinking a large amount of sugar that is easily absorbed into your blood stream, leading to the hypoglycemic roller coaster I have mentioned before. This is covered in more detail in the "Anatomy and Physiology" chapter, but suffice it to say, consuming a glass of milk can be as disruptive to blood sugar as eating several handfuls of candy.

In addition, the protein in milk (casein) is a common allergen. Allergies are hard on the adrenals and therefore place further stress on people with low adrenal function. Like many mild allergens, it temporarily stimulates adrenal function but then leads to further adrenal fatigue. If you like the taste of milk and the nutrients in milk, a much better alternative is fresh goat's milk.

Goat's Milk - Goat's milk is a much better choice than cow's milk. It is more similar to human milk, lower in lactose and very much less likely to cause allergies. In fact, I have used goat's milk successfully to replace of cow's milk with hundreds of babies and young children who are allergic to cow's milk. These infants often came into my office with diarrhea and a rash. Switching them to goat's milk not only made their diarrhea and rash disappear, but also increased their immune function. In many states it is possible to get unpasteurized goat's milk from certified goats. This is the best form of goat's milk. One thing to note about goat's milk is that the longer it stands in the refrigerator, the stronger the taste. Therefore, the fresher the goat's milk, the milder the taste and the more you will enjoy it, so buy only the quantity you will use up within 3 or 4 days. Goat's milk is a rich source of many nutrients and is usually available through health food stores and local farmers. Several national supermarket chains now also carry a pasteurized form in the dairy section. Goat's milk is a healthy, nutritious choice.

Rice Milk - Rice milk can be made at home or is available commercially from health food stores and most grocery stores. Rice milk can be used in place of regular milk in most instances, although its nutritional content is not the same. We use it on cereals, in cooking, baking, shakes, and smoothies; there is even rice milk ice cream. Rice milk varies quite a bit among commercial manufacturers, therefore look at the ingredients and taste test different brands to choose the one you like the best. Rice milk does not contain the variety of nutrients found in goat's milk, but the calcium-fortified version does provide a comparable amount of calcium. It has the advantages of being more widely available and it can be made at home.

To make your own rice milk, put 2 cups of organically grown short grain brown rice in a 3 quart stainless steel or glass cooking pot with a tight fitting lid. Rinse rice with tap water until the water is clear and drain. Pour 4 cups spring water in the pot with the rice, add ½ teaspoon of sea salt and bring to a boil, uncovered. As soon as it comes to a boil turn down heat to a low simmer, place the tight fitting lid on pan and cook for 1 hour. Do not lift the lid or stir the rice. It will cook fine without being stirred and looked at. After cooking, let it cool. Place 2 cups cooked rice with 8 cups water, 2 tablespoons sesame oil and 1 tablespoon of unfiltered honey in the blender and blend for 2-3 minutes. Strain through three layers of cheesecloth into a sterile container, squeezing the cheesecloth to express as much liquid as possible. The brown rice solids can be used to make rice pudding, rice bread or other nice tasting items. The brown rice mixture can be mixed with nuts (almonds are especially good) to make a drink containing a complete protein (nuts and grains). The portion of nuts to be cooked with brown rice is approximately 4:1 rice to nuts.

Soy Milk – Soy milk is now widely available in most grocery and health food stores. Like rice milk it can be used in place of regular milk but is more difficult to make at home. It is higher in protein than rice milk and the calcium-fortified version has about the same amount of calcium as cow's milk. Soy milk comes in several flavors and is also made into ice cream. Try different brands to find one you like. Note, however, that soy is becoming one of the most common allergens, so proceed slowly with it and pay attention to how you feel after eating or drinking soy products.

Nut Milks – Nut milk can be easily made in a blender with almost any kind of nut and water. My two favorites are almond milk and cashew milk, or a combination of almond and cashew milk. Nut milks are a pleasant substitute for people who are sensitive to cow's milk and are looking for an alternative that they can make themselves. Milks can also be made from certain seeds, such as sesame seeds and pumpkin seeds, using the same procedure. It should be noted that both the nut and the seed milks are an excellent source of essential fatty acids and are a welcome addition to North American diets.

To make nut and seed milks, place in blender:

1 cup of your favorite raw nuts and seeds
4 cups of warm spring water
1 tablespoon unfiltered honey diluted with ¼ cup warm water ¼ teaspoon
of sea salt

3 capsules (400 IU) Vitamin E (mixed tocopherols) - open and squeeze oil into mixture, discard capsule.

Blend together for 2-3 minutes on medium high speed. Strain through 3 layers of cheesecloth into a sterile container, squeezing the cheesecloth to express as much liquid as possible. Store in the refrigerator. The nut residue can be mixed with cooked rice or other ingredients like dried fruit to make bars, cookies and desserts.

Carob - Carob can be used as a chocolate substitute and is preferable to chocolate in its physiological activity in the body. For example, whereas chocolate aggravates hypoglycemia and over stimulates the adrenals, carob normalizes hypoglycemia and does not contain stimulants. Carob comes in the form of powder, bars, or chips that can be used in baking instead of cocoa powder or chocolate chips. The powder makes a delicious hot or cold beverage that is a favorite at our house. To make a carob drink mix one heaping teaspoon of carob with one teaspoon of honey diluted in one teaspoon of warm water, then stir this syrup into six to eight ounces of hot or cold goat, nut or rice milk. You can find carob in all health food stores and in the specialty section of some supermarkets. Carob is great for people who are allergic to chocolate, because carob tastes a lot like chocolate, but does not produce the allergic reactions like chocolate. Because it stabilizes blood sugar and contains several nutrients, carob is a healthy alternative to chocolate and as a stand-alone favorite beverage.

Don't Drink Me
Chocolate - Hot cocoa, and other chocolate beverages are too likely to drive your adrenals with the combination of caffeine and sugar that they contain. Play it safe and avoid them.

Caffeine - *"Forbid adrenal stimulating foods and drugs, especially coffee... The adrenals are already over stimulated." (Harrower, '29, pg. 86)*
There has long been convincing evidence about the adverse effects of caffeine and caffeine like substances on your health. My advice is to avoid them altogether. Read the labels to make sure that what you drink or eat does not have coffee, chocolate, black tea, or added caffeine (like

many soft drinks) as one of the ingredients. Coffee, black tea and chocolate all contain various quantities of caffeine and also a substance similar to caffeine called theobromine that further interferes with adrenal function. Therefore even decaffeinated coffee and tea are not recommended for people with adrenal fatigue. Another reason to avoid coffee is that as coffee is roasted and then ground; the oils in coffee become rancid much more quickly after roasting or grinding and these rancid oils have detrimental effects of their own. A certain percentage of people are sensitive to the rancid oils contained in foods and beverages, often without realizing it. If you still need another incentive to leave that coffee on the shelf, let me tell you that coffee is also a strong pro-oxidant, greatly increasing oxidation within the cells. Simply put, this causes you to **age faster**.

Because coffee contains all these undesirables that affect your adrenals and your overall metabolism, it makes sense to eliminate coffee completely. However, knowing that industrialized nations drink tons and tons of coffee per day, it is likely that some of you, even though you know that coffee is not good for you, will occasionally have a cup of coffee. If you embark on this dangerous route, here are some pointers. (1) Understand that what you are doing is not good for your body; it only makes you more tired in the long run and there are other ways to feel better. (2) Never have coffee by itself; always have it with some good quality food. (3) Get the freshest and highest quality coffee possible. (4) Drink coffee with cream as the oils in the cream slightly mitigate the negative effects of the caffeine. (5) Do not drink coffee late in the afternoon because it interferes with the formation of the alpha rhythm in the brain necessary for sound sleep. (6) Take extra magnesium, calcium, B complex, vitamin C and antioxidants when drinking coffee, to help detoxify the pathways that coffee impairs. (7) Instead of consuming a full cup of coffee, only have one to two sips and leave the rest of the cup. (8) Take several doses of homeopathic chamomile (12x potency) to help counter the negative effects of coffee. 9). Remember that even when you do all these things, and even though you may feel better initially after a cup of coffee, the upside of coffee is always followed by a down side. The downside is usually felt in the morning and lasts much longer than the upside.

Alcohol - Alcohol is a special kind of poison for the adrenals that should not be consumed by people suffering from hypoadrenia. Alcohol is a naked carbohydrate in an extremely refined form (more refined than white sugar) that quickly finds it way into the cells of your body, forcing them to make energy at a rapid rate. This sets off the blood sugar roller coaster described earlier in the section "What not to eat" and uses up a large number of your body's nutrients that are not replaced by the alcoholic beverage. Tintera in his excellent 1955 article on hypoadrenia, comments on two kinds of alcoholism related to the adrenals. In one, the alcohol craving is driven by the body's desperate need for quick energy that results from weak adrenals. The alcohol temporarily compensates for the signs and symptoms of hypoadrenia but leads to further adrenal fatigue after the effects of the alcohol have worn off, thus producing a further need for alcohol. In the other, the person becomes hypoadrenic as a result of alcohol consumption.

If, despite these warnings, you are going to consume alcohol, follow these pointers. 1) Consume it only in small quantities and on a full stomach. 2) Have alcohol with meals that are high in fats or oils as the fats and oils help inhibit the absorption of alcohol and moderate its sudden impact on your cells.

If you are using liquid herbal extracts, look for ones that are in a non-alcohol base. Tinctures use alcohol as the solvent and although this is normally an excellent method for extracting the active elements in herbs, the amount of alcohol in the tincture can offset the benefit of the herbal product when your adrenals are low. It is better to use either a water-soluble preparation or one in a glycerin base. If this is not possible, either let the herbal mixture sit after it has been mixed with juice or whatever. Some of the alcohol will evaporate while it is sitting. Better yet, heat the mixture. After about 5-15 minutes of steeping, the alcohol will evaporate and the mixture will become relatively alcohol free. Cool and drink.

Soft Drinks - Colas and other carbonated beverages should also be avoided. All contain sugar or artificial sugar, and most contain caffeine. Artificial sweeteners are themselves a becoming a major concern as their side effects and possible hazards to health are getting more recognition.

Do yourself a favor and do not be lured into drinking them. They may taste good, but are only a detriment to your health.

It is as important to know what to avoid as it is to know what foods and beverages to eat and drink. Make regaining your health a major priority and do not sacrifice it for the cheap gratification of a favorite, but unhealthy, food or drink. In order to heal and maintain your health, you need to stack as many things in your favor as possible. Another factor you can stack on your side is eating in a way that facilitates digestion.

Chapter 14

Food Allergies and Sensitivities

Role of Allergies in Adrenal Function

Most allergies involve the release of histamine and other pro-inflammatory substances (substances that produce inflammation). Cortisol is a strong anti-inflammatory (a substance that reduces inflammation). Your circulating level of cortisol is the key factor in controlling the level of inflammatory reactions in your body. For this reason your adrenal glands play an important role in mediating the histamine release and inflammatory reactions that produce the symptoms experienced with allergies. It is therefore not surprising that people with food and environmental allergies commonly have weak adrenal function.

- The more histamine that is released, the more cortisol it takes to control the inflammatory response and the harder the adrenals have to work to produce more cortisol.
- The harder the adrenals have to work, the more fatigued they become and the less cortisol they produce, allowing histamine to inflame the tissues more.
- This vicious circle can lead to progressively deeper adrenal fatigue as well as to larger allergic reactions.
- Anything that you can do to break this cycle will help your adrenal glands and reduce the effects of allergies.
- Eliminating foods that you are allergic or sensitive to from your diet is one of the best and easiest ways to decrease the demands on your struggling adrenals.

Allergic Reactions to Food Vary

Responses to particular foods and drinks vary from person to person but there are some food substances that tend to produce allergies more frequently. The most common allergens are milk, wheat, corn, soy, chocolate, peanuts, tomatoes and beef. Sugar is not a common allergen, but it can greatly increase an allergic reaction. If you find yourself feeling odd or experiencing more of the signs and symptoms of adrenal fatigue after eating, think of allergies or food sensitivities. The foods listed above are the ones that are most likely to be a problem, but food allergies and sensitivities can be very individualistic. You can be allergic to just about anything. Food allergies and sensitivities also vary in severity quite a bit. For example, people who are sensitive to corn range in their sensitivity from those who can eat corn once or twice a week without problems, to those who are so sensitive that even eating poultry or meat from an animal fed on corn gives them a reaction. These reactions also vary in magnitude, even within the same individual. At one time an allergen may produce only a small response and at other times be incapacitating. Most symptoms of allergies or food sensitivities are first felt between thirty minutes and three hours after the meal, but some may be delayed as long as two to three days.

Food allergy reactions vary from person to person even when they are caused by the same food because different physiological systems in different people may be affected by the same allergen. For example, the same food affecting the skin of one person may affect the nervous system of another or the digestive system of someone else. One of the most common types of allergies is called a "cerebral allergy" because it primarily affects your brain and nervous system. Because of the abundance of histamine receptors in your brain, an allergen will often cause a greater reaction in your nervous system than it does anywhere else. Ranging from subtle to profound, these cerebral allergy reactions can include such symptoms as a cloudy head, confusion, sudden awkwardness, loss of consciousness, coma and occasionally death. Food allergens can interfere with your daily functioning and become a profound stress on your adrenals. It is important to track down and eliminate these food sensitivities and allergies in order to help your adrenal glands recover. Getting an Elisa IgE food allergy test is the best place to start.

Tracking Hidden Food Allergies and Sensitivities
Laboratory Tests
Elisa Tests - Tracking your food allergies can be a tedious and time-consuming process. Fortunately, this process has been made much easier these past few years by the advent of the Elisa (enzyme-linked immunosorbant assay) food panels tests. The Elisa panels can pinpoint the foods you are allergic to much faster and more easily than trying to figure it out yourself. Usually only one blood sample is needed to test a

large number of foods. The basic panel covers 90 - 100 foods and the more comprehensive panels cover about 175 foods, including spices, herbs,condiments and uncommon foods. For about 50% of people taking this test, the Elisa will be all that is needed to uncover their significant food allergies. Just eliminating the foods it flags will improve adrenal function and remove a major body burden. The resulting report is a printout in an easily understandable format that shows your particular food allergies and your degree of reaction to each food. The results will be sent to the physician who requisitioned the test. Most labs send 2 copies, one for the doctor and one for you. Be certain to get copies of this and all lab test results for your personal health records to keep at home. These simple blood tests are available from most alternative and some standard physicians. In some states, chiropractors and nurse practitioners can order them. Unfortunately, many practicing physicians are still unaware of these Elisa food panel tests, so you may have to shop around to find a doctor who will order them for you.

Despite the usefulness of the Elisa tests there are certain kinds of food reactions that they do not pick up. For these the Cellular Immune Food Reaction Tests may be more useful.

Cellular Immune Food Reaction Tests - Cellular Immune Food Reaction Tests, also known as delayed-type hypersensitivity reaction tests (DTH) or activated cell tests (ACT) are less common blood tests that can be very valuable in detecting subtle or delayed allergies not caught by the Elisa. These tests look at the part of the immune system's response to food that can be delayed by up to 3 days after eating the food. Such food allergies are seldom discovered by observation and are not picked up by the usual food panels. Although more costly, the Cellular Immune Food Reaction Tests have helped many people solve their food allergy riddle.

Combined Food Tests
Some labs combine the Elisa and ACT tests into a very comprehensive test known as an Elisa/ACT test. If you can afford it, this is the best way to detect food allergies.

After Getting Your Results
After getting your results using any of the above tests, make a list of the foods you are sensitive or allergic to and carry it around with you until

you are familiar with them and learn to avoid them. Eliminate for 2 weeks all foods that showed a reaction on the panel. If you are allergic to one of the common allergens given above, you need to find out all the foods that contain that allergen. Sometimes the lab results include a list of the foods containing the substances you tested positive for. If not, go to our website at **www.adrenalfatigue.org** and print out a copy of the lists of food items containing these ingredients. Our website will show you a separate list of foods for each substance. Keep a copy as your reference because certain prepared foods often contain allergic substances that one would not suspect. For example, many canned soups contain wheat or wheat gluten. Texturized vegetable protein (TVP), another common food additive, may contain up to 50% monosodium glutamate (MSG), yet MSG is not mentioned on the label. Having a list of foods that contains the substances you are allergic to will make it much easier to avoid adverse reactions and to detect their source when they occur.

If your food sensitivities do not show up on lab tests
If your food sensitivities do not show up on any of these lab tests, more detective work is needed. Below are some excellent tools to help you uncover your hidden allergies and sensitivities. Select the one(s) that seem most appropriate and follow the instructions given in that section. If you need more help check our website for a list of recommended books and other information on the subject.

If you cannot afford lab tests
Even if you cannot afford the lab tests for food allergies, you can still use one or more of the methods below to discover your food allergies and sensitivities. The main advantage of laboratory tests is that they provide a lot of information quickly about food allergies. But before they were available, physicians had their patients use the tests given below with a good success. With some determination, careful observation and good record keeping, you can detect most of your food allergies using the methods below.

Methods for Detecting Food Sensitivities You Can Do at Home
If you have eliminated all the foods you tested positive to but are still reacting, you may have some additional food sensitivities that do not cause an actual allergic reaction. Food sensitivities can affect your life in subtle ways. They can manifest by increasing your fatigue, clouding

your judgment, intensifying your anger and other emotional reactions, or just make you feel bad for no apparent reason. To help you discover your subtle food sensitivities, read all of the methods below and determine which one(s) is most appropriate for you.

Picking the Right Method

Four different methods are given here to help you identify your food sensitivities: Observation Method, Reflective Diary Method, Food and Reaction Diary and the Cocoa Pulse Test. One of these methods will usually ferret out the culprits with the bonus that you will feel better, stay more clear-headed and have better energy with each food sensitivity discovered and removed. More importantly, you will have a significant leg up on how to relieve your body's stress and speed your adrenal recovery time.

Observation Method - Use the observation method when you know you are reacting to one of several foods but are just not sure which one. Observe your reactions to various foods and then simply do not eat the food that you suspect for two weeks. After two weeks reintroduce that food and watch your response. Pay attention because it is often after the food is consumed the second or third time that the reaction is experienced. Write down your responses in a notebook. If your results are inconclusive but there is another food you suspect, you can repeat this process with the other food or go on to one of the methods described below to help you zero in on the problem.

Reflective Diary Method - The reflective diary method is an excellent way to track food sensitivities that occur soon after eating but only occasionally (less then twice per week). In this method, when you do experience a reaction within a few hours of a meal, record your symptoms, reactions and what you ate or drank at that meal in a written diary to help you reflect on the cause of your problem. After 8 to 10 entries, review and check them for common foods and/or ingredients in foods. Occasionally it is not what you eat, but where you eat. For example, some restaurant salad bars use potassium bitartrate to keep items fresh but others do not. You may not be reacting to the food itself, but to an ingredient that has been sprayed on it at a particular place. One restaurant may use an oil or a spice you react to. Sometimes you will not be able to determine the exact cause, but will be able to determine that it only happens at Jack's Restaurant or only when you eat the grilled salmon at Jack's. Below is an example of the reflective method. If you still cannot trace and identify the culprit(s) with this method, go on to the next method.

Reflective Diary

Date	Food/Beverage item	Place	Reactions/Comments
Jan 1	Tomato, Avocado San Macaroni Salad Pickles Carrot Sticks red pepper slices' Green tea with ginseng	Moms	Sleepy, cannot keep track of football scores, or concentrate playing cards* Fighting off a cold
Jan 3	Coffee	Albert's Rest	Increased coughing, swollen eyes next AM
Jan 7	Tuna salad, cheese crackers, green tea	Home	After meal- felt dull headed, sleepy all afternoon*
Jan 10	Chicken salad san. Fruit salad W Wheat bread/butter	Marios Rest	Could not think well and memory dull- 3 hours*
Jan 14	BLT San Garden Salad	Home	Foggy headed, mild stomach discomfort*
Jan 17	Red wine- Herkamers'94 Cabernet	Sandra's	Hands slightly swollen; increased coughing] Sulphites??/Alcohol/ Red wines
Feb 2	Ham san/mayo, mustard Totilla chips Pickle barley tea	Home	Could not think well most of afternoon*
Feb 10	Lean beef san Potato salad Carrots Jicama Sparkling water		Felt worse after lunch fuzzy head, dopey*
Feb 15	Reviewed notebook from Jan 1		Could cloudy thinking be something common to lunch? Suspect: Mayo – in some foods where I am cloudy headed (those with *) Watch Red wines - coughing
Feb 16	Tomato, Avocado San	Moms	Same meal as Jan except no Mayo -

Food and Reaction Diary - The food and reaction diary is an excellent tool for detecting subtle and/or multiple food sensitivities or allergies. This is the method to use when you cannot see much of a pattern or there seems to be a pattern but you cannot put your finger on it. It is very useful for uncovering and learning about the subtle behavior problems (of which there are many) that can be produced by food sensitivities. With the food and reaction diary method you keep track of everything that goes into your mouth, food (including gum) and drink (including water). You also keep track of any signs or symptoms that occur during the day or night. Initially, you simply act as a recording secretary, just writing down everything that goes in your mouth and any sign or symptom you experience, without trying to correlate symptoms with foods or beverages. The recording of symptoms and the recording of food intake are not related. For example, if you wake up at 7:00 AM with a headache in the front part of your head, list that. If you eat breakfast at 9:00 AM, record what you eat and drink. If you have water at 10:30 AM, record it. If you get mad and yell at someone or become clumsy for no reason at 11:00 AM, record it. List the date and time of each item you ingest and each reaction in the appropriate column. Every seven days review your symptoms and your food intake. If you notice any associations or patterns, then circle the signs and/or symptoms with the food or drink you suspect, drawing a line between the two to connect them. When you suspect a substance, make a note of your suspicions, e.g. "Most of the time when I eat cheddar cheese, I feel a little off the next day." If after seven days there are no clear connections, continue this procedure until a pattern emerges. This is a detailed method that requires discipline to keep up, but it is the best tool you or your doctor can use to unravel the mysteries of your hidden food sensitivities. Below is an example of one morning's entries in a food and reaction diary.

Food and Reaction Diary

Date/Time	Item	Signs & Symptoms
Jan 20		
7:00 AM		Woke with headache – front and left side
9:00 AM	Whole wheat toast	
	Mint tea w cream & honey 1 cup	
9:30 AM		Headache gone
10:30 AM	Glass of water	
11:00 AM		Lost it and called neighbor names for making noise while emptying garbage - felt out of control
11:30 AM	Chicken salad san – ww bread, mayo mustard	
	Vegetable soup – 1 cup	
	Barley tea – 1 gl	
	Water – 1 gl	
12:00		Felt much better after lunch

Food Related Morning Hangovers - One thing I have found to be especially valuable is to watch how you feel in the morning. If you feel like
you have a mild hangover but did not consume any alcohol the day before, it is likely that something in your previous day's food or beverages
is toxic to you. Immediately drink a glass of water with 1/2 teaspoon of
salt. If after twenty to thirty minutes you feel yourself starting to come
around and the hangover symptoms are going away, this is a further indication that what you consumed yesterday is probably affecting you today. This "hangover" effect is not the usual fatigue felt in the morning
from low adrenals but rather comes most often from liver congestion.
When you have this mild hangover, go back and list everything that you
put in your mouth the previous day. If it happens frequently, you should
use the food reaction diary. However, if you experience this effect only
occasionally, simply write down everything you ate and drank the day
before and keep these records in a notebook. After this has happened
four to five times, go through this list and circle the items common to all
of these days. These are the substances you can suspect of causing the
problem. Then try eating the very same meal again but omitting the suspect food or drink. Note whether or not you have that hangover feeling
the next morning. If you do not, chances are you have isolated one of
your food sensitivities. Write this down in your notebook so you will not
forget it over time. If there is more than one food item that bothers you,
keep a list in the notebook of any foods you have discovered you are
sensitive to or any foods you suspect, and date your entries.

Cocoa Pulse Test - A number of years ago Arthur Cocoa wrote a very
valuable book on using the Cocoa Pulse Test to track hidden food allergies.
It is a simple test that anyone can easily learn to do and is based on the
fact that when you are allergic to a food, you have an adrenal response
that causes an increase in your heartbeat. Therefore, taking your pulse
before you eat and again at 15 minutes and 30 minutes after you eat will
give you almost immediate feedback about the presence of an allergen in
what you just ate. If you do not know how to take your own pulse, see
Appendix D for complete instructions. Record the date, the time, your
pulse rate before eating, the food or drink you consume, and your pulse
at 15 and 30 minutes after eating for each meal or each time you eat or
drink.

This is an excellent way to uncover hidden food or beverage allergies, although it does have a few drawbacks. If you are suffering from moderate to severe adrenal fatigue you may not generate an increased pulse rate after eating something you are sensitive or allergic to because your adrenals are too fatigued to respond to the food allergy. You may experience increased symptoms after eating even though your pulse rate stays the same because of adrenal fatigue. In this case you should go by your symptoms rather than by your pulse rate. As your adrenal health improves, you will find the same foods you suspected eventually will raise your pulse rate.

Elimination/ Provocation Confirmation Test
Once you have determined that a particular food or drink is bothering you, it is time to test it by doing an elimination/provocation test. To do the Elimination/ Provocation Confirmation Test (the test is simpler to do than to say), you simply eliminate that food from your diet completely for at least 3 weeks and then reintroduce it. This requires total elimination of the suspect food, drink or substance to get definitive results. When you eliminate something from your diet you have to be sure that you do not eat anything at all that contains the suspected substance. For example, if you think that corn might be the problem you must remove all products containing or made from corn, cornstarch, corn oil and corn syrup (even the glue on envelopes and stamps often contains corn) from your diet. You will have to read the ingredient labels on everything, and if you cannot find out what is in something, it is better not to eat it at all during the elimination period. If you suspect wheat, corn, soy, milk products, egg or yeast containing foods, it is best to go to our website where you will find lists you can print out of all the foods and beverages that contain each of these. These substances are hidden in so many food products, you may be surprised by what you find.

When you start the elimination, write the date on a calendar. After you have not consumed (or even tasted or chewed) the suspect food, beverage or substance for at least three weeks, reintroduce it. Choose a weekend or a time you are not in great demand and are able to observe your reactions for the reintroduction. Also allow for the possibility that you might need to rest because sometimes the offending food has a larger impact than you expected. This may not be the time when you will be at your peak.

The first time you reintroduce the food, beverage or substance it is best to have only a small amount (one or two mouthfuls). The clearest way to test it is to drink or eat the substance by itself. That is, do not eat or drink anything but water for approximately 1 hour before and 2 hours after you consume your test item. Take your pulse sitting quietly before eating the food and every 15 minutes after, for an hour. Keep a notebook handy to write down your symptoms. Record any emotional swings, mood changes, or alterations in mental clarity. Note if your energy level goes up or down. One of the most common reactions found in food allergies/sensitivities is to feel especially good, almost giddy, for 30-45 minutes after you ingest the test item and then to fall into a real low. If this or any other noticeable physical, emotional or mental change happens to you, write it down in your notebook.

Sometimes, it is during the second or third reintroduction rather than the first that the changes become apparent. You should eat the same food substance the next day to see if a reaction occurs. If no reaction occurs on the first or second day, try it one more time on the third day so that you have ingested the suspect food or drink three days in a row. If you still do not notice any detectable difference in your pulse, energy level, mental clarity, mood or in any other way physically, mentally or emotionally, you are probably not sensitive to that food or perhaps you are only sensitive to it under certain conditions. If you do notice such changes, you are probably sensitive to that food substance. You can do a repeat of the elimination provocation test again for that same food or beverage if you are at all unsure. Detail all your results in your notebook, including your pulse test, any changes you observed and when those changes occurred.

If you are mildly sensitive, meaning you had only a slight reaction to the item when it was reintroduced, you may be able to have it once every four to five days. However, if you find the food or drink you tested gave you a significant reaction, a reaction you do not want to experience in your daily life, then eliminate this item completely.

The elimination/provocation test is an accurate, inexpensive and easy way to confirm suspicions about food sensitivities/allergies. It lets you know with relative certainty which foods, drinks or substances are the offending agents. Before reliable laboratory tests were available, progressive doctors used to have their patients test all suspect foods like this.

The Problem with Skin Tests for Food Allergies

Many dermatologists and allergists still use skin tests as a way of determining food allergies even though they are probably the most unpleasant and imprecise approach. Although the skin tests do detect some food allergies, they produce too many false positives (a skin wheal appears, but for a different reason than a food allergy) and false negatives (no wheal or only a small wheal appears even though there is a food allergy). They are also relatively expensive. Most doctors who have kept abreast of the information on allergy testing use blood tests in preference to skin tests.

Combining the Use of Food Allergy Tests and Diaries

The most effective way to detect food allergies is to use the Elisa test first and eliminate any indicated foods from your diet. Then, if that does not completely clear up the problem, go through the methods for tracking down food allergies and sensitivities yourself: observation, reflective diary, food reaction diary, Cocoa pulse test, and elimination/ provocation test. Finally, if you still have not located all the culprits, do the cellular immune food reaction test, ACT or Elisa/ACT. Using the Elisa test first allows for rapid detection of food reactions and saves a lot of time. Following it with one or more of the food allergy tracking methods provides a lot of information without further costs. That way you only have to do the more expensive ACT or Elisa/ ACT tests as a last resort. By eliminating those food items you are allergic or sensitive to, you will not only increase your adrenal strength, but your overall level of health and well being.

Food Sensitivities That Are Not Allergies

As mentioned above, you do not have to have a true allergy to a food for it to make you feel bad and really interfere with your life. Below are two actual case histories that illustrate the profound effect certain foods can have on your ability to function, even when these reactions are not considered to be real allergies.

Cerebral Milk Sensitivity

Sandy was a 30-year-old woman with periodic depression that had begun after puberty. Milk especially increased her depression and yet she had a compulsive desire to drink milk. She would drink it a quart at a time. When she was 28 she developed bronchial pneumonia and after approximately two weeks, she slowly began to recover. However, her fair skin was even paler and her energy was much slower. Her deep fatigue continued and two years later she was still suffering considerable fatigue, lack of stamina, and an inability to concentrate. She said that after the pneumonia, her depression had gotten worse, and had only marginally improved as her stamina increased slightly. Closer examination of Sandy's case history revealed that she had been mildly hypoadrenic for most of her teenage life. It turned out that milk was contributing not only to her depression but also to her adrenal fatigue and low energy level. The pneumonia had simply been an additional stress on her already somewhat depleted system. Happily, with proper treatment and the complete elimination of milk from her diet, the outcome was successful. When she learned how to care for her adrenals and reduce stress, she was able to carry on a life that was more active and fuller than she had ever experienced.

Sensitivity to Rancid Oils

Sam, a young medical student was taking a final exam in the CPR (Cardiac Pulmonary Resuscitation) course required as part of his internship program. Because of their medical background, this multiple choice exam, is usually a slam-dunk for medical students. However, Sam failed the exam. The instructor was very surprised, as Sam was one of the top students in the school, and so called him to the front of the room and asked him how he could have possibly failed the exam.

Sam explained to the instructor that he was sensitive to rancid oils and that he had accidentally consumed some rancid oils in the fish and chips he had eaten in the school cafeteria at noon, just before he had taken the test. He further explained that rancid oils rendered him unable to think clearly for a number of hours after their consumption. However, he had learned from experience that an apple helped counteract the effects of rancid oils in his body, so he asked the instructor if he could go to the cafeteria, eat an apple, and retake the test. The instructor looked incredulously at him, but because he was one of the top students and his test score was so out of line with his usual performance, he granted this unusual request. The student ate the apple, took the test, and made 100% on the same test he had failed ½ hour earlier. The difference was that the effects of the rancid oil on his brain had been neutralized by something in the apple.

At other times this young man became nearly comatose if he consumed rancid oils. At first he would just become very sleepy, but as the rancid oil reaction progressed, he would find himself unable to move, although he remained aware of everything that was happening around him. To others, it appeared that he was sleeping, but he was in fact temporarily paralyzed by the rancid oil's effect on his brain. His friends had learned to ask him if he wanted an apple whenever he seemed suspiciously sleepy and to put a piece of apple in his mouth if he did not answer them. In this state he was sometimes unable to even move his mouth to chew the apple slice, so they would move his jaw up and down to help him chew the apple. After only a few moments, he would go from being unable to move to being normal once again. If left on his own, he would sleep for two to three hours and wake up with a hangover that would last for approximately twenty-four hours.

This is another example of a food sensitivity that would not be detected by any laboratory test. It is also a good example of the subtle effects rancid oils can have in a person's life. As you can imagine, rancid oils are not only tough on the brain, they interfere with adrenal function as well.

Food Addictions

People can be addicted to certain foods just as surely as they can be addicted to other substances. If you have strong cravings for a particular food but after eating it you feel worse, you are probably suffering from an addiction to that food or a substance in that food. This usually means that this food contains both a nutrient you need more of and a substance you are sensitive or allergic to. It is important to try to discover what nutrient your body needs more of but, at the same time, you should avoid this food because the damage it does to you is usually greater than the benefit. If there is a food you cannot stop eating, do not start. Do not fall for that "only one bite" or "one bite isn't going to hurt me" trap. Addictions always win. If you were addicted to peanut butter last week, you can be almost positive that you are still addicted this week. So save yourself an experience in failure by completely eliminating those foods you simply cannot leave alone.

Keep a list of the foods that push your addiction button so you can see if they share any common features, as well as to remind you to avoid them. There are books and computer programs that list the nutrients in various foods. Check these and, if you have more than one craving, compare the nutrients in the foods you crave to see if there is one that is high in all of them. If there is, you can try adding that nutrient as a dietary supplement to your diet and then waiting to see if the craving goes down after a few days or weeks. Patients often express their gratitude not to be "hooked" on a food anymore once they discover this solution.

Addiction can also be due to body states like hypoglycemia (low blood sugar). In this type of addiction, the body is missing something (energy) and it craves something (sugar) that can quickly provide energy, although this is only a temporary solution. Two examples of food addictions created by hypoglycemia are given below. Both are true incidents.

Examples of food addiction without allergies or food sensitivities
Hypoglycemia Can Make You Lose Control
Neil was trying to eat only foods he thought were good for his health. However he continually got up late, and rarely had time for breakfast. But because he was hypoglycemic, by mid-morning he was so hungry he was desperate. One morning after missing breakfast yet again, he learned that work had been canceled because of rain. Neil went straight to a donut shop and in less than 10 minutes had crammed down four doughnuts and three cups of coffee with double cream and triple sugar in them. Two friends of his were driving by and saw him through the window. Surprised to see Neil in a donut shop and knowing how detrimental coffee and doughnuts were to his health, they stopped their car, ran into the shop, paid the bill and physically dragged him out of the establishment while onlookers stared. He was so addicted to coffee and doughnuts that he screamed and yelled and tried to order more as they pulled him, one on each arm, outside and into their van. Once he was in their van they sat on him to keep him from running back inside, until he came to his senses. Although this was a very humorous event for onlookers, it was a serious event for his metabolism.

Luckily, it was dramatic enough that he realized just how addicted he was to sugar, white flour and caffeine products. He took definite steps to make sure he did not find himself in this situation in the future by eating regular, high quality meals and, of course, by avoiding coffee and white flour or sugar products. His friends were happy because he was much more even tempered and a more able-bodied worker. His addiction was a result of neglecting his hypoglycemia and hypoadrenia. Once he began eating well-balanced breakfasts and other meals regularly and avoiding his addictive foods, his body was not as stressed and his addictions disappeared.

Charlene, the manager of a health food store talked each day to customers about all the right foods to eat but unfortunately neglected to take time to eat lunch and dinner. So when the store closed at night, she dove into the pastry counter and consumed several dollars worth of pastries. Even though these were "health food" baked goods, they were still sweet enough to cause her blood sugar to spike and then to crash. Charlene's erratic blood sugar levels made it so difficult for her to concentrate that after her pastry binge, it sometimes took her 2-1/2 to 3 hours to count the cash and do the bank deposit after closing, instead of the 30 minutes it should have taken. Often she could not even balance the cash and left it for the morning person, claiming there was something wrong with it. Yet the morning manager would find that everything balanced perfectly. This woman, even though she worked in the health food store and was conscious of many aspects of health, was helpless to control her own predicament. It was only when she explained what was truly happening to her boss that her boss saw the problem and ordered her to take time to eat lunch and dinner. After she started doing that her cravings disappeared, her head was a lot clearer, and her adrenals began to recover.

Environmental Toxins Can Make You Eat In A Bizarre Way
Environmental toxins such as perfumes, polluted air, or airborne chemicals can affect your taste buds and brain to make you eat in a bizarre way. These same toxins can also increase your adrenal fatigue. One true anecdote from my case histories will illustrate this point.

Will was in his mid 20's. He was just moving into a house with seven other friends. During the past six months, Will had been on a very strict vegetarian eating regimen for his health and was conscious of every bite that went into his mouth. Just after they moved in, the group decided that the wooden floors in the new house needed refinishing. As Will was the only person in the group with any manual labor experience, he volunteered to refinish the floors to save them all money. Early the following Saturday morning Will began sanding the floors, exposing the beautiful oak wood below the wax and grime. By Saturday evening, he had finished sanding and had added the sealer and the first coat of spar varnish. Because it was February, he had kept the windows closed to keep the house warm and help the floors dry faster.

Will suddenly became aware that he felt tense, angry, hostile, and a little erratic. Thinking he needed a break, he stepped outside for a breath of fresh air and noticed he was ravenously hungry. He went to the bar next door and in a matter of moments had consumed three hot dogs and four beers.

After this unusual supper, Will return to the house for a meeting. Two other members of the house told him he was acting strange and they didn't like it. His sudden anger and verbal lashing out was very atypical for him, but he shrugged it off and laid the blame on a hard day's work. The next morning he awoke feeling extremely tired and had a headache.

Reflecting on the day before, he realized how bizarre it was for him, as a strict vegetarian and non-drinker, to even consider a bite of a hot dog or taste of beer, yet he had gobbled down several of each, as though he was starving for them. Will realized then that he was a victim of environmental toxins. Being in a closed room with all the volatile fumes from the varnish and sealer had temporarily made him nearly crazy. It took about three days before he felt normal once again.

Environmental pollutants can have a dangerous and deleterious effect on your health, without you knowing it. Avoid exposure to as many fumes and airborne pollutants as possible. If you live or work in a neighborhood with these substances in the air, strongly consider moving. Until you move, take extra antioxidants and other dietary supplements that will support your liver such as milk thistle (silymarin), burdock and lipoic acid.

Eliminate All Foods to Which You Are Allergic, Sensitive or Addicted

If you think that a particular food substance interferes in any way with achieving your optimum health, then eliminate it immediately. If you suspect, but do not know which foods or beverages you are allergic, sensitive or addicted to, then it is important to find out. One of the above methods will definitely allow you to do this. Use them and be certain to write down your results because memory fades with time. Writing down the foods and beverages you react to will save you from the unpleasant experience of rediscovering your sensitivities over and over again. The adrenals are extremely important in all allergies, including food allergies and sensitivities. As your adrenal function improves, you will be less prone to allergies and will be able to eat more things. However, for the first three months, do not push the envelope. Completely eliminate all the foods you are sensitive to or suspect you are sensitive or allergic to. The idea is not to see how far you can test the limits; the idea is to get yourself well. If you need more information check our website for recommended books and other information on the subject.

The next chapter explains which nutritional supplements and herbs, out of the thousands that are available, are the best ones to take to help rebuild your adrenal glands.

Chapter 15

Dietary Supplements

Dietary supplements play a very important role in healing from adrenal fatigue. They not only speed your recovery but are also often necessary for complete recovery to take place at all. The supplements described in this section are chosen specifically for their restorative effects on the adrenal glands. The significance of each will be briefly explained because you need to understand why these nutritional supplements are included as part of your rehabilitation program and the absolute necessity of taking them regularly.

Vitamin C

Of all the vitamins and minerals involved in adrenal metabolism, vitamin C is probably the most important. In fact, the more cortisol made, the more vitamin C used. Vitamin C is so essential to the adrenal hormone cascade and the manufacture of adrenal steroid hormones that before the measurement of adrenal steroid hormones became available, the blood level of vitamin C was used as the best indicator of adrenal function level in animal research studies. Vitamin C is used all along the adrenal cascade and acts as an antioxidant within the adrenal cortex itself.

Vitamin C, as it occurs in nature, always appears as a composite of ascorbic acid and certain bioflavinoids. It is this vitamin C complex that is so beneficial, not just ascorbic acid, by itself. Bioflavinoids are essential if ascorbic acid is to be fully metabolized and utilized by your body. The ratio of bioflavinoids to ascorbic acid should be approximately 1:2, that is 1 mg. of bioflavinoids for every 2 mg. of ascorbic acid. Bioflavinoids basically double the effectiveness of ascorbic acid in your body and allow its action to be more complete. The kind of vitamin C you use makes a difference. Vitamin C is much more than ascorbic acid.

Most ascorbic acid in supplements is synthesized from corn syrup, and some from cane sugar or beet sugar. This does not mean that corn syrup and sugar contain any vitamin C, they do not. It simply means that these are the raw materials most commonly used to commercially manufacture vitamin C. Some people are sensitive to the source from which the vitamin C supplement has been derived. If you are sensitive to corn, try taking a vitamin C supplement derived from sago palm or beets instead. Sago palm and beet sources of vitamin C seem to be tolerated well by most people.

I have designed a specific vitamin C supplement for those suffering from adrenal fatigue that contains enough bioflavinoids, magnesium, pantothenic acid and other nutrients needed to metabolize and potentiate vitamin C. This supplement is available from suppliers listed on the website.

Because vitamin C is water-soluble and quickly used up or excreted from your body, it should be consumed several times per day. This is particularly true when your body is under any kind of physical, emotional, environmental or infectious stress. The quantity of vitamin C required varies by person and by stress level. As stressful events increase, the need for many nutrients, but especially vitamin C, also increases. To help provide this, some companies make a time-release vitamin C. A time-released vitamin C is fine except that most of them do not contain enough bioflavinoids.

To find out how much vitamin C your body requires, try a very simple test called the **Vitamin C Loading Test**. On day one take 500 mg. of ascorbic acid with 250 mg. of bioflavinoids. Increase your ascorbic acid by 500 mg. and your bioflavinoids by 250 mg. every hour until your bowel movements become somewhat loose and runny. Once you have achieved this level, then reduce your ascorbic acid by 500 mg. and your bioflavinoids by 250 mg. This is usually the amount of vitamin C your body needs at this time. The most common point for this to occur is about 2,000 to 4,000 mg. (2-4 grams) for people with adrenal fatigue, but I have known people that required 15,000 to 20,000 mg. (15-20 grams) a day in order to reach this point. Typically, the more chronic and severe your illness, the more vitamin C is necessary.

Vitamin C not only increases adrenal function, but also stimulates the immune system. If you feel yourself starting to come down with a cold or respiratory infection, start taking vitamin C at the first signs of distress. This not only aids your immune system in fighting the infection, but it helps your adrenals to respond to the stressful situation in your body created by the infection. If you know you are going to be up late, take extra vitamin C. If you are stressed for an examination or work event, take more vitamin C. If you are going through an emotional crisis or have to push yourself, take vitamin C. If you have eaten food that is bad for you, take additional vitamin C. If you do not make vitamin C available to your body through supplementation and diet, the adrenal hormonal cascade cannot begin or continue. When your adrenal glands cannot make the additional adrenal hormones required to maintain you during stressful times, you will feel worse and be slower to recover. Because there are so many other tissues in the body that also need increased vitamin C during any kind of stress, an adequate supply of it is vital to your body's ability to respond properly.

Humans do not have the ability to convert blood glucose into vitamin C as do most animals. Therefore, we must obtain our vitamin C from an outside source. Food sources of vitamin C include colored vegetables and fruits such as green leafy vegetables, tomatoes, peppers and oranges with the highest amounts of vitamin C found in sprouts (sunflower sprouts, alfalfa or clover sprouts, and all the sprouts of any seed or grain). In most plants, the younger the plant, the more vitamin C it contains per milligram of plant material. However, the amount of vitamin C available in foods is not sufficient to support the adrenals during stress or during the recovery phase. So if you are hypoadrenic, it is essential that you take a supplement containing sufficient vitamin C during the whole recovery period and extra vitamin C when you start to become fatigued or ill.

There is a myth about the amount of vitamin C in oranges. Not only have there been questions about the actual content of vitamin C contained in the juice compared to label claims, but the amount of vitamin C contained in the orange dissipates with time. Oranges are typically harvested in the United States in the late fall and early winter. By February, after two months of storage, only a small percentage of the original amount of vitamin C remains. In addition, the bioflavinoids in the fruit are found mostly in the white part on the inside of the rind that is usually not eaten rather than in the juicy part of the fruit that usually is consumed. There are two ways of making orange juice commercially, with and without the rind. Those made without the rind lack the appropriate amount of bioflavinoids. Orange juice made with the rind, (the most common method) contain chemical residues and sprays used on the fruit. I have had many patients who were sensitive to these chemical residues.

Orange juice is specifically not recommended for people suffering from adrenal fatigue because few substances drive the blood sugar up so quickly and drop it so abruptly. Orange juice in the morning is frequently a tragic start to the day for people with hypoadrenia. To test this, take a large glass of orange juice by itself in the morning and see how you feel and function during the rest of the morning. If you do this test, be sure it is not during a day you need to be clear headed, well spoken, well coordinated, or doing anything dangerous.

Cautions with Vitamin C - As you take more vitamin C your body adapts to this higher level of vitamin C. Therefore, when decreasing your vitamin C intake, do it gradually. A sudden drop in vitamin C intake can lead to symptoms of scurvy (severe vitamin C deficiency) even when your actual vitamin C levels are well above the recommended levels. Decrease your intake by 500 mg. every three to five days. Gums that bleed during tooth brushing, swollen gums, or bruising easily are signs of vitamin C deficiency. If you begin experiencing any of these symptoms it means you are decreasing your vitamin C intake too fast. You should temporarily increase the amount of vitamin C and bioflavinoids you are taking, and then step down the dosage more slowly. Just as the body adapts to an increase in vitamin C, it will also adapt to a decrease in vitamin C. However, it takes about twice as long for the body to get used to the decrease as it does to the increase.

This is true too for nursing babies or babies in utero whose bodies also adapt to whatever level of vitamin C their mothers are taking. If a mother has been taking high doses of Vitamin C during her pregnancy, the newborn should be given gradually decreasing amounts of vitamin C/bioflavinoids. This should be done from birth if the baby is not nursed or at weaning if the mother continued to take high doses of vitamin C while nursing.

If you are on blood thinners, monitor your blood clotting. The increased vitamin C may require you to lower your anti-coagulation medication. Vitamin C works with Vitamin E and other antioxidants to decrease blood clotting and coagulation. Therefore, if your blood clotting time increases on blood clotting tests, it may be possible to decrease or eliminate your anti-coagulation medication while taking adequate amounts of Vitamin C by itself or with other antioxidants. As a patient of mine once said, Doctor, I would much rather take antioxidants than rat poison. As a farmer, he recognized that the substance given to rats to poison them was the same substance given to humans as a blood thinner.

Vitamin E

Vitamin E is a very interesting vitamin in adrenal fatigue. Technically speaking, vitamin E is not required for any part of the adrenal hormone-manufacturing cascade, yet it is essential, indirectly, in at least six different enzymatic reactions in the adrenal cascade. This is because the manufacture of adrenal hormones generates substances called free radicals that can create great damage inside the cells if they are not controlled. An excess number of free radicals slow down the enzymatic reactions and, carried to the extreme, can do physical damage to the adrenal cell structure. Vitamin E absorbs and neutralizes these damaging free radical molecules inside the adrenal glands and elsewhere. Vitamin C enhances vitamin E's activity inside the cell by regenerating the capacity of vitamin E to sequester the free radicals. These two work hand in hand to keep the adrenal cascade functioning. Therefore, high amounts of vitamin E are necessary in order for the adrenals to maintain high levels of steroid production and recover adequately.

It is important to choose the right vitamin E supplement. Vitamin E, in chemical terms, is a "tocopherol." Most vitamin E supplements sold in health food and grocery stores are in the form of d-alpha-tocopherol. Although this is a natural form of Vitamin E, it is only a fraction of the complete vitamin E complex. It is the least expensive to manufacture and the most profitable. Therefore, it is not surprising that the majority of companies promote this type of vitamin E, making it the most available type of vitamin E on the market.

However, the vitamin E necessary for adrenal regeneration is a mixed tocopherols supplement, specifically one high in beta-tocopherols. Recent studies have shown that too much d-alpha-tocopherol can actually suppress the beta and other tocopherols necessary for adrenal rejuvenation. So taking a mixed tocopherols vitamin E is critical if you want to restore adrenal health. Have **800 IU of mixed tocopherols vitamin E** per day with meals. You must take this vitamin E for at least three months in the quantities given before you can expect to see any significant improvements in your adrenals. Even though you may not notice any difference when you start taking the vitamin E every day, it is so important to your adrenal health that it is essential to continue taking it consistently, probably for the rest of your life. Vitamin E is not only valuable in healthy adrenal function, but has many anti-aging properties as well. This means that while you are nourishing your adrenals with a mixed tocopherols vitamin E, you are also nourishing the rest of your body, slowing down the aging process, and facilitating a number of other essential functions in your body.

Cautions with Vitamin E - Like vitamin C, vitamin E is a natural blood-thinning agent. If you are taking a blood thinner, monitor your blood clotting. It may be necessary to cut back on your medication. Blood thinning medications often have a caution that Vitamin E may interfere with their action. This is not quite accurate. As mentioned earlier, Vitamin E and other antioxidants can be used to normalize the clotting mechanism, making the consumption of both the antioxidant and the drug unnecessary. Comparing the benefits and risks of both would make me want to choose the natural alternative, but whatever your decision, if you are taking blood thinners, monitor your clotting regularly.

B Vitamins

Pantothenic Acid: Pantothenic acid, one of the B-complex vitamins, is another essential contributor in the adrenal cascade. Like magnesium, it is important for energy production. Pantothenic acid is converted into acetyl CoA, a substance critical to the conversion of glucose into energy. It is present in all cells but in higher quantities in the adrenals because so much energy is needed to produce the adrenal hormones. The combination of pantothenic acid with magnesium, vitamin E and vitamin C increases energy production and takes much of the fatigue out of the adrenals, without over stimulating them. The quantity of pantothenic acid recommended is typically **1,500 mg.** per day. Tablets of 500 mg. can usually be purchased in health food stores. Therefore, three tablets per day at this strength are adequate.*

* I have designed an "Adrenal Exhaustion Formula" that contains correctly balanced proportions of B vitamins, including a non-flushing niacin, combined with more vitamins, minerals and other nutrients balanced to work in synergy to optimize adrenal function. Check the adrenal website for details.

Niacin: Niacin, in addition to pantothenic acid, is one of the most important of the B vitamins to the adrenal cascade. Large amounts of niacin are necessary to form the molecular structure of certain niacin dependent coenzymes critical for several steps in this cascade. Therefore, a B complex that is high in niacin is important in facilitating some of the crucial enzymatic reactions that take place during the adrenal cascade. If you cannot find a B complex vitamin that contains more niacin than it does the other B vitamins, you may need to purchase a separate niacin supplement. When you are recovering from adrenal fatigue, **25 to 50 mg.** niacin a day is recommended. If niacin's tendency to make people flush (turn red and tingle) bothers you, buy a "non-flushing" type, such as niacin hexanol.

Vitamin B6: Vitamin B6 is also a co-factor in several of the enzymatic pathways in the adrenal cascade. One easy test for vitamin B6 deficiency used by alternative doctors is to ask patients if they can remember their dreams. If they have trouble recalling their dreams, then they often need vitamin B6. When adequate Vitamin B6 is added as a dietary supplement they usually begin to remember their dreams. Typically **50 to 100 mg.** a day is plenty. If you find that even with 100 mg. a day of vitamin B6 you still cannot remember dreams, then you may need a special form of vitamin B6 called Pyridoxyl 5 Phosphate (P5P). A small percentage of the population has difficulty metabolizing the regular vitamin B6 supplement (pyridoxine HCL) and as a result requires a P5P vitamin B6 supplement to fully activate these enzymatic pathways. P5P is the natural form of vitamin B6 and can be purchased in health food stores, and some pharmacies and grocery stores. Although it is somewhat more expensive than regular vitamin B6, P5P ensures adequate utilization of vitamin B6.*

B Complex: The entire B complex is needed in small quantities throughout the adrenal cascade. All the B vitamins work together in concert with each individual B vitamin while it does its "job." Therefore, a small amount of all the other B vitamins are necessary to help the actions of niacin, vitamin B6 and pantothenic acid. Most vitamin B supplements contain synthetic B vitamins. Even though the natural forms are preferred, the synthetic can be used effectively to help restore adrenal function. When buying a B complex vitamin supplement, the key is to look for one that has the B vitamins in the proper proportions for the human body to utilize. For example it should have **50-100 mg of B6, 75-**

125 mg of B3, and 200-400 mcg. of B12. The stress formulas that are composed of equal amounts of most of the Bs are not formulated for the human body to metabolize properly. If you find a B complex from completely natural sources, it will contain much lower amounts of each B vitamin or the individual amounts will not be listed. However, smaller amounts are required when the B vitamins are in their natural form. Food sources of B vitamins include the following: whole grains, brewer's yeast, miso (a Japanese soup stock), Marmite (a vegetable concentrate paste), liver and rice bran syrup. These all contain natural forms of B complex.

Minerals

Magnesium: Magnesium acts like a spark plug for your adrenals and for the energy portion of every cell in your body. It is essential to the production of the enzymes and the energy necessary for the adrenal hormone cascade. Several of the steps that create energy in all of your cells, but especially in your adrenal glands, are so dependent on the presence of magnesium that it is a specific for adrenal recovery. Approximately **400 mg. of magnesium citrate** is the recommended daily dosage for the average person and it is absorbed best when taken at night, before bed. Magnesium works in concert with vitamin C and pantothenic acid to potentiate the action of the adrenals. During times of stress, always increase your intake of vitamin C, magnesium and pantothenic acid. You may also need to do this two to four times per day or even hourly if the stress is severe. Although magnesium is absorbed better after 8:00PM, for best absorption then and at other times of the day, always take magnesium and all other minerals and trace minerals with an acid like tomato juice or apple juice, at meals with whole grapes or meats, or with digestive aids. Food sources of magnesium include brown rice, beans, nuts, seeds and sea vegetables such as kelp (the highest source).

Calcium: Calcium helps settle your nervous system and create inner calm, among other important functions. Although calcium is also absorbed best after 8:00PM, it is better not to take calcium and magnesium together. You can take them on alternate evenings or, if you take them at separate times in the later part of the same day, take the magnesium closer to bedtime. Look for calcium citrate or calcium lactate (if you are not sensitive to milk). The typical recommended amount is **750 to 1,000 mg.** per day.

Cow's milk and dairy foods are commonly considered to be good sources of calcium. However, commercially available cow's milk presents two problems in this regard. 1) The process of pasteurization changes the calcium complexes in the milk, making them less suitable for your body. 2) The addition of synthetic Vitamin D2 (irradiated ergosterol) to the milk produces a tendency for the calcium in the milk to be deposited in your joints and other areas of your body instead of being taken up by the cells where it is needed. Certified raw milk and goats milk do not have these problems.

There is also the substantial problem of sensitivity or allergy to milk and dairy foods. Other good food sources of calcium include sesame seeds (unhulled) and products made from them such as tahini and humus; deep green vegetables such as kale, collard, swiss chard, parsley and broccoli; beans; nuts; and sea vegetables such as kelp. Fish and meat stews where the bones are cooked in the dish are also excellent sources of calcium.

Trace Minerals
Trace minerals occur only in very small amounts in your body and in food but are very important for your overall health. These include *zinc, manganese, selenium, molybdenum, chromium, copper, iodine* and a host of other minerals in micro amounts. They also typically have a calming effect on the body and are especially valuable if you are jittery, nervous, or easily frightened or upset. When your adrenals fatigue, you may become extremely edgy and trace minerals can help you feel more tranquil. Trace minerals are absorbed and utilized better when they are taken in the evening and/or with an acidic food or drink. Therefore have them with meals when your body's digestive juices are secreted or with something acidic such as tomato juice or vitamin C. If needed, however, trace minerals can be taken throughout the day as a calming influence.

Trace mineral supplements vary in the quality and quantity of each mineral they contain. Generally, liquid trace minerals are easiest to absorb but you should be careful of so called "colloidal" preparations. They often contain toxic trace minerals including lead, mercury, cadmium and arsenic. The best sources of trace minerals are sprouts, young plants, algae and sea vegetables and the trace mineral supplements made from them.

A hair analysis is an inexpensive and fairly reliable way to determine your mineral and trace mineral deficiencies and toxicities. Sources for hair analysis are listed on the website.

Fiber

When you are experiencing adrenal fatigue, mild constipation is sometimes present. Increasing the amount of fiber in your diet not only improves bowel motion and re-establishes normal bowel function but also helps strengthen your adrenal function.

As your adrenals begin to heal and your body's responses become more efficient, your liver often begins to detoxify more rapidly. This means that more toxic constituents are contained in the bile that is secreted by your liver and emptied into your intestinal tract for elimination. Fiber prevents bile from becoming toxic in your large intestine by binding with it and moving it along the digestive tract. In this way, fiber helps eliminate fat-soluble toxins from your body. Without sufficient fiber present, these poisons may be released from the bile and reabsorbed through your intestines.

Several different kinds of fibers such as cellulose, hemi-cellulose and pectin are necessary for good health. They all work together to provide many benefits to your whole body, although their primary site of action is in your digestive tract. To make certain that you get a sufficient quantity and variety of fiber each day, include fiber sources in every meal. Fiber comes from plants and good sources include most vegetables, legumes, fruits, seeds and whole grains (not refined grains).

Some dietary supplements are excellent sources of fiber such as psyllium seed, multi fiber mixtures and a preparation I designed called "Squeaky Clean"* that contains 8 different types of fiber combined with other factors necessary to the health of your digestive tract. However, be cautious of the commercial brands of fiber (bulking agents) available in grocery and drug stores. They may contain artificial colors and flavorings, and large amounts of sugar or sugar-like agents such as maltodextrin (a sweetener derived from corn), sucrose, corn syrup solids, and dextrose which can stimulate Candida (yeast) growth, upset blood glucose and undermine your adrenal recovery. Even the "sugar free" forms of these products can contain maltodextrin and artificial sweeteners. It is important to read the ingredient label on any product before you use it. Check the website for recommended brands and products.

Herbs

Certain herbs can be beneficial in your recovery from adrenal fatigue. However, other herbs can be quite detrimental, delaying or preventing your progress. The six best herbs to help support your adrenals and assist in their recovery are listed below. Following that are a few words about herbs you should avoid.

Licorice Root (Glycyrrhiza glabra) - The herb best known for supporting adrenal function is licorice. Yes, the ingredient that gives that common black twist of candy its flavor is beneficial for your adrenal glands. Licorice is an anti-stress herb known to increase energy, endurance and vitality and act as a mild tonic. It has been used to ease drug withdrawal and stimulate the hormones for anti-inflammatory action. It is known to naturally fortify cortisone levels, arguably the most important hormone in stress and adrenal fatigue. Licorice has also been used to help decrease symptoms of hypoglycemia, a common side effect of decreased adrenal function. Wound healing, which can be slowed down by stress, has been improved by using licorice. Licorice can also soothe nervous stomachs, a common occurrence in people under stress. Both blood circulation in the heart and arteries and production of interferon-like substances by the immune system are stimulated by licorice

There has been some concern that licorice increases blood pressure. This is because licorice partially blocks the conversion of cortisol into cortisone, which can produce higher amounts of circulating cortisol. Cortisol slightly increases contraction of the medium arteries and heart muscle causing blood pressure to rise. However, according to Dr. Jonathan Wright, you would have to consume approximately one-quarter pound of licorice candy per day in order to produce any elevation in your blood pressure. In any case, people who suffer from hypoadrenia typically have low blood pressure, so this is not usually a concern. Simply monitor your blood pressure and if you find it rising to levels above 140/90, or if you do happen to be one of the few who have both high blood pressure and low adrenal function, then limit your intake of licorice to less than one-quarter pound a day.

It is best to take licorice as a tea, with a little honey if desired, rather than by eating the candy. The candy usually contains too much sugar and may only contain licorice flavoring and not any actual licorice. Some authentic natural licorice candy, however, is always good to keep on hand in case you suddenly feel your adrenals giving out and need to temporarily boost yourself.

Licorice is available in capsules, as a liquid herbal extract, and in the original dried root which can be chewed or made into a tea.* For dosage, see the section at the end of the list of herbs.

Ashwagandha Root and Leaf (Withania somnifera) – Ashwagandha is an ancient Indian herb with a history of therapeutic use dating back to at least 1000 BC, probably because of its direct beneficial effects on adrenal tissue and function. Although it is also known as Indian ginseng, it is not related to ginseng. Traditionally, ashwagandha has been pre-scribed as a tonic for all kinds of weaknesses, as well as to promote strength and vigor. It has long been regarded as a rejuvenator and mild aphrodisiac. Because of its ant-inflammatory action, Ayruvedic physi-cians use it as the treatment of choice in rheumatic pains, inflammation of joints and other related conditions that are commonly seen in states of adrenal fatigue.
Ashwagandha is considered to be an adaptogen. An adaptogen is any substance that helps the body function more towards its normal level, for example if cortisol is too high, it lowers it, and if it is too low, it raises it. Studies have shown Ashwagandha is capable of normalizing cortisol lev-els, whether they are too high or too low. Although ashwagandha is not well known in the United States, my prediction is that in the future many people will be using this very valuable herb for its multiple health ben-efits. It is especially useful in treating adrenal fatigue and is included in my herbal formula for adrenal support and recovery.** However, in very high doses (above 35 gms/day) ashwagandha can actually inhibit adrenal function.

Korean Ginseng Root (Panax Ginseng) – Panax ginseng is an herb more suitable for men than for women. Although it has been shown to help increase cortisol levels, my experience is that while men can usually take Panax ginseng with mild to significant benefits, women should be careful in its use. This type of ginseng, especially Korean Red, can have adverse effects in some women, similar to the adverse effects they experience with excess DHEA. These can include an increase in facial hair and acne. In men increased aggressiveness, irritability, or sexual excesses are signs that they are taking too much and should cut down or stop taking it. My advice to men is to use it in small doses at first and build up gradually. I recommend that women avoid its use altogether.*

Siberian Ginseng Root (Eleutherococus senticosus) – Siberian ginseng, although not from Siberia and not strictly a ginseng, is good for women as well as men. It has a wide range of activities that help support and rejuvenate adrenal function, increase resistance to stress, normalize metabolism, and regulate neurotransmitters (which are important in modifying the stress response). It counteracts mental fatigue and is known to increase and sustain energy levels, physical stamina and endurance. With its antidepressant properties, Siberian ginseng has demonstrated its ability to calm anxiousness, improve sleeping, diminish lethargy, lessen irritability and induce a feeling of well-being. It has been used by Russian workers, deep-sea divers and Olympic athletes for better performance and by cosmonauts for stress and disease resistance, increased vitality and to counter depletion of the adrenal stress hormones. In addition it has been shown to normalize blood sugar, stimulate antibodies to bacteria and viruses, increase resistance to environmental pollutants, improve absorption of some B vitamins and decrease vitamin C loss. Although it has been shown to normalize blood pressure, do not use it if your blood pressure is very high. Siberian ginseng is more normalizing than stimulatory in its effects on your adrenals and, as you can see by its actions, it can be an important healer for anyone trying to recover from adrenal fatigue.*

Ginger root (Zingiber officinale) – Ginger root is another adaptogen for the adrenals that helps modulate cortisol levels, normalize blood pressure and heart rate; burn fat; increase energy and metabolic rate, and stimulate digestive enzyme secretions for proteins and fatty acids. Ginger is great for nausea of any kind and has been used historically for morning sickness during pregnancy. It also decreases lethargy during convalescence from an illness and has been used for centuries for many different health purposes.*

Fresh ginger root is available in the produce section of most grocery stores. You can easily make a pleasant spicy tea by following the instructions below in the section on the preparation of herbs.

Ginkgo leaf (Ginkgo biloba) – The adrenals suffer tremendous oxidative stress when under stress themselves, especially when producing excess cortisol during the stress response. This leads to a significant increase in free radicals within the same adrenal cells that make the needed hormones. If free radicals generated in this process are not neutralized, the production of hormones is slowed and tissue damage increases within the adrenal cells. Ginkgo is a powerful anti-oxidant that sequesters free radical production, thereby protecting the adrenal glands, the brain and the liver from free radical damage.

It also contains several bioflavinoids that improves blood flow to the brain, ears, eyes, heart and extremities. Ginkgo has been shown to lessen tissue damage from inflammation and shock, elevate mood in people prone to depression, and decrease mental fatigue. Its unique qualities make it valuable to any adrenal recovery program. Follow the instructions below on how to take herbal preparations.

The above herbs can be obtained and taken singly or together, in liquid or dry forms. I have designed a liquid formula called "Herbal Adrenal Support Formula"* combining these herbs in the proper portions to support your adrenals. The typical dosage of the liquid extract is 10-15 drops, 2-4 times daily, and of encapsulated powder is 2-4 capsules per day.

How to take herbal preparations
Always take the usual precaution of starting with low doses, and increasing the dosage slowly when using herbal preparations. Because of the varying strength of herbal preparations, it is best to follow the instructions on all packaged herbs. If there are no instructions, a general rule for preparation of herbs is as follows:

* A list of supplement manufacturers and suppliers is given in a constantly updated list on our website

Tincture (alcohol extracts) – 10-15 drops in liquid 3 to 4 times per day. Unfortunately, some of the most active ingredients in these herbs can only be extracted using alcohol. Water extractions or glycerin-based preparations may not have the potency of alcohol extracts. Many people with low adrenal function are sensitive to alcohol. Therefore, the liquid preparations containing alcohol should first be simmered in tea or water to evaporate the alcohol before taking them.

Fluid extracts – 5-10 drops in liquid 3 to 4 times per day.

Leaves - Steep (cover with boiling water) 1 teaspoon of dry leaves per cup of water for 15 minutes. Strain and drink. Honey or other natural sweeteners can be added to taste.

Root – Simmer (heat in water kept below boiling) 1 teaspoon of grated dry or fresh root for each cup of steaming hot water for 15 minutes. Strain and drink. Honey or other natural sweeteners can be added to taste.

Herbs to be cautious of

Just as there are herbs that are beneficial and restorative to the adrenals, there are herbs you should avoid if you have adrenal fatigue because they can worsen your symptoms, increase your recovery time, or prevent your recovery by further exhausting your adrenals. These herbs include Ephedra, (or Ma Huang), cola nut or strong black teas. Also avoid any herbs or teas containing stimulants, sedatives, or hallucinogenic substances, and any teas that over stimulate the nervous system or the adrenals. Just because it is natural does not mean it is good for you. Strychnine, arsenic, aflatoxin and mercury are also all "natural" substances, but I would not want them in my body. So avoid these herbs.

Chapter 16

Adrenal Cell Extracts

Adrenal extracts have been recommended and successfully used for a variety of conditions that involve low adrenal function, including asthenia, asthma, colds, burns, depletion from colds, coughs, dyspepsia (poor digestion), early Addison's disease, hypotension (low blood pressure), infections, infectious diseases, depletion from infectious diseases, convalescence from infectious diseases, neurasthenia (low energy/weakness), tuberculosis, light-headedness and dizziness, and vomiting during pregnancy. (Harrower, '39, pg. 19-22)

History of Adrenal Cell Extracts

The earliest, and still probably the most reliable, way of rebuilding the adrenals from adrenal fatigue is the use of extracts from liquid or powdered bovine adrenal glands. Historically and in many modern clinics, preparations using adrenal cell extracts have been used extensively and are considered to be the most important aspect of the treatment. The first recorded use of an adrenal extract was in 1898 when Sir William Osler administered a crude preparation of adrenal cells to a person with Addison's disease. Since 1918, when they became commercially available, adrenal cell extracts have been a valuable and powerful form of therapy and have been used by thousands of medical doctors in the treatment of non-Addison's type of hypoadrenia.

Their first claim to fame in the United States occurred with the epidemic flu virus of 1918. Respiratory infections are especially hard on the adrenal glands and fatigue them rapidly. This effect was shown by Lucke and his associates at Camp Zachary Taylor in 1919, when he found that adrenal exhaustion was present in 103 of 126 autopsied cases of mortality from the flu epidemic. In 3 other cases he even found adrenal hemorrhages and enlargement of the adrenal glands to twice their size. This means that in 106 of 126 patients who died from influenza, the adrenals were actually damaged by the infection. It is not that the adrenals were infected per se, but that the effort they made to try to restore balance to the body led them to a degree of exhaustion that was physically detectable upon autopsy (Lucke, B., et al., Archives of Internal Medicine, August 1919, XXIIII, pg. 154).

While this flu epidemic was debilitating and even killing thousands around the world, a few hundred of its victims were given a formula containing liquid adrenal cortical extracts (extracts from the adrenal cortex) combined with small amounts of thyroid and gonadal extracts. The formula was found to be unusually effective in overcoming many of the asthenic (weak) and depleted states that were so common to those afflicted with this deadly flu. It also effectively reduced the serious sequeli that usually followed this particular infection. The benefits of this adrenal cell extract formula dramatically drew attention to its practical use. The quick and uneventful recovery experienced by those taking it contrasted to the long period of recuperation normally seen in this flu epidemic. These results made many physicians aware of the possibility for recovery from less severe forms of hypoadrenia as well. It was known even in 1919 that the early functional endocrine disorders, especially adrenal fatigue, are infinitely more common and far more likely to respond to therapy than extreme endocrine diseases such as Addison's (Harrower, '39, pg. 17).

By the mid 1930's, adrenal cell extracts in liquid and tablet forms were produced by several companies. By the late 1930's, they were being used by tens of thousands of physicians. As recently as 1968 they were still being made by some of the leading pharmaceutical companies (Upjohn and Eli Lilly, among others).

However, in the early 1950's synthetic cortisol became available. Because the synthetic hormone produced effects that seemed, at first, so much more dramatic than the effects of adrenal extracts, many physicians switched to synthetic cortisol and its derivatives to treat conditions they had previously treated with adrenal cell extracts. Unfortunately for patients, the profit margins were also more dramatic for the synthetic corticosteroids. This quickly made the synthetics the unquestionable favorite of the pharmaceutical industry. Within a few short years, the many detrimental side effects of the synthetics started appearing, but the pharmaceutical industry had made its profitable choice and would never turn back. In fact there has been a concerted effort to discredit adrenal and other cellular extracts and to remove them from the market. Luckily, these valuable cellular extracts, which provide more true benefits to your body without the damaging side effects of synthetic corticosteroids, are still available from a few sources.

Adrenal Cortical Extracts

Also known as adrenal cell extracts, adrenal cortical extracts are the liquid or powder extracts of the adrenal cortex. Their action is to support, fortify and restore normal adrenal function, there by enhancing adrenal activity and speeding recovery. Adrenal cell extracts are not replacement hormones, but instead provide the essential constituents for adrenal repair. They include all the adrenal cell contents, such as nucleic acids (adrenal cell RNA and DNA) and concentrated nutrients in the form and proportion used by the adrenals to properly function and recover, but contain only tiny amounts of the actual hormones in the adrenal gland. Adrenal cortical extracts have been used orally and as injectables since the end of WWI and have only rarely produced unwanted side effects.

These extracts have been the cornerstone of effective therapy for adrenal fatigue since they were first developed. There are several brands available in both tablet and liquid form. The liquid is generally more powerful than the tablet, however it is more costly. I usually use the liquid in moderate to severe cases, and tablets in milder cases. Dosage for the adrenal cortical extract tablets is 6-12 per day, depending upon severity, taken in three to four intervals throughout the day. Dosage for the liquid form is usually one vial under the tongue 2 to 3 times weekly or as directed by your physician. In severe cases, it may need to be more frequent. Although these extracts are classified as dietary supplements, they must usually be purchased through a physician. Check our website for present suppliers of liquid and tablet forms of adrenal extract. A few sell directly to the public, but it is usually much better to work with a physician familiar with the treatment of adrenal fatigue.

Most medical doctors are unaware of the existence of this type of therapy and do not know how to use it. Because it is a departure from their usual thinking and protocol, they are often reluctant to even explore it. If a patient asks about cell extracts, they are typically negative about the subject. But as my friend, Dr. Leo Roy, the first holistic physician of

Canada, said, "Doctors are down on things they are not up on." This is especially true of live cell substances and their use.

The doctors who are up on treating adrenal fatigue find significant value in adrenal extracts for alleviating all levels of adrenal fatigue. Today, by combining our knowledge of adrenal cortical extracts with lifestyle modifications, dietary supplements and herbal formulas, we can stabilize people with adrenal fatigue and accelerate their recovery more efficiently than ever before. Adrenal extracts have been and continue to be a fundamental part of the treatment protocol for adrenal fatigue used effectively for over 80 years.

Cortisol vs. Adrenal Cell Extracts
It is important to understand the difference between adrenal cell extracts and natural or synthetic cortisol and cortisol type steroids such as cortisone, prednisone, prednisolone and many other forms of adrenal steroid hormones. Adrenal cell extracts nourish and help rebuild your adrenal cells. As these cells recover, they can once again produce the proper amount of the various hormones needed for the many functions

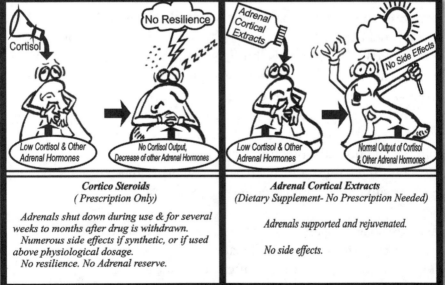

CORTISOL VS. ADRENAL CORTICAL EXTRACTS

performed by your adrenal glands. By this means they tend to normalize adrenal function. In contrast, corticosteroids, whether natural or synthetic, tend to reduce or shut down the activity of your adrenal glands. This happens because your brain senses the presence of these cortisol substitutes and, in response, withholds the signal (ACTH) it would otherwise send to your adrenal glands to make more adrenal hormones. (See illustration – "Cortisol vs. Adrenal Cortical Extracts"). Thus corticosteroids suppress the functions of your adrenal glands, over-riding the normal feed back loops that regulate and balance adrenal hormones. In spite of the fact that this action can produce dramatic initial improvements in your symptoms, these symptomatic improvements come with a heavy price.

Although corticosteroids are replacement hormones; that is, they replace the natural hormone (cortisol) they are designed to mimic, they do not function exactly the same as natural cortisol because they are not identical to it. For one thing, synthetic corticosteroids are up to 17 times more powerful than the natural form of cortisol. If taken in excess of the physiological needs of the body (above the equivalent of 20 mg of cortisol per day), which many prescriptions are, their unfortunate side effects are many and far-reaching. Even after a course of just a few days of corticosteroid medication, it takes several days to several weeks for adrenal function to return to normal. When taken for a long period of time, the adrenals may require anywhere from several months to 2 years to revive and produce their own cortisol again. Sometimes they never fully recover.

This is why it is so difficult to get off a corticosteroid drug once you have been on one for a while. You get caught in the "catch-22" that if you stop taking the corticosteroids, you crash and your symptoms return worse than ever because your adrenal activity is suppressed. So you keep taking them, but the longer you take them the harder it is for your adrenals to regain proper function.

Because corticosteroids mask the symptoms of adrenal fatigue and, when used in excess, depress immune function, the person taking them is at greater risk from stress and infection. Such therapy can become more hazardous than the original disease. Corticosteroids may have quick and dramatic symptomatic results, but unless they are used in their natural form and in physiologic doses that mimic the natural secretion of cortisol, they make the adrenals weaker rather than stronger. In addition, the list of their side effects is sobering for those who care to look them up in the Physicians Desk Reference (PDR). They range from rash to sudden death.

If corticosteroid therapy is necessary, it is best to use the natural form of cortisol, hydrocortisone, available by prescription. Even though this natural hormone also diminishes or shuts down the adrenals while it is being taken and for several weeks after it is discontinued, it can be used effectively as a therapy for severe adrenal fatigue. When administered in physiological doses of approximately 20 mg per day to emulate the natural daily secretion of cortisol, it can give the adrenals a rest for a period of time, thereby providing an opportunity to recover. This is described in the next chapter.

"I am 47 years old . . . I was first diagnosed with asthma at age 3 and spent the first 20 years of my life on a continuous regime of prednisone (I was actually addicted for 2 years, ages 11 & 12, because my adrenals had shut down), weekly allergy shots, frequent antibiotics due to multiple upper respiratory infections (supposedly) and all the asthma drugs on top of that (theophylline, isuprel inhalers and more). Also multiple epinephrine injections due to frequent trips to the ER with many resulting in hospitalizations .... My health is actually improving, slowly but surely. My single biggest problem now is a constant weariness, frequent exhaustion, and a seeming inability to get ahead and on with my busy life. (Oh, and I'm also addicted to my one cup of strong coffee a day which I rationalize because it's organic ....) So I think adrenal supplementation is the key at this point. I feel like I'm at the end of my rope and that the only thing that will help is a year alone in the tropics somewhere so I can sleep and be warm. Of course, the other thing would be to address my adrenals."

Mrs. DN - Source: quote from letters received.

Elaine was a bright, energetic and athletic young girl with a true desire for competition. However, during a basketball tournament in her junior year, she slammed into a wall. The accident was traumatic both physically and emotionally. Following the accident, Elaine experienced fatigue, decreased stamina, and a loss of focus that negatively affected her academic, athletic and social activities. About six months after the accident, Elaine developed swollen joints that were very pain-ful upon movement, especially in the later part of the day. In addition she had an intermittent fever with no detectable cause. This continued for several years, perplexing her doctors, until finally Elaine was diag-nosed with rheumatoid arthritis.

She was placed on corticosteroids, which decreased the inflammation and increased her stamina to some degree so she could function better. The price for her improvement was the development of some common side effects of corticosteroids such as a moon face and buffalo hump, along with some thinning of her skin. After just a couple of occasional rheumatoid arthritis flare-ups, the doctor increased the strength of the corticosteroids and had her take it continuously. For several years Elaine was able to manage successfully. However, one Friday night while she was out at a local restaurant, she experienced severe diar-rhea with a 105° temperature and was taken to the hospital. At the hospital, her kidneys shut down, her blood pressure dropped to 60/30, her liver function diminished and she was placed in ICU. Miracu-lously, the doctors were able to reverse the systemic shut down of Elaine's body and she was sent home to recover after four days. The diagnosis was toxic shock syndrome precipitated by corticosteroid therapy.

This is an excellent illustration of what happens when someone has ad-renal fatigue produced by a sudden trauma and it goes undiagnosed and untreated. The low cortisol levels resulted in too little anti-inflamma-tory activity in Elaine's joints and she experienced a mild form of rheu-matoid arthritis. The over-treatment with ever increasing doses of corti-costeroids shut down her adrenal function even further, as well as se-verely suppressed her overall immune function. She had been able to manage up until that evening at the restaurant because she had not been exposed to any infectious agents. However eating contaminated food at the restaurant, something that would typically have made someone sick for a day or two, became a life-threatening event for Elaine. She no longer had adequate adrenal or immune function to fight the infection.

Possible combined therapy of cortisol and adrenal cell extract in severe adrenal fatigue. There have been a few reported cases of Addison's disease that showed some improvement when adrenal cell extracts were used in conjunction with small amounts of hydrocortisone. Any program for Addison's disease should be instituted and monitored by a physician who is familiar with this disease and with the use and properties of both these substances. If you need to use some form of cortisol, see the sections "Cortisol as a Treatment Option" and "Cortisol Combined with Adrenal Cell Extracts" in the next chapter.

Chapter 17

Replacement Hormones

Cortisol as a Treatment Option

As I mentioned in the previous chapter, in a few cases of severe hypoadrenia that border on actual Addison's disease, a short therapeutic course of natural cortisol may be needed. Jeffries gives an excellent account of how to use the natural hydrocortisone in therapy in his book, "Safe Uses of Cortisol", (Jeffries, 1998). He also does a nice job of covering the historical aspects of the development of the synthetic corticosteroids and the disadvantages of using them. Briefly, if this therapy is necessary, it should be confirmed by special tests such as the combined 24-Hour Urinary Cortisol & ACTH tests mentioned in Chapter 11. In addition, it is important to remember that corticosteroids suppress adrenal function in proportion to the dosage. For this reason it is important that treatment should be withdrawn slowly, never abruptly.

There are many types of corticosteroids on the market but the only type that should be used is the natural form of hydrocortisone. The commercially available hydrocortisone, although essentially the same as the cortisol your body produces, also contains unnecessary ingredients some patients react to. To make certain you are getting pure cortisol without additives, it is best to have a compounding pharmacist prepare your prescription.

Although there are different therapeutic regimens for taking natural hydrocortisone, most conform to the normal 24-hour cortisol secretion of approximately 20 mg of cortisol. Jeffries recommends 5 or 7.5 mg. orally before each meal and at bedtime (Jeffries, '98, pg. 43). Other alternative physicians use an initial dose of 12, 5, 2, and 1 mg. at 8:00 AM, 12:00, 3:00 and 6:00 PM respectively. If sleep disturbances are part of the syndrome, 1 mg. before bedtime may be helpful.

After approximately 6 months most doctors try to gradually decrease the dosage. If the adrenal glands have recovered sufficiently, they will pick up the slack and begin to respond normally. If not, they may need the same or a reduced dose for awhile longer. Most patients will only need hydrocortisone therapy for a temporary time. It is seldom necessary to go beyond 2 years.

It goes without saying that if steroid replacement therapy is needed, blood and urine tests should be completed regularly to monitor progress. Although the administration of cortisol will produce fast, almost immediate relief, it should not be used except in the most severe cases. Again, this is because the cortisol shuts down the adrenals and as such, may not be substantially therapeutic in the long run.

Cortisol Combined with Adrenal Cell Extracts
In several cases, natural cortisol has been taken simultaneously with adrenal cell extracts. This regimen for severe hypoadrenia often allows the adrenals to rest and rebuild much faster than with either therapy alone. After 2-3 months on both cortisol and adrenal extracts, the daily dose of cortisol is slowly withdrawn while a vitamin C complex, the adrenal cell extracts and other supplements (as described in Chapter 15) are increased. This allows the adrenal glands to recover more quickly and to strengthen enough that when the cortisol is discontinued, the adrenals can function adequately on their own. For people with severe adrenal fatigue, and even some cases of Addison's disease, this can be a very satisfactory combination therapy.

Naturally, if you are going to use cortisol, you will need the help of a physician because it is by prescription only. The physician needs to have an in depth knowledge of adrenal function and how to use adrenal extracts and cortisol together for optimum benefit. If you consult a physician, do not be afraid to ask what experience and training she or he has had in restoring adrenal function.

DHEA
DHEA is one of the androgen hormones secreted by the adrenal glands and is the precursor to several other sex hormones. DHEA levels often become depressed during adrenal fatigue. Even though DHEA is a hormone, it is considered a dietary supplement in the United States and can be purchased at a reasonable cost in health food stores and other supplement outlets. A saliva test will determine whether your DHEA levels are below normal (see section on Saliva Testing). When it is low, it is a good

idea to supplement with DHEA if you are a male. Approximately 25 mg. to 200 mg. is the accepted and normal dosage range for men. Typically older men need more than younger men, although this varies with the individual. People often see improvement within 2-3 weeks of beginning DHEA. Be careful of overdosing with DHEA; more than 200 mg. for men can create hostility, aggression and make you unpleasant to be around. There are also some minor concerns in some alternative medical circles about the possibility that DHEA may represent a threat to health because it can be converted into dihydro-testosterone, which has been linked to prostate cancer. However, there are other studies that show that men with higher DHEA levels are actually protected against prostate cancer, so the jury is still out. If you take DHEA for more than three months, it is also good to have your PSA (prostate serum androgen) level checked every six months, as a precaution. If it begins to rise, you should decrease or eliminate the use of DHEA until the cause of the rise is found.

It is my clinical experience that women often do not do well on DHEA unless their adrenals are very fatigued. Levels as low as 10-25 mg. have produced symptoms of excess DHEA such as facial hair and acne. A safer and more successful way of raising DHEA levels in women is to have them take either progesterone or pregnenolone, although some studies of women with chronic fatigue syndrome or lupus have found benefit from using 200 mg. of DHEA/day.

Progesterone and Pregnenolone
Progesterone and pregnenolone are hormones that are manufactured in the adrenal cascade as well as in the ovaries and testicles before they are metabolized into DHEA. In the adrenal cascade, pregnenolone is the first hormone to be made from cholesterol and progesterone is the second. Both can be converted into several other adrenal hormones besides DHEA, including the sex hormones, aldosterone and cortisol. Thus, taking replacement hormones like pregnenolone and progesterone that occur early in the adrenal cascade lets your body's wisdom choose which other hormones it will make from them, according to your body's needs. With adrenal fatigue, the sex hormone levels often fall because your adrenal glands are not able to manufacture adequate levels of hormones. One function that sex hormones serve is to act as antioxidants that help prevent the oxidative damage caused by cortisol. So the lower the sex hormones,

the more damage there is to tissues, especially when you are under stress. This oxidative damage is one of the key factors in rapid aging. Either pregnenolone or progesterone can better be used to raise the hormonal levels in both men and women, and decrease some aspects of adrenal fatigue. By bypassing the very complex and energy consuming steps required of your adrenals to make pregnenolone or progesterone from cholesterol, your adrenals do not have to work nearly so hard to keep your hormone levels adequate.

Besides helping fatigued adrenals, both these hormones have been used very successfully to diminish premenstrual syndrome (PMS). This is not surprising considering that the most common cause of PMS seems to be too little progesterone and/or too little magnesium. Progesterone is made in both the ovaries and the adrenal glands. Women suffering from adrenal fatigue often have lower saliva progesterone levels and increased PMS. The addition of oral pregnenolone or natural progesterone cream is often needed for relief of PMS and female complaints common in adrenal fatigue. With pregnenolone 10-40 mg. per day is usually sufficient, taken orally, and 20-30mg. (1/4 – ½ tsp.) per day of progesterone when applied as a cream to the skin. More specific instructions are given below.

Both pregnenolone tablets and progesterone cream are available from many health food stores and some pharmacies. If you cannot find them or want immediate sources, check our website for a list of suppliers.

It is important to note that we are speaking of the natural progesterone and not the synthetic progestins in tablet form usually prescribed by your doctor for hormone replacement therapy. The synthetic progestins can have many side effects and should be avoided. The various progestins exist because drug companies need forms of progesterone different enough from their competition to be patented and controlled by the company. The reason all progestins have side effects is that none of them are exactly like the natural progesterone your body makes. Unfortunately, most doctors only know about products made by pharmaceutical companies, and the bulk of their information about therapeutic substances comes from these same companies. Because the large drug companies do not produce natural progesterone creams, many doctors are not knowledgeable about them and are unaware of the difference in safety between the synthetic progestins and the natural progesterones. They further complicate the issue by referring to the synthetics as progesterone, when they should be called progestins. Progestins are the synthetic altered forms of progesterone that are responsible for most of the negative side effects experienced by women taking them.

The progesterone contained in progesterone cream, however, is usually a natural plant progesterone (phytoprogesterone) that has been converted into exactly the same molecule as the progesterone in your body. It can be used safely by most women. You do not need a prescription for it and it is available from many health food stores and on the internet. Rub 1/4 to 1/2 teaspoon cream into the tender areas of your skin (swimsuit areas plus the inside of thighs and arms) each morning and evening. Pre-menopausal women should apply it from the 12th day of the menstrual cycle to the 26th day (the first day of bleeding is counted as the 1st day). Post-menopausal women can use it for 21 days each month. An excellent book that covers this topic is by Dr. John Lee, <u>What Your Doctor May Not Tell You About Menopause</u>.

Using hormone replacement therapy for adrenal fatigue is an area that requires skill. Although some of the hormones mentioned in this chapter can be purchased without a prescription, I highly recommend using a physician familiar with hormone replacement in cases of adrenal fatigue. If you cannot find one in your area, check our website for physicians within driving distance or who do telephone consults. Hormones work together in symphony to perform in the concert of life. To throw in a hormone here and another there in a haphazard way is like having a heavy metal band thrown in with an orchestra. Hormones are powerful engineers of body processes and balancing them calls for delicate precision. The timing, the quantity and the form of hormone used are all critical. It is best to work with an expert who will monitor your progress using laboratory tests. If you do embark upon this yourself, use caution: start low and go slow.

Chapter 18

Daily Program for Adrenal Recovery

The following is a sample daily program for recovering from adrenal fatigue. It is meant to be a flexible general model that you can adapt to your own individual needs and lifestyle, but try to include all of the therapeutic elements.

7:00 AM - Get up (only if you need to get up by this time in order to get to work on time). Otherwise sleep in until 9:00 AM or so, every chance you get.

7:15 AM – Drink one 8oz glass of water with ½ teaspoon sea salt stirred in.

7:30 AM – Do light work out or relaxation and breathing techniques. Shower.

8:15 AM – Breakfast: include protein, fats (oils) and a small amount of starchy unrefined carbohydrates, 1 cup green tea, mint tea with cream and honey (if desired) or other beverage; (no coffee, black tea or colas). Chew well.
    Supplements – 2 capsules Adrenal Exhaustion Formula*
             2 capsules Adrenal C*

10:15 AM – Break: snack (a few bites of a food that contains protein, fat (oils) and an unrefined, starchy carbohydrate; no caffeine or refined carbohydrates, rest lying down after snack; use breathing or relaxation techniques if needed (whatever makes you feel good that does not harm your body).

11:45 AM – Lunch: include protein, a small amount of starchy unrefined carbohydrates, fats (oils) and vegetables; no caffeine or refined carbohydrates. Chew well.

2:00 PM - Break: snack (same general constituents as morning break); no caffeine or refined carbohydrates, rest lying down after snack; use breathing or relaxation techniques if needed.
    Supplements – 1-2 caps. Adrenal Exhaustion Formula*
             2 capsules Adrenal C*

5:30 PM – Supper: include protein, starchy unrefined carbohydrates, fats (oils), 3-4 vegetables and possibly some fruit; no caffeine or refined carbohydrates. Chew well.

Supplements – 1-2 caps. Adrenal Exhaustion Formula*

2 capsules adrenal C*

7:00 PM – Do relaxation and breathing techniques.

9:30 PM – Have a small healthy snack if you usually have difficulty sleeping.

10:00 PM – Bed

On weekends, or any day possible, sleep-in until 9:00 AM or later. Take a nap in the afternoon and even in the morning if you feel draggy. In the evening time, enjoy yourself. Read entertaining books, rent funny movies, make a point of laughing as much as possible. At first, laughing may seem insincere and may take some effort, but with practice, laughing and enjoyment will be refreshing, not tiring. Once or twice per week, spend time with friends as long as it is not tiring. Keep the visits relatively short (under 2 hours), do not associate with any energy suckers, and only stay as long as you are enjoying yourself.

* These are formulas I designed specifically for people suffering from adrenal fatigue. Check our website for a list of suppliers. These high quality formulas bring together in one supplement all the nutrients necessary in the proper proportions to support the adrenal glands in their many functions. If you would rather take the nutrients individually, make a list of what you need from the nutritional supplement sections in this book and substitute them at the indicated times for taking supplements.

General Rules for Adrenal Fatigue

Below are some general rules to follow and things to avoid to help you recover from adrenal fatigue. Use the list as a reference guide after reading the preceding chapters.

Do These Things

- Be in bed before 10:00 PM.
- Sleep in until 9:00 AM whenever possible.
- Look for things that make you laugh.
- Eliminate the energy robbers (things in your life that drain your energy).
- Make your lifestyle a healing one
- Do something pleasurable every day.
- Whenever you are not enjoying your life, go back to the "Three Things You Can Do" section and take action.
- Notice at least one small, everyday thing that you are grateful for each day.
- Take your dietary supplements, regularly.
- Move your body and breathe deeply
- Believe in your ability to recover
- Use your mind as a powerful healing tool
- Keep a journal – jot down your experiences each day.
- Eat the foods your body needs
- Learn which foods make you feel bad (keep a list of them)
- Re-read this book as often as you need.
- Try having a glass of water in the morning containing ½ to 1 teaspoon of salt stirred in until dissolved.*
- Salt your food; salt your water.
- If you are to have fruit, have something with salt before or after the fruit and chew very well.
- Combine starchy carbohydrates, protein and fats at every meal.
- Eat an abundance of whole foods – those foods which are eaten like nature grows them
- Eat lots of colored vegetables.
- Chew your food well.
- Take the power and responsibility of your health into your own hands.
- Make whatever lifestyle changes you need to make to regain your health
- Laugh several times per day.
- Enjoy your recovery.
- Take 1,000 mg. of Vitamin C complex with 200 mg. magnesium and pantothenic acid at approximately 2:00 PM every day along with a small snack in order to help avoid the 3:00 to 4:00 PM low.

---

* If this makes you feel better, continue doing it. Note - on mornings when you exercise fully, you may not want as much salt. Be mindful of your cravings for salt and potassium containing foods during the day. These desires may serve as rough indicators of adrenal function during the day.

Avoid These Things

- Getting overtired.
- Caffeine, sugar, alcohol, and white flour products.
- Coffee, even decaf
- Staying up past 11:00PM
- Pushing yourself
- Energy suckers
- Being harsh or negative with yourself
- Feeling sorry for yourself
- Foods you are addicted to
- Foods you suspect an allergy or sensitive to.
- Foods that make you feel worse, cloud your thinking or pull you down in any way.
- Never skip breakfast.
- Avoid fruit in the morning.
- Never eat starchy carbohydrates (breads, pastas) by themselves.
- Do not eat foods that adversely affect you in any way, no matter how good they taste or how much you crave them.

Chapter 19

Trouble-shooting
What To Do If You Still Need Help

Even when you have faithfully followed the adrenal recovery program in this book, there are several factors that can prevent it from working completely. So if you have been using this program for more than 2 months but you are still having difficulty recovering, read this chapter and take the steps recommended here. As a first step, review the recovery program you have been following for the past two months, using the following as a guide.

1) Re-examine your overall lifestyle – especially consider the balance of demands on your mind/body system and replenishment to your system. Make certain you have eliminated the energy robbers, as well as the largest negative aspects in your life that you circled in the "Health History Timeline" and "Locating the Energy Robbers" sections. If you have not, do it now.

2) Have you incorporated the major lifestyle changes you circled in the sections "Separating the Good from the Bad and the Ugly" by using the methods in the "Three Things You Can Do" section? If not, make these changes now.

3) Are you using the exercises in the "Reframing" and "Relaxation" sections to learn to change how you respond to the stress around you?

4) Re-examine your exercise program. Are you moving your body in enjoyable invigorating ways at least three times a week? Are you breathing deeply every day for 20 minutes or more?

5) Are you getting enough sleep?

6) Re-examine your food and beverage choices. Are they from good quality sources?

7) Have you checked yourself for food allergies and sensitivities and eliminated everything you are sensitive, allergic or addicted to?

8) Are you taking the dietary supplements and other substances described in chapters 15-17 that support your adrenals?

9) If you have followed all of the above suggestions, go on to the next step on body burdens to see what else you can do.

Body Burdens

A body burden is any problem that negatively affects your body and continues to drain your overall health. An undiscovered body burden is the most likely culprit when you are not progressing as well as you should in your program and can be one of the largest obstacles to full recovery. Body burdens originate from many different internal or external sources ranging from a chronic, untreated sub-acute infection, to a poorly ventilated work place. (See illustration "Body Burdens Related to Adrenal Fatigue"). Generally speaking, your adrenals have difficulty recovering when you have any significant physical or emotional body burden because they are sensitive glands that are especially vulnerable to the biochemical imbalances caused by such stresses.

BODY BURDENS RELATED TO ADRENAL FATIGUE

NO RELAXATION
INADEQUATE SLEEP
HYPOGLYCEMIA
INADEQUATE SALT INTAKE
ALLERGIES
ENERGY ROBBERS
INTESTINAL PROBLEMS
ALCOHOL   ANEMIA
LACK OF ENERGY
POOR DIGESTION
HEAVY METALS BURDEN
(Aluminum;Mercury;Lead;Cadmium)
PESTICIDES & HERBICIDES IN FOOD & AIR
DECREASED IMMUNITY
CHRONIC INFECTIONS
SELF DEGRADING ATTITUDES
CHEMICALS IN WATER
CONGESTED LIVER
PROCESSED FOODS
DRUGS   COFFEE
LACK OF FRESH FOOD
POOR TEETH   RANCID OILS
CHRONIC ILLNESS
TOOTH & GUM DECAY

Finding the body burden(s) requires you to become like a private detective looking for clues. Begin by reviewing the events listed in your "Health History Time Line" around the onset of your adrenal fatigue. Recall how you felt after each event, writing down the specific signs and symptoms. Compare those with the ones you are experiencing now. The event(s) that produced the symptoms and signs most similar to those you are currently suffering from is the likeliest source of the body burden(s), especially if you did not fully recover from that event. Below are some examples of body burdens.

Recurrent respiratory infections - Although this has been mentioned in previous sections, recurrent respiratory infections are one of the most significant body burdens hampering recovery from adrenal fatigue. It is often necessary to treat the respiratory infection as well as the adrenal fatigue before the adrenals can recover. When the adrenals have recovered, immune resistance increases enough to decrease or eliminate the recurrent respiratory infections. To support your adrenals and help your immune system overcome its susceptibility to respiratory infection, follow the guidelines in Chapter 15 on dietary supplements, with special attention to your vitamin C intake. The "Taz" soup given on page 93 was specifically designed to help people with adrenal fatigue recover from an infectious illness. In addition, there is a unique product called Nat-Stim™ that was developed in Bulgaria that is especially valuable in this situation. Check the website for sources.

Dental problems – Another common source of body burdens is the mouth. This includes tooth abscesses, cracked or decayed teeth, root canals with sub-acute infections, periodontitis, gingivitis and other gum infections, improperly extracted teeth with smoldering infections in the socket where the tooth used to be, mercury fillings leaking into the body (mercury directly suppresses cortisol levels), dental materials that provoke sensitivities, and poor dental work that irritates the teeth, gums or inside of the cheek. Unresolved dental problems are common but often unrecognized sources of stress and adrenal fatigue. The use of mercury amalgams has been a continual, yet vehemently denied, source of toxicity. Mercury is a specific toxin of the adrenals, directly suppressing adrenal hormone output. If you see in your history that your symptoms started within a few months of having particular dental work, the dental work might be an important factor in restoring your health, as any one of these dental problems can hamper your ability to heal. It would be best to have your teeth checked by a dentist who does not use amalgam (silver) fillings and who practices dentistry with an awareness of the importance of the mouth and teeth to overall health. Unfortunately, most dental schools do not provide much training in the specific ways and means by which your mouth tremendously influences your total health or in methods of inspecting and treating your mouth and teeth within this total body context. They also do not typically include instruction about individual sensitivities to dental materials or the use of alternative safe materials. To find out more about the importance of your teeth and gums to the health of your whole body or for a list of some holistic dentists check our website.

Rick was a man in his mid 70's who had suffered a myriad of health problems for several decades. He was forced to change dentists because he moved. Upon his initial examination, the new dentist told him he thought Rick's teeth were causing or adding to many of his health problems. They agreed upon an extensive therapy that included removal of cracked teeth, treating diseased gums and removing the silver fillings under his gold crowns. Each time he came home from the dentist, Rick saw positive changes. His foggy thinking cleared, his memory improved, his writing went through a transformation of lucidity he had never experienced. Rick reported his energy was back to what it had been 20 years ago. Removing the body burdens in his mouth brought new life into this man.

Kristin was a woman in her mid 40's who was suffering from mild adrenal fatigue. Knowing quite a lot about adrenal fatigue, she de-cided that an infection below one of her wisdom teeth was producing a body burden. She consulted a dentist who agreed that the area needed surgery. The area below the tooth was indeed infected and the surgery successfully cleared the infection. Although the surgery was success-ful, Kristin was knocked flat by the trauma of the surgery. Her adrenals were in no shape to support this kind of stress on her body. When she first consulted me, it had been over two years since the dental surgery and she still had not recovered. Kristin's case is a good example of the reduction in ability to handle stress experienced by people already suf-fering from adrenal fatigue. Any major additional stress (such as sur-gery) can pull them down further and keep them there until the right therapy is applied.

Jackie was a woman in her mid 40's who suffered from adrenal fatigue for many years. During our initial consult, Jackie told me that her symptoms of adrenal fatigue and migraines started almost 20 years ago. Upon examining her case history more closely, she realized her symptoms started within 2 months after a very painful and slow healing wisdom tooth extraction. Jackie was referred to an alternative minded dental surgeon who detected a chronic but subtle infection at the site of the extraction. The dentist reopened the smoldering wound, cleaned the site and closed the wound. Within a month Jackie was a different person. Her adrenal fatigue and migraines were gone. Her life had taken a sudden leap forward and she never looked back. Tissue samples of the area revealed good cause for her suffering. Two different kinds of bacteria were growing in the old socket. Eliminating this body burden changed her life.

Intestinal Dysbiosis - An imbalance in the microorganisms of the intestines called intestinal dysbiosis is another common body burden. The healthy intestines normally contain over 400 different kinds of microorganisms, all living in a delicate balance within their own ecosystem. This balance can become disturbed and produce symptoms ranging from vague and mild intestinal upsets to debilitating fatigue and intolerance to food and/or environmental substances. The use of antibiotics and other antimicrobial medications is frequently the immediate trigger for such imbalances. The antibiotics kill not only the disease causing bacteria, but also the good bacteria in your intestinal tract that are a necessary part of intestinal health. When the good bacteria are killed, harmful bacteria, fungi, yeast, and other ill doers have the opportunity to move in and take over. It is the abundance of these detrimental microorganisms growing out of proportion that creates the problem. A lack of vegetables, fruit, and fiber combined with an over abundance of fats, sugary products and refined foods in the diet of the industrialized nations have predisposed us to intestinal dysbiosis. This kind of diet creates an internal intestinal environment that favors the growth of harmful bacteria, fungi, mold, and occasionally parasites that are detrimental to the body. In such an environment, unwanted microorganisms such as Candida albicans become dominant in the intestines, overwhelming the friendly bacteria. This imbalance in the intestinal microorganism can exist for years, creating vague intestinal symptoms, but also many symptoms of adrenal fatigue, particularly mental depression, fatigue and foggy memory. Friendly bacteria are necessary and are responsible for breaking down bile from the gall bladder, metabolizing some food stuff, and manufacturing certain vitamins like vitamin K and some of the B vitamins (especially vitamin B12). They also help keep the pH of the bowel at the right level for continued growth of friendly bacteria.

Several special, relatively inexpensive urine, bowel, breath and blood tests detect intestinal dysbiosis. Usually these tests can determine both the microorganisms causing the problem, and the most effective natural and pharmaceutical treatments to eliminate them. There are an increasing number of alternative and main stream physicians who have become aware of this common problem. I have found the best way to find a doctor experienced in treating intestinal dysbiosis is to call and simply ask if the doctor has had training in treating intestinal dysbiosis. If you get a vague or indefinite response, keep looking for one that responds with an unequivocal "yes" to your question. If you cannot find a doctor in your area, there is now a significant amount of information on the Internet. Our website has some specific information on the diagnosis and treatment of this problem.

Lack of Fresh, Good Quality Food – The lack of good quality food in your diet is most definitely a major body burden. There is no vitamin pill that is an adequate substitute to provide all the building blocks from which your cells are made. Food is the beginning and the sustaining element of adrenal recovery. Without it your recovery will be slower or in complete, no matter what else you do.

Food Allergies and Sensitivities – One reason so much space in this book was devoted to food allergies and sensitivities is because they represent such a common, but unrecognized, body burden. I have seen people lose jobs, destroy relationships or sink into chronic poor health because of food sensitivities. Only after they came into my office and used my diagnostic protocol did they realize that the reasons for their bad temper, intolerance, anti-social tendencies, general malaise or health problems were due to food sensitivities and adrenal fatigue. Food allergies and sensitivities are easily treated and their remedy can result in dramatic improvement in adrenal function. However, subtle food allergies and sensitivities can be difficult to find unless you are willing to take the time and make the effort to really look. All the tools you need to do this are in Chapter 14.

Sub-acute or Chronic Sub-clinical Infections – A tip-off to the presence of sub-acute infections is that none of the therapies that should work are working. If this is true in your case, you will probably find a clue to the origins of the infection in your "Health History Timeline" around "the last time I felt well" entry. Over the years I have seen a variety of patients who were suffering from what are termed sub-acute or chronic sub-clinical infections. These are infections that remain below the point of causing overt illness but continually smolder and chronically pull down the health of their host. The appendix, tonsils, gall bladder, gums, teeth, intestinal tract and areas that are tender or remain tender after surgery (including dental surgery) are the most common foci of sub-acute infections. The blood picture sometimes shows a mildly elevated (11,000-15,000 cu.mm.) or decreased (< 3,000 cu.mm) number of white blood cells.

The following is a list of blood test results that may indicate the presence of a sub-acute or chronic sub-clinical infection (if they are present in repeated blood tests over several weeks or month). You can ask your doctor to have these tests run and, although they need to be interpreted by a knowledgeable physician, you can obtain your own copies of your results to look at yourself.
Increased or decreased white blood cell count
Mildly increased sedimentation rate (ESR)
Increased total serum globulin
Increased lymphocytes
Increased LDH isoenzyme #1

Decreased lymphocytes with neutrophils increased = chronic bacterial infection
Increased lymphocytes with neutrophils decreased = chronic viral infection

Incomplete Recovery from Anesthesia - I have had a number of patients come in for a consultation because they never felt the same again after having surgery, especially gall bladder surgery. Early in my practice, I discovered that the anesthetics used in surgery can be especially debilitating to some individuals. The liver seems to suffer the most in these sensitive people. In each case, I had the person do a liver cleanse and take large amounts of deodorized Kyolic garlic for 2 to 3 months. All fully recovered. Once the liver was attended to, they were on their way to a healthier life. Some of these patients had been functioning at "half mast" for more than ten years, but after only a few weeks of a simple treatment directed towards the cause of their problem, they were able to fully recover.

Lack of Sleep - Lack of sleep is a common sign of both low and high cortisol levels. It can be a significant body burden. In fact it ranks with diet and regular exercise as an essential component of a healthy life. Chronic lack of sleep is now regarded as a health hazard and has been associated with several health conditions. These include decreased immunity with increased susceptibility to infections, impaired glucose tolerance, and decreased morning cortisol levels that cause cravings for carbohydrates even when enough calories have been consumed. Lack of sleep can also increase circulating estrogen levels, upsetting the hormonal balance. This is in addition to the decreased alertness and concentration that most people experience when missing an inordinate amount of sleep. Lack of sleep can slow healing and prolong the period of recovery. The bottom line is that it is necessary to sleep an average of eight hours per day. Some of my patients have needed even more in the beginning phases of recovery. If you have difficulty sleeping, consult the section in Chapter 12 on sleep again.

"Sick Building" Syndrome - This term, coined a number of years ago, refers to buildings that make people sick due to characteristics of their construction. It may be the building materials, the lighting, the heating, the cooling or the ventilation, but what ever the cause, an inordinate number of people who live or work in the building become ill. These are often illnesses with rather nondescript or vague symptom pictures. Note the date your symptoms started and compare it to the date you moved into a building, began working in a new building, etc. If your symptoms began or increased within 6 months of being in a new environment, be suspicious of the building as a possible cause. If you discover that a number of people have also become ill, suspect sick building syndrome or a related cause. If you notice that you feel especially tired after being in a particular building, such as where you live or work, it may also be due to "sick building" syndrome. OSHA is aware of this phenomenon as are some unions. There are sometimes relatively simple and inexpensive solutions such as increasing the number of green plants in the work area, or placing negative ion generators either in the work area or in the ventilation system. The amount of fresh air or the number of times the exchange of air takes place per hour in the building can also be increased. But most of the time it is easier to leave if you are suffering from "sick building" syndrome than to go through the hassle and red tape of making the building "people friendly." Sometimes it is just not feasible. If you are also suffering from adrenal fatigue, the last thing you need is a new battle. Leave the sick building, get yourself well and then see what you can do about the building.

Living or Working in Toxic Fumes – If you are living or working in an area where you are breathing toxic fumes, this can be more than an unpleasant inconvenience. Buildings with poorly ventilated gas furnaces or stoves, paint or chemical fumes, carbon monoxide from auto exhaust, industrial pollution, petroleum plants, or pesticide and herbicide sprays are examples of toxic environments. These problems are not just found in the large cities. Part of the reason for the high cancer rates and other health problems in farmers is the number of toxic chemicals they expose themselves to in tending to their crops. If you find yourself in a toxic environment, leave the environment. The average business is too invested in saving money to do much to help clean up the air. Once again, save yourself first. After you are breathing fresh air and have recovered your health, then you will be in better shape to help change the air. If you think you have become ill by living or working in a toxic environment, seek the help of a clinical ecologist (a doctor who specializes in recovery from toxic substances). A good place to start is to contact the American Academy of Environmental Medicine (AAEM) (**www.aaem.com** or 316-684-5500).

Lack of Fresh Air – If you live or work in an environment that does not provide a continual source of fresh air, it will constantly pull your health down and keep you from full recovery. Increased ventilation, negative ion generators, ozone generators, increased turnover of air, opening windows, and placing green plants in the work place can greatly increase the quality of air. Stale air usually has decreased oxygen content. Everyone knows we need oxygen to live. The less oxygen you have, the less efficient are your body processes. Many of the reactions in the biochemical cascade of adrenal hormone production require a rich source of oxygen. It is now possible to obtain personal fresh air generators designed to sit on an office desk. These generators filter the air and inject it with ozone and negative ions, making the area around you much more pleasant to be in and furnishing better air for breathing. They are definitely worth getting, especially if you are in a poorly ventilated or polluted environment. But if possible, change where you work or live to somewhare that provides fresh air.

The Thyroid - Adrenal Connection - It has been known for over half a century that about 80% of those suffering from adrenal fatigue also have a number of symptoms of low thyroid. If your adrenal fatigue has a thyroid component, it is usually necessary to strengthen both the adrenals and the thyroid simultaneously for full recovery to take place.

The thyroid is another endocrine gland sensitive to the effects of stress. Unlike the adrenals that have many functions, the thyroid has one major function, to control the rate at which energy is produced in the individual cells of the body. However, getting your thyroid function tested has the same disadvantages as testing for adrenal function using blood tests; marginally low thyroid function does not show up on these standard tests. Compounding the problem, insurance companies have limited thyroid testing to only one test (the TSH) instead of allowing a wider range of thyroid blood tests that could give more information.

There are some observations, though, that you can make yourself to determine if your thyroid may be low. Although these are not precise or conclusive, I have found them valuable clinical indicators that make me suspect thyroid function to be lower than optimal. A list of these follows:

1) Your basal body temperature, taken before rising in the morning, is below 98.2°F (oral) or 97.2°F (underarm).

2) Your stamina or capacity does not improve with increased exercise. (Typically, as you exercise, your stamina and capacity increase with repeated exercise, even if you have adrenal fatigue).

3) At 9:30 PM you hit a wall and are ready for bed but there is no 11:00 PM second wind (as is often seen in pure adrenal fatigue).

4) Reaction time is slightly slower than you know it should be when you are driving a car, engaging in sports or operating equipment.

5) You gain weight easily, especially around your hips and thighs, even when eating the right foods in normal portions.

6) The outside of your eyebrows are much thinner than normal.

7) You feel sluggish and not fully awake much of the day. (Those with pure adrenal fatigue usually feel awake by 10:00AM, or if not by 10:00AM, after the noon meal.)

8) Your energy does not noticeably improve after your evening meal or after 6:00PM.

If approximately half of the above indicators are present, then you may have a low thyroid component to your adrenal fatigue. If so, there are several possible solutions. Both your adrenals and thyroid are ultimately regulated in similar ways by a gland called the hypothalamus (see Chapter 22 for the relationship of the adrenals to the hypothalamus). Taking a hypothalamus extract may help normalize your thyroid as well as your adrenal function when they need a little fine-tuning. Sometimes your thyroid only requires the addition of a nutritional supplement containing the proper nutrients in a form that can be easily absorbed and utilized efficiently by the thyroid. This usually allows the thyroid to rebound in 2-3 months. Check the website for suggestions on natural thyroid supplements.

Note that both of these glands are very sensitive to and easily undermined by body burdens. If low thyroid seems to be a factor in your adrenal fatigue, check for body burdens again before doing anything else.

The above are only some of the body burdens that can continually compromise your health without your knowledge. Once again, the key to determining underlying body burdens is to look at your "Health History Time Line". Note any things that occurred within a few months of the onset of your adrenal fatigue. Once the body burden is discovered, find a way to limit or remove it. Just because they are sometimes difficult to isolate or treat, does not mean they are not important. The real detective never gives up until the crime is resolved.

Chapter 20

The Road to Recovery

What to Expect

The process of healing from a lingering health problem is like a journey down the road of recovery. It presents many challenges for each person who embarks on it, but outweighing the challenges is the wonderful reward of discovering how much power you have to affect how you feel, physically as well as emotionally and mentally. This is especially exciting if you have been living with the sense of frustration and helplessness that plagues most people with adrenal fatigue. Often after reading self help books such as this, people start out doing the program with enthusiasm. Then, as soon as they come across a few frustrations or setbacks, they quit and go on to something else, some other "quick fix." I cannot emphasize enough how critical it is that you see the program all the way through to recovery, reassessing yourself occasionally so that you can adjust and continue. My 24 years of clinical experience as an alternative physician have brought me many very ill patients. With rare exception, when recovering from a long illness there are setbacks, frustrations, and periods of discouragement (see illustration - "Road to Recovery").

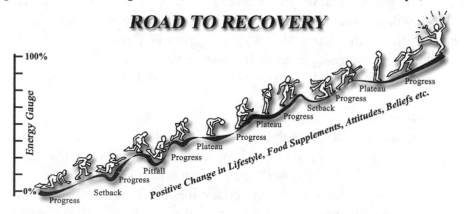

This by no means indicates that therapy is not working or that you are not progressing. In most instances, nothing could be further from the truth. It is simply a setback. Getting well is very much like the adage, two steps forward and one step back. The step backwards can be as valuable as the step forward. Therefore, as you go into this program, it is important to keep perspective and realize that there will be setbacks, there will be delays and there will be disappointments, but there will also be progress. The progress will outweigh the setbacks and will be well worth the effort.

Frustration and Discouragement in Adrenal Fatigue

It is especially important to re-iterate this point to you because frustration and discouragement are experienced intimately by most people suffering from adrenal fatigue. When you start on the road to recovery and have a setback, you may become discouraged and frustrated even more easily than someone recovering from a different illness because frustration and discouragement are part of the adrenal fatigue syndrome itself. But do not give up! Even when things are not going like they should and you have tried everything, do not despair. Often, it is the next thing you do, or sometimes it is just the amount of time needed for the program to work. If you keep trying, there is hope. If you give up and quit doing the things that make you better, you can be sure your chances of healing are slim to none. So the first and last rule of this program is never give up.

How Long Will This Take?

No restorative therapy can work unless you stick to it long enough to see if it is going to be effective. For example, adrenal recovery will take at least three months, and may take up to two years. That does not mean that you will not see any improvement in that time. Some people start feeling better in the first week, especially if they dramatically improve their diet or make changes in their lifestyle that greatly reduce stress. But typically you should not expect changes before at least three weeks.

Keep a Journal

The changes often come so subtly that they are not always recognized, so I advise patients to keep journals in which they jot down notes daily about how they are feeling, what they are able to do, and their general overall symptoms. On days when you are feeling discouraged, you can go back to the early journal entries and note that you have made progress even though it does not feel that way at the moment. As you get better you will find that you are able to do and complete more things, your frame of mind is improving, generally things are going more smoothly in your life (see illustration –"Recovery from Adrenal Fatigue"), and you are better able to handle the rocky times. Like the illustration shows, you will begin to trade the heavy lead ball that holds you back for the things that lift you up. You will even have happy days or nearly happy days, replacing all those bleak ones that came before. Note the happy days in your journal. They will serve as landmarks and as inspiration on other days when you need encouragement.

RECOVERY FROM ADRENAL FATIGUE

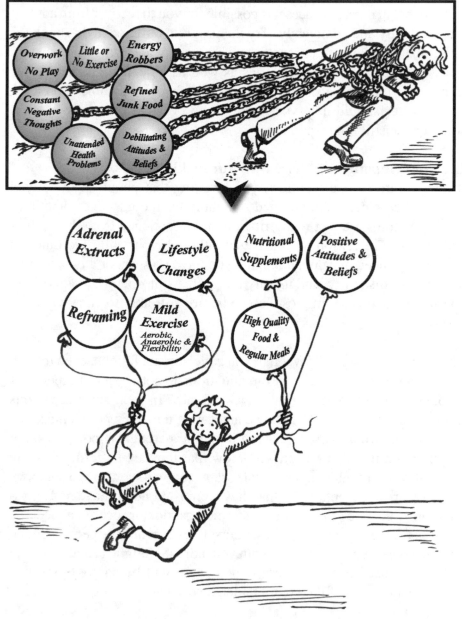

Most health problems can be overcome with natural therapies. With the right natural therapy there can actually be cure, not just symptomatic relief or temporarily feeling better. I once had a nurse who came to work in my office after being employed for many years in a typical medical office. During her 90-day review, I asked her if she liked working in my clinic and she responded with enthusiasm that she did. When I asked her why she quickly replied, "Because people actually get well here!" Be assured that in most instances it is possible for you to recover from adrenal fatigue totally and completely. Try the program outlined in this book for three months. If after three months you have not made significant progress as assessed by your journal entries as well as objective and subjective signs and symptoms, go back to the previous chapter "Trouble-shooting." This chapter should help you uncover the possible reasons why your adrenals are still not responding.

Lack of Sympathy for Those with Adrenal Fatigue
It may comfort (or discomfort) you to know that people with adrenal fatigue often receive only limited sympathy from others and sometimes their symptoms are met with irritation and impatience from themselves and others. The reason for this is that although your ability to function has been reduced by adrenal fatigue, you have no scars or any other visible sign of disability, and usually no lab tests or doctor's diagnosis to confirm your illness. In most cases you are still able to carry on some sort of life.

Therefore, once you discover that you have adrenal fatigue, even though the diagnosis gives you a sense of validation, do not expect a tremendous amount of understanding from other people. In fact, several patients have commented to me that they cannot wait until this book comes out because they want to give a copy of it to their parents or spouse or other loved one so that that person will know that they are suffering from an actual illness. In other cases, people want a copy to confirm to someone that they are not mentally ill, that they were right not to have had a hysterectomy or some other therapy their medical doctor recommended as a solution for their symptoms. Trust yourself, even when the people around you do not see what is going on with you, adrenal fatigue is real and what you experienced is real. These same people will be happy to see you getting better, even if they don't understand what is wrong.

As you improve you may hear comments about looking better, being more pleasant to be around, or other compliments. After several months, people you have not seen for a long time may remark on how different you seem. Take these comments as favorable indicators that your program is working and that you are indeed recovering.

Reclaiming Your Life

The road to recovery needs constant fine-tuning. As you improve, new health problems may be uncovered, and as you resolve those, a greater level of health overall will be achieved, specifically adrenal health. It requires a general vigilance and awareness about yourself, your responses to things, your growing awareness of attitudes and beliefs that limit your recovery, your improved lifestyle and your conviction to stay on the road to recovery. Writing these observations in a journal works well because sometimes such insights are fleeting even when they seem unforgettably obvious at the moment. If you write them down as you experience them, not only will they will be available to you at a later date but you may gain a clearer understanding of their significance and their place in your own personal health puzzle.

Although regaining your health and vitality is very important and re-quires considerable commitment and persistence on your part, do not to wrap your entire life up into getting well. This creates a compulsiveness that is not usually conducive to restoring health. It causes you to be driven by the effort to get well which then becomes just another source of stress draining your adrenals. Simply work out your program, do your program consistently with awareness, and live your life day by day. Each day is a new opportunity to be kind to yourself and your body.

Suffice it to say that the road to recovery is one that each person must take by themselves and for themselves. It is one of the best, most educa-tional, revealing and rewarding roads you will ever travel as your level of health increases. So do not be discouraged by temporary setbacks, there are always some of those along the way. Be encouraged instead by the possibility you now hold in your hands of truly recovering and feel-ing well for perhaps the first time in a long time. Every step you take along this road is a step closer to reclaiming your life and soon you will be able to enjoy the benefits of bathing in the "Fountain of Recovery."

FOUNTAIN OF RECOVERY

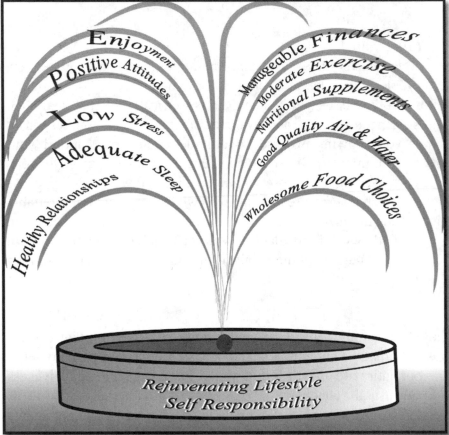

Chapter 21

Questions and Answers

This chapter is a series of questions and answers related to adrenal fatigue. It is meant as a review, and as a way of answering questions that may not have seen obvious to you when reading the other chapters. Hopefully, this chapter will fill in gaps in your understanding and answer most of your questions about adrenal fatigue.

What is adrenal fatigue?

Adrenal fatigue is any decrease (but not failure) in the ability of the adrenal glands to carry out their normal functions. The chief symptom of adrenal fatigue is, indeed, fatigue, but is accompanied by many other signs and symptoms. Adrenal fatigue occurs when stress from any source (physical, emotional, mental, or environmental) exceeds, either cumulatively or in intensity, the body's capacity to adjust appropriately to the demands placed upon it by the stress. When this happens, the adrenals become fatigued and are unable to continue responding adequately to further stress.

Who suffers adrenal fatigue?

Anyone, from birth to old age and from any race or culture, can suffer from adrenal fatigue. People vary greatly in their ability to respond to and withstand stress. However, those suffering from serious or repeated injury, illness, infectious disease, allergies, inadequate nutrition, intense social, emotional or physical pressures, or who are exposed to a toxic environment are most likely to suffer from adrenal fatigue. Unfortunately many of these factors are common in modern life.

What causes adrenal fatigue?

There are multitudes of individual causes of adrenal fatigue but they usually stem from one of four common sources that overwhelm the body.
  1) disease states such as severe or recurrent pneumonia, bronchitis or flu, cancer, AIDS, auto-immune and other illnesses

2) physical stress such as surgery, poor nutrition, addiction, injury, exhaustion, etc.
3) emotional stress, usually arising from relationship, work or psychological origins
4) continual and/or severe environmental stress from toxic chemicals and pollutants in the air, water, clothing or food

Where are the adrenal glands?
The adrenal glands are two small glands, each about the size of a large grape, which sits over the kidneys. They are located in the back, near the bottom of the ribs on each side of the spine.

Is adrenal fatigue common?
Yes, adrenal fatigue is a common disorder, estimated to affect many millions of people in the United States and other industrialized nations.

Once I have adrenal fatigue, can I ever recover?
Yes, with proper treatment, most people can fully recover from adrenal fatigue.

Can children suffer from adrenal fatigue?
Yes, especially children born to parents suffering from adrenal fatigue themselves. These children are often more sickly, have less ability to handle stressful situations, and take longer to recover from illnesses.

Is adrenal fatigue common in someone with cancer who is going through chemotherapy?
Yes, the extreme fatigue of this and any other chronic illness is often the result of decreased adrenal function. Chronic illness and toxic treatments like chemotherapy are both large stressors for the body and the adrenals are intimately involved in trying to balance these stresses.

Does adrenal fatigue affect the thyroid gland?
Yes. Approximately 80% of the people suffering from adrenal fatigue also suffer some form of decreased thyroid function. Often people who are shown to be low thyroid and are unresponsive to thyroid therapy are suffering from adrenal fatigue as well. For these people to get well, the adrenals must be supported in addition to the thyroid.

Am I more prone to infections if I have adrenal fatigue?

Yes. Adrenal fatigue often goes hand in hand with decreased immune function, which makes someone more prone to illnesses. There is a special association between adrenal fatigue and respiratory infections, such as bronchitis and pneumonia.

My ankles swell after a long hard day on my feet. Is this due to adrenal fatigue?

There are many causes of ankle swelling, but one of the causes is adrenal fatigue. Your ankle swelling is more likely related to it if you have many other signs of adrenal fatigue.

Does anyone ever go through life without adrenal fatigue or adrenal fatigue problems?

Yes. Many people go through life with only a temporary decrease in adrenal function after an infection, the death of a loved one, loss of a job or other severe stress, but their adrenals are able to bounce back and they recover. Someone with adrenal fatigue is overwhelmed and is very slow to recover from these same kinds of problems.

I'm highly allergic now but didn't used to be, is this change due to adrenal fatigue?

It has been long observed that people suffering from adrenal fatigue have a definite increase in allergic responses or become allergic to things that previously did not bother them. This is because cortisol, the major adrenal hormone, is the most powerful anti-inflammatory substance in the body. When the adrenals fatigue, cortisol levels drop and make it more likely that the body will have allergic (inflammatory) reactions and that these reactions will be more severe.

What is the difference between adrenal fatigue and hypoadrenia?

Hypoadrenia, as it is used in a medical sense, refers to adrenal failure or the extremely low adrenal function which is called Addison's disease. Although hypoadrenia, in actuality, occurs in a spectrum ranging from almost normal to Addison's, only the most extreme low end is recognized and called hypoadrenia in medicine. The less severe forms of hypoadrenia are referred to as adrenal fatigue.

Are there laboratory tests that detect adrenal fatigue?
Yes. The most accurate and valuable test for detecting adrenal fatigue is
a saliva adrenal hormone test. This is a simple and relatively inexpensive test and has been unavailable until recently. There are other lab
tests but they need special interpretation by physicians trained to recognize and treat adrenal fatigue.

Is age a factor?
Any age can suffer from adrenal fatigue but both the very young and very
old are more vulnerable to stress and therefore to adrenal fatigue.

How often can I have a bout of adrenal fatigue?
It varies with the person. Some people have only one episode of adrenal
fatigue during their lifetime, some have several, and others experience
chronic adrenal fatigue from which they never fully recover. The most
common ways in which adrenal fatigue develops are described in the
section on "Human Response Patterns to Stress" in Chapter 23.

Can adrenal fatigue become chronic?
Yes, in some people the adrenal glands do not return to normal levels of
function without help, either because the stress was too great or too prolonged, or because their general health is poor. However, when adrenal
fatigue becomes chronic it is almost always because of factors that can
be changed. That is why I wrote this book, to provide the knowledge
people need to recover from adrenal fatigue.

How can I keep my adrenal glands healthy?
The guidelines for keeping your adrenal glands healthy are very similar
to the overall principles of good health. A moderate lifestyle with high
quality food, regular exercise and adequate rest, along with a healthy
mental attitude to the stresses of life go a long way towards keeping your
adrenal glands strong and resilient. However, because modern life is so
stressful, certain nutritional supplements are also important to both maintaining healthy adrenal glands and helping depleted adrenal glands recover. These supplements, which are listed in Chapter 15, can be taken
individually, but it makes more sense to simply take a nutritional supple-

ment designed specifically for the adrenals that combines all the necessary nutrients. Sources for these nutritional supplements are listed on our website.

Can adrenal fatigue affect my sex life?

Yes. A common complaint from people suffering from adrenal fatigue is decreased sex drive. This is because some of the sex hormones are manufactured in the adrenal glands, as well as in the sex organs themselves. Low adrenal function can lead to low performance or low desire. Both usually return to normal as the adrenals recover.

How do doctors diagnose adrenal fatigue?

Most medical doctors are not aware of adrenal fatigue or the syndrome. They only recognize Addison's disease, which is the most extreme end of low adrenal function. Astute doctors who are familiar with the varying degrees of decreased adrenal function usually test the adrenal hormone levels in the saliva. This is an accurate and useful indicator of adrenal fatigue. There are other common lab tests that can be used more indirectly to detect adrenal fatigue, but the majority of medical doctors are unaware of how to interpret these tests for indications of adrenal fatigue. Many doctors who are aware of adrenal fatigue syndrome use some form of questionnaire to help make their diagnosis.

Can I pass the tendency of adrenal fatigue genetically to my children?

It is not known if there is an actual genetic predisposition to adrenal fatigue. However if one or both parents suffer from adrenal fatigue, either chronically or during the time of conception, and if the mother has adrenal fatigue during gestation, there is a greater than 50% chance that their children will also suffer from adrenal fatigue. This may be seen as a child with a weak constitution, early allergies, a propensity towards lung infections, and a decreased ability to handle stress who takes longer to recover after illness. Although these children will never have exceptionally strong adrenal glands, much can be done to help them recover by the use of adrenal extracts and other remedies given in this book.

Is adrenal fatigue related to fibromyalgia or clinical depression?

Yes, adrenal fatigue can be related to both. Most people who suffer from fibromyalgia have a form of adrenal fatigue. Sometimes the adrenal fatigue comes before the fibromyalgia. A mild depression is also a chief sign of adrenal fatigue and although there are other conditions that cause clinical depression, if clinical depression is present, a saliva test for adrenal hormones will determine whether the adrenals are involved.

Is adrenal fatigue related to chronic fatigue syndrome?

Yes, adrenal fatigue is a common, but usually unrecognized, component of chronic fatigue syndrome (CFS). The most likely connection between them is that the infectious agent(s) that lead to the development of CFS also set up conditions that foster adrenal fatigue. The direct effects of a smoldering pathogen in the body as well as the systematic stress the infection creates put the adrenals on overload. With new diagnostic procedures available for detecting the specific infectious agent(s) responsible, there have been encouraging results using a combination treatment that eliminates the specific pathogen(s) while strengthening the adrenals.

Is adrenal fatigue involved in people with HIV or Hepatitis C?

Yes, adrenal fatigue is a common factor in people with Hepatitis C and HIV. Unfortunately one of the treatments for Hepatitis C is the administration of corticosteroid drugs. This suppresses both the adrenals and the immune system, and causes a more rapid death. With HIV, a relationship between survival and cortisol levels has been shown.

Will I need prescription drugs to treat adrenal fatigue?

Most cases of adrenal fatigue can be remedied without prescription drugs. The treatments given in this book are natural, inexpensive and effective, and most have been used by many aware physicians to help people recover from adrenal fatigue. The most severe cases may need prescription drugs in the treatment.

My doctor says there is no such illness as adrenal fatigue. What should I do?

Unfortunately, this is the view of many conventional doctors, but they are not as well informed as they believe. Adrenal fatigue was first diagnosed over 100 years ago and has been successfully treated for decades. However, for various reasons that largely have to do with the close association between medicine and the pharmaceutical industry, the medical community has ignored the existence of adrenal fatigue syndrome over the past 40 years. The best thing to do is to switch to a doctor who is familiar with adrenal fatigue syndrome. If you want to keep the same doctor, give him/her a copy of this book, but do not get your hopes up about him/her having a change of position.

My doctor has never heard of adrenal fatigue. How do I convince him/her that I might have it?
Unless your doctor is more open than most, you probably will not convince him or her that you have adrenal fatigue. My only suggestion is to give your doctor a copy of this book. The other solution is to wait ten years. By then most doctors will probably have heard of it, and hopefully many more will know how to recognize and treat it.

Does smoking increase my chances of adrenal fatigue?
Yes. Anytime you place a stress such as smoking on your body, it is more difficult for your adrenals to function. Smoking by itself does not lead directly to adrenal fatigue, unless the adrenals are already weak. However, smoking is one of the body burdens that accelerate adrenal fatigue and keep complete recovery from occurring.

Do athletes or very fit people have the same risk as the rest of us of developing adrenal fatigue?
Athletes and very fit people can also suffer from adrenal fatigue under certain circumstances. If they push themselves too hard, skip meals, take drugs (e.g. steroids), and have a lifestyle that is otherwise not conducive to their health, they can lead themselves into adrenal fatigue, the same as anyone else. Relentlessly pushing themselves, as some athletes do, is also a significant risk factor. Also, severe injuries, illnesses and emotional stresses can debilitate the adrenal glands of athletes the same as they can in other people. Just because someone is an athlete does not necessarily mean they are in excellent health. The better overall health someone has, the less they will experience adrenal fatigue.

Does diet have anything to do with adrenal fatigue?

Yes. Diet has a lot to do with adrenal fatigue, both in its cause and in its recovery. The phrase "garbage in, garbage out" aptly describes the relationship between what we eat and adrenal fatigue. If we eat garbage, our bodies eventually become trashed and one of the common results is adrenal fatigue.

I am disabled and cannot exercise. Will that make my chances of getting adrenal fatigue even higher?

Not necessarily. There are a variety of factors in addition to exercise that influence your adrenal resiliency. It all depends on how many things you stack in favor for your own health. Read the chapters in Part III of this book, "Helping Yourself Back to Health" and use this information to do all that you can to make your adrenals strong. This will allow you to maximize your adrenal strength.

Are Americans more prone to adrenal fatigue than people from other nations?

Despite a relative abundance of resources, Americans have increased their likelihood of suffering from adrenal fatigue because of their hectic lifestyle, poor food choices, lack of exercise, and drug, alcohol and caffeine consumption. People of less wealthy nations may be subject to other factors that are individually worse than those Americans experience, but their overall lifestyle and social structure help counterbalance these.

Does adrenal fatigue affect a woman's menstrual cycles?

Yes, adrenal fatigue can affect menstrual cycles. PMS, altered menstrual flow and difficult menopause can definitely be related to adrenal fatigue.

Does pregnancy set off adrenal fatigue?

No, usually pregnancy helps adrenal fatigue because the fetus produces a greater amount of natural adrenal hormones than the amount in the non-pregnant female. However, if the pregnancy is very stressful, it can lead to or increase adrenal fatigue.

If I already have adrenal fatigue, how likely am I to get worse or to even acquire Addison's disease?

The answer to this question largely depends upon you. The more things in this book you do to recover, the less likely you are to go down that path. Approximately 70% of cases of Addison's disease are actually an auto-immune disease, but the rest (about 30%) are precipitated by things that happen in people's lives. Your lifestyle, food choices, exercise patterns, attitudes and how you teach yourself to respond to stress all have a tremendous impact on whether you recover from adrenal fatigue or continue to progress downhill.

Are there any precautions I need to take before surgery to protect my adrenal glands?

Yes. Increase your intake of magnesium, pantothenic acid and ascorbic acid with bioflavinoids according to the directions in Chapter 15. Eat only high quality foods, especially good quality proteins and lots of dark green vegetables. Use self-hypnosis, visualization and/or relaxation methods to prepare yourself mentally and emotionally to remain calm and positive throughout the procedure to heal more quickly afterwards.

What can I do to prevent adrenal fatigue?

Read Part III of this book, "Helping Yourself Back to Health" and faithfully follow the instructions. Whenever you get sick, dramatically increase your intake of vitamin C, bioflavinoids, magnesium and pantothenic acid. Better yet, use a customized formula for adrenal fatigue such as those listed on the website. Often tonics are valuable, especially the herbal formulas for adrenal fatigue. Adrenal cell extract, by itself or as part of a formula, is also very beneficial. After you have an illness, do not try to hit the floor running, Instead take an extra day off work in order to rejuvenate. If you are still tired after an illness, emotional shock or other event that produces adrenal fatigue, sleep in late, be especially conscious of eating high quality foods, and avoid caffeine and alcohol. In addition, saunas can be great for detoxifying and unwinding, thus lessening the stress load on your adrenals.

The next section, "Part IV – Functions of the Adrenal Glands," contains some very interesting and important information that you may not find anywhere else. If you would like to understand why and how your adrenal glands are so vital to your physical and psychological well-being.

Part Four

Functions of the Adrenal Glands

In Part IV we will briefly look at the major functions of the adrenal glands and how these are related to adrenal fatigue. Physiology is the study of function and so a large part of this section has to do with the physiological processes connected with adrenal function. To me, this is one of the most exciting sections of the book and anyone who loves to understand how things work should find it fascinating.

In the pages that follow, I have tried to present a brief overview that will give you an overall understanding of the workings of the adrenals as they relate to adrenal fatigue, while avoiding most of the technical words and more complex interactions. This part is designed to be read from front to back, but if you want only specific information about a particular hormone or process, most of the sections can be read independently of the others.

Even this cursory glimpse at the incredible balancing act your system maintains moment by moment should give you an appreciation and new respect for your own body. So get ready to jump into the anatomy and physiology of the adrenals and be amazed at what your body is doing for you every minute of every day.

Chapter 22

Anatomy and Physiology of the Adrenal Glands

Anatomy of the Adrenal Glands
Location

The adrenal glands sit on top of the kidneys near the spine, just underneath the last (twelfth) rib and extending down about an inch. The right adrenal is shaped something like a pyramid, whereas the left is shaped more like a half moon. Each is only about 1" high by 1¼" to 2" wide by ¼" thick, and weighs just 3½ to 5 grams (about 1/8 to 1/4 ounce), with the male's adrenals usually being slightly larger and heavier than the female's (see illustration "Location of the Adrenal Glands").

LOCATION OF THE ADRENAL GLANDS

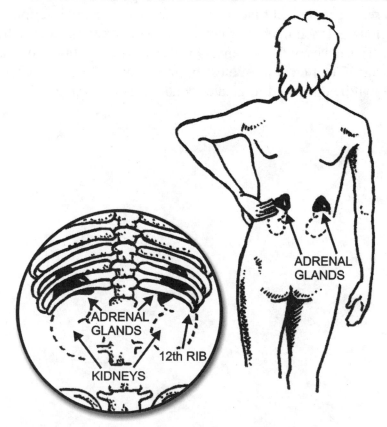

Both adrenal glands are only a very short distance from the aorta, the major artery of the body, and the vena cava, the major vein. This strategic placement allows for a very rapid adrenal response to hormonal messages transported via the blood. For example, Adrenal Corticotrophic Hormone (ACTH) is a hormone messenger from the pituitary gland that tells the adrenal glands how much cortisol to secrete. Within a few seconds of receiving this message the correct level of cortisol is on its way from the adrenals to the rest of the body. In the tremendous wisdom of the body, the adrenals are also placed in close proximity to the liver, pancreas, major fat storage areas and the kidneys, as these are the organs that need rapid communication with the adrenals in situations requiring their immediate response to adrenal hormones.

Regions of the Adrenal Glands
Each adrenal gland is composed of a medulla (inner part) and a cortex (outer part). The cortex consists of three or possibly four zones. The medulla and each of the zones in the cortex each produce different hormones that serve a variety of functions in your body. A brief description of these regions and their major hormones follows and can be seen in the illustration "Hormones of the Adrenal Glands and Their Actions" on the following page. The functions of these hormones as they relate to adrenal fatigue will be discussed in greater detail in the "Physiology" section.

HORMONES OF THE ADRENAL GLANDS AND THEIR ACTIONS

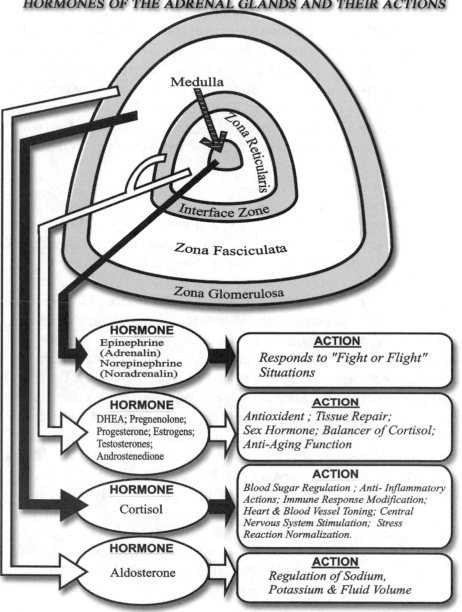

The Adrenal Medulla

The medulla produces the adrenal hormones, epinephrine (adrenaline) and norepinephrine (noradrenalin). Epinephrine and norepinephrine are important mainly in crisis situations. During a crisis, they work together to dilate bronchi (air passages of the lungs) and blood vessels to the muscles, increase heart beats and strength of contraction, and cause other physiological changes to help the body respond to the stressful situation via "fight or flight." These adrenal hormones are responsible for the superhuman efforts such as the lifting of a car by a small woman that occasionally occur during a crisis. The medulla is involved in extreme stress and, within this context, epinephrine and norepinephrine both work with cortisol from the adrenal cortex. It is the cortex that is the main concern of this book.

The Adrenal Cortex

Most of the ongoing daily regulation and modification of bodily processes arises from the adrenal cortex. The adrenal cortex is divided into three or possibly four zones which each secrete different hormones that carry out specific functions throughout your body. 1) The outermost zone is the *zona glomerulosa* from which the hormone *aldosterone* is secreted. 2) The next zone is the *zona fasciculata* in which *cortisol* is produced. 3) The innermost zone is the *zona reticularis* where progesterone, *DHEA-S* and *DHEA* are produced. In humans and other primates, between the zona fasciculata and the zona reticularis, there is a narrow space called the *interface zone*. Although the zona reticularis has traditionally been thought to produce the *sex hormones* such as the estrogens and testosterones, it has recently been proposed that this interface zone is the actual site of production of most of the sex hormones (Roberts, '99). Because most adrenal research uses rodents (mice and rats) and other non-primate mammals, little attention has been paid to this interface zone until recently. These three (or four) zones of your adrenal cortex collectively produce over fifty hormones. Most of these are intermediary hormones that only act as bridges to form other adrenal hormones. However, about a dozen hormones end up in your circulation and actively affect the rest of your body.

Zona Glomerulosa and Aldosterone - The zona glomerulosa secretes the hormone aldosterone. Aldosterone is the major hormone controlling the sodium and potassium levels, and thus the fluid balance, within your bloodstream, cells and interstitial fluids (the area between the cells). The connection between aldosterone levels and symptoms of adrenal fatigue will be covered in the section "Adrenal Fatigue and the Cravings for Salt."

Zona Fasciculata and Cortisol - The zona fasciculata secretes cortisol. It is by far, the largest part of the adrenal cortex. Cortisol controls or greatly influences the metabolism of fats, proteins and carbohydrates to maintain blood glucose within a narrow optimal range and keep it there even under stressful conditions. Cortisol also has many other important functions, as we will see in the "Physiology" sections related to cortisol in this and the following chapter.

Zona Reticularis and the Sex Hormones and Their Precursors - Although the sex hormones are made primarily by the gonads (ovaries and testes), the adrenal zona reticularis manufactures an ancillary portion of sex hormones for each sex and also produces male hormones in women and female hormones in men to keep the effects of the dominant sex hormones in balance. DHEA and its relatively inactive precursor, DHEA-S, are two other major hormones that are manufactured and secreted by the zona reticularis. Nearly all of the DHEA-S in circulation is manufactured by the adrenals, which is why DHEA-S blood or saliva levels are excellent indicators of adrenal function. The functions of these hormones as they relate to adrenal fatigue will be covered in the Physiology section of this chapter.

Physiology of the Adrenal Glands

The Regulation of Cortisol

Although cortisol is secreted by the zona fasciculata in the adrenal glands, it is regulated primarily from the brain. Cortisol is responsible for many of the life sustaining functions attributed to the adrenal glands.

The HPA Axis - The amount of cortisol circulating at any particular moment is regulated by a complex interaction between the hypothalamus (a regulatory part of the brain), the pituitary gland at the base of the brain, and the adrenal glands. This regulatory trio operates through a negative feedback system and is referred to as the Hypothalamus/ Pituitary/Adrenal (HPA) Axis or HPA System [see illustration "Hypothalamus – Pituitary – Adrenal (HPA) Axis"].

HYPOTHALAMUS - PITUITARY - ADRENAL (HPA) AXIS

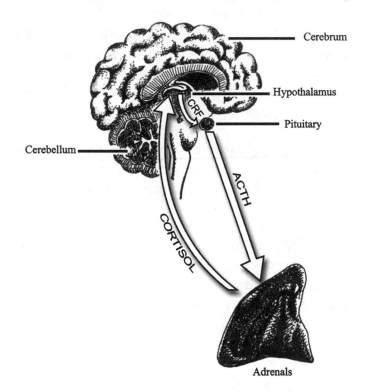

Cerebrum

Hypothalamus

Pituitary

Cerebellum

CRF

ACTH

CORTISOL

Adrenals

The HPA Axis is the primary regulator of Blood Cortisol Levels

A negative feedback system works like the thermostat in a house or apartment. The thermostat senses the heat in the room and compares it with the desired temperature it has been set to. When the heat gets too low, the thermostat signals the relay switch to tell the furnace to ignite, sending out hot air into the room and raising the heat. When the heat has risen to the desired level, the thermostat signals the furnace to quit until more heat is needed. This cycle is called a negative feedback system because when enough heat is released, a negative signal is sent to slow or stop the input.

In your body, your hypothalamus is analogous to the thermostat, your pituitary to the relay switch, your adrenals to the furnace, and your body to the room (see illustration "The Regulation of Cortisol"). The amount of cortisol released is comparable to the heat released from the furnace. To a large extent you control the thermostat through the demands you place on your body. These demands arise from the physical situations your body has to deal with (diet, exercise, work, climate, etc.) and your reactions (emotional and physiological) to them. This negative feedback system is described below in the language of physiology.

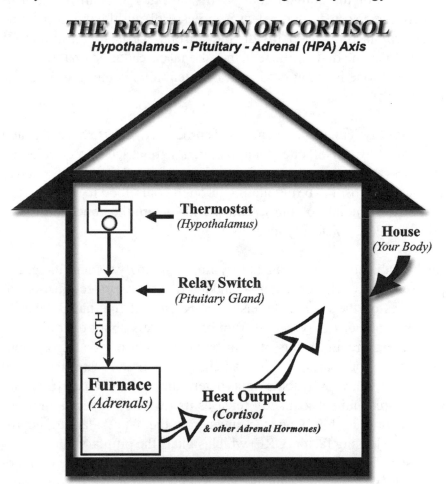

THE REGULATION OF CORTISOL
Hypothalamus - Pituitary - Adrenal (HPA) Axis

Thermostat
(Hypothalamus)

House
(Your Body)

Relay Switch
(Pituitary Gland)

ACTH

Furnace
(Adrenals)

Heat Output
(Cortisol
& other Adrenal Hormones)

The physiology of cortisol regulation - The HPA Axis is one of the most important elements of the whole body process known as homeostasis, the process that maintains a steady internal biochemical and physiological balance in your body. The HPA Axis adjusts cortisol levels according to the needs of the body, under normal and stressed conditions, via a hormone called the Adrenal Corticotrophic Hormone (ACTH). ACTH is secreted from the pituitary gland in response to orders from the hypothalamus and travels in the bloodstream to the adrenal cortex. There it activates cells in all three (or four) zones to produce their various hormones (see previous illustration - "Hormones of the Adrenal Cortex and Their Actions"). Each zone generates different hormones as end products, but the process of making all hormones in all zones begins with ACTH binding to the walls of the adrenal cells. This initiates a chain reaction of intracellular enzymes that release cholesterol within the cell. The cholesterol is then used inside the adrenal cells to manufacture pregnenolone, the first hormone in the adrenal cascade. No matter which adrenal hormone is being produced, pregnenolone is the first hormone formed in the series.

In the zona fasciculata, pregnenolone is processed to form cortisone and then cortisol. Cortisol, once manufactured, is released into circulation. It takes less than a minute after the initial stimulation by ACTH for newly synthesized cortisol to be circulating through your blood to every part of your body, including to your hypothalamus where the concentration of cortisol is being constantly measured.

Your hypothalamus, in its regulatory function, analyzes and integrates input from many different external and internal sources (see illustration- "Influences on the Hypothalamus - The Keeper of Internal Balance"). This input includes information from brain centers about overall excit- ability, energy requirements of your body, and sensory data from your brain centers for hearing, seeing, smelling, touch and taste. Based on this information, your hypothalamus determines how much cortisol your body requires and subsequently releases its own hormones as messen- gers. The primary hormone messenger from the hypothalamus is corti- cotrophin releasing factor (CRF) which signals the pituitary gland to se- crete a specific amount of ACTH. Thus ACTH is sent from the pituitary to your adrenal glands to begin the process described above all over again. Alterations in ACTH levels, and hence cortisol levels, are made minute by minute using this negative feedback loop, modulated by other infor- mation received by the hypothalamus as shown in the illustration.

INFLUENCES ON THE HYPOTHALAMUS
THE KEEPER OF INTERNAL BALANCE

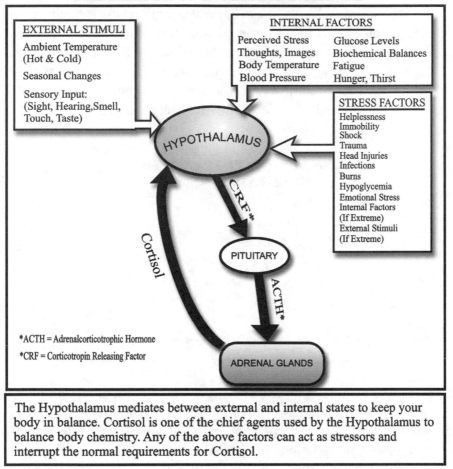

EXTERNAL STIMULI

Ambient Temperature
(Hot & Cold)

Seasonal Changes

Sensory Input:
(Sight, Hearing, Smell,
Touch, Taste)

INTERNAL FACTORS

Perceived Stress   Glucose Levels
Thoughts, Images   Biochemical Balances
Body Temperature   Fatigue
Blood Pressure   Hunger, Thirst

STRESS FACTORS

Helplessness
Immobility
Shock
Trauma
Head Injuries
Infections
Burns
Hypoglycemia
Emotional Stress
Internal Factors
(If Extreme)
External Stimuli
(If Extreme)

HYPOTHALAMUS

CRF*

Cortisol

PITUITARY

ACTH*

*ACTH = Adrenalcorticotrophic Hormone

*CRF = Corticotropin Releasing Factor

ADRENAL GLANDS

The Hypothalamus mediates between external and internal states to keep your body in balance. Cortisol is one of the chief agents used by the Hypothalamus to balance body chemistry. Any of the above factors can act as stressors and interrupt the normal requirements for Cortisol.

The Circadian Rhythm of Cortisol - Cortisol, ACTH and aldosterone are not secreted uniformly throughout the day, but rather follow a diurnal pattern with the highest levels secreted at approximately 8:00 AM and the lowest between midnight and 4:00 AM. As a matter of fact, it is the rising cortisol level that helps us wake up in the morning. After its peak at approximately 8:00 AM, it downtrends through the rest of the day, often with a small dip in the afternoon between 3:00 and 5:00 PM. This curve of cortisol secretion however, is not a nice smooth curve, but is filled with episodic spikes that generally fit into an increasing and a decreasing pattern throughout the day and evening. Eating something, even a little snack, causes a small burst in cortisol levels. This is shown in the illustration "Circadian Rhythm of Cortisol," where the episodic spikes have been averaged to give a more understanding picture of this daily cycle of cortisol levels. Note in the illustration how regular snacks and meals keep cortisol at higher levels for more of the day compared to people who do not snack. This is another reason to have regular snacks in addition to regular meals if you have adrenal fatigue. Exercise also elevates cortisol levels similarly to food, so the combination of regular meals, small snacks and exercise can do a lot to enhance depressed cortisol levels.

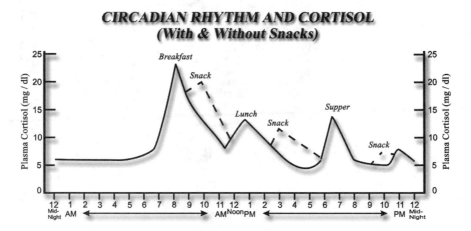

CIRCADIAN RHYTHM AND CORTISOL
(With & Without Snacks)

In people with adrenal fatigue this daily cycle of cortisol secretion may be irregular. Just as there are several long-term patterns of adrenal fatigue (described in a later section "Human Response Patterns to Stress") there are circadian variations in adrenal fatigue as well. Some people with adrenal fatigue have an overall low pattern of cortisol secretion with circulating cortisol levels lower than normal at every point of the cycle. Others spike to the normal level at 8:00 AM, but by 10:00 AM their cortisol levels have fallen below normal. Some exhibit the normal pattern and levels through most of the cycle but have a severe drop below normal between 3:00 and 5:00 PM. Still others fluctuate throughout the day and can even vary from day to day so that their cortisol levels are unpredictable. Whether these variations are a function of their overall stress level, adrenal health, food or environmental sensitivities, or other factors, it is important to be aware that in some people cortisol levels are very erratic during a twenty-four hour period. They may go through part of their day with elevated cortisol levels, part of the day with low levels and part with normal levels.

Although cortisol has its diurnal pattern of variations each day, it remains at an amazingly consistent level throughout your lifetime, under normal conditions. In later life, some people actually experience a small rise in cortisol. If this rise is excessive it may be related to some disorder. However, a rise in cortisol in response to stress is a natural reaction that actually protects the body in several ways. Below are some of the protective actions of modest rises in cortisol.

Actions of Cortisol

How Cortisol Protects the Body from Stress

Many of the symptoms of adrenal fatigue arise from decreased cortisol levels in the blood or inadequate levels of cortisol during times of stress when more cortisol is needed. Below and in the illustration entitled "Actions of Cortisol" is a brief summary of some of the actions of cortisol and the price your body pays when your cortisol levels are too low.

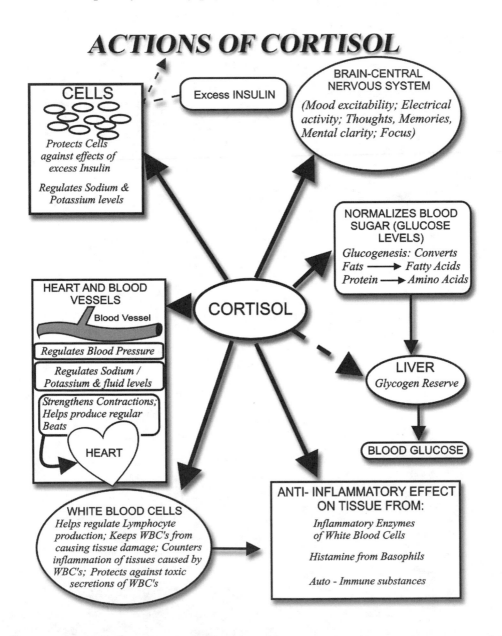

ACTIONS OF CORTISOL

Normalizes blood sugar (glucose) levels – Cortisol is essential for maintaining blood sugar (glucose) levels in the proper balance. A drop in blood sugar triggers the adrenals to make more cortisol. The cortisol increases blood sugar levels by converting fats and proteins into energy in a process called gluconeogenesis. In this energy production process first fats are broken down into fatty acids and proteins into peptides and then these are converted into the needed blood glucose. This process is vital to keeping the blood glucose levels relatively constant throughout the day. Your body depends upon glucose as its most consistent form of energy. Cortisol works in tandem with insulin from the pancreas to provide adequate glucose to the cells where it is burned for energy. Cortisol ensures adequate levels of glucose in the blood while insulin unlocks the cell membranes to let glucose into the cells.

When your body is under stress from any source, there are more demands placed upon its various tissues and organs, requiring more available glucose to fuel more energy production in the cell. As you can see, cortisol plays an important role in making glucose available to these different tissues and organs so that they can adequately respond during stressful situations. What happens to this process when cortisol levels are low because of adrenal fatigue is described in the section "Low Cortisol, Adrenal Fatigue and Hypoglycemia" later in this chapter.

Anti-inflammatory Effects of Cortisol - Cortisol is a powerful anti-inflammatory, even when secreted at normal levels (Munck, '95). It acts quickly to remove and prevent redness and swelling of nearly all tissues. These anti-inflammatory actions keep mosquito bites from flaring into giant wheals, bronchial tubes and eyes from swelling shut from allergens, and mild scratches from looking like you have just had a close call with Jack the Ripper. Cortisol maintains the balance through the unwritten law that "for any physical body to remain in homeostatic equilibrium every inflammatory reaction must have an opposite and equal anti-inflammatory reaction." Although there are other anti-inflammatory responses occurring at local sites, cortisol is the main anti-inflammatory agent circulating naturally in your body. You can assume that almost any time you have an inappropriate amount of redness and/or swelling, there is too little cortisol in circulation.

Cortisol has similar anti-inflammatory control over auto-immune reactions. In auto-immune reactions white blood cells attack parts of your body as if they were the enemy. These reactions can range from mild to life threatening. In most auto-immune reactions cortisol levels are inadequate for the degree of reaction taking place in particular tissues or locations in the body. This is one of the reasons why strong corticosteroids (prednisone, prednisolone, etc.) are used with all diseases involving inflammatory processes, including auto-immune diseases. They imitate the anti-inflammatory effects of cortisol, although unfortunately with some very serious undesirable side effects. Cortisol not only affects the redness and swelling but also the actions of the white blood cells, as described in the next section.

The Effects of Cortisol on White Blood Cells - Cortisol influences most cells that participate in immune reactions and/or inflammatory reactions, especially white blood cells. It specifically regulates lymphocytes, the commanders of the white blood cells. Cortisol and corticoids (cortisol like substances) also affect the actions of other white blood cells with names such as natural killer (NK) cells, monocytes, macrophages, eosinophils, neutrophils, mast cells and basophils. These white blood cells gather in defense of the body at places of injury or perceived invasion and some flood the area with very powerful chemicals to attack the invaders. Although they are a great defense, these chemicals irritate the surrounding tissues, causing redness and swelling. Cortisol is like a fire truck rushing to the site to put out the fire made by the lymphocytes and other white blood cells. It keeps the local white blood cells from sticking to the site and releasing their chemicals and also controls the number of circulating lymphocytes and other white blood cells, so there are fewer white blood cells available. This prevents an overreaction by the immune system and controls the irritation and tissue destruction that takes place at the site of congregating white blood cells.

Cortisol also reduces the rate at which lymphocytes multiply and accelerates their programmed cell death to further protect the body from this overreaction. In fact, when cortisol is elevated during the alarm reaction (see "The Alarm Reaction" in chapter 23), there is almost a complete disappearance of lymphocytes from the blood. That is why your immune system is suppressed when you are under stress or taking corticosteroids. On the other hand when circulating cortisol is low, its moderating effect on immune reactions is lost and lymphocytes circulate in excess. In this situation inflammation is greater with more redness and swelling, and it takes a longer time for the inflamed tissue to return to normal. So, directly and indirectly cortisol dramatically influences most aspects of immune function.

The Effects of Cortisol on the Cardiovascular System - Cortisol has complex and sometimes opposing effects on the cardiovascular system. The most significant of these effects is probably the control of the contraction of the walls of the arteries in regulating blood pressure. The more circulating cortisol, the more contracted the mid-sized arteries. Thus, people who are deficient in cortisol usually have pervasive low blood pressure (hypotension) and reduced reactivity to other body agents that constrict blood vessels.

Cortisol also directly affects the heart. It helps regulate sodium and potassium in the heart cells and increases the strength of contraction of the heart muscle. Sodium and potassium levels are critical for normal heart function. Cortisol also tends to increase blood pressure, but this hypertensive effect is moderated by calcium and magnesium. These minerals are required to prevent the heart muscles from cramping when they contract, thus keeping the heart beating smoothly. They also help relax the walls of the arteries, counteracting and balancing the increase in smooth muscle contraction produced by cortisol.

The Effects of Cortisol on the Central Nervous System - Cortisol influences behavior, mood, excitability and even the electrical activity of neurons in the brain. Behavioral changes frequently occur in cases of excess and deficient cortisol levels, for example, sleep disorders are common with both high and low cortisol. Many of the signs and symptoms of adrenal fatigue involve moodiness, decreased tolerance, decreased clarity of thought, and decreased memory. These occur because the brain is affected by both too little and too much cortisol. The right amount is needed for proper function during stress.

The Effects of Cortisol on the Physiology of Stress - An intimate association between stress and cortisol is manifested in several ways (see illustration "Adrenals' Role in Stress"). No matter what the source of stress, most challenges to homeostasis (internal body balance) stimulate the HPA axis, resulting in increased secretion of cortisol. In animal experiments, the animals with weakened adrenals died in response to even mild stress. However, when animals with weakened adrenals were given cortisol or similar agents, they survived those same kinds of stress. People with adrenal fatigue can often tolerate mild stress, but succumb to severe stress. As stress increases, progressively higher levels of cortisol are required. When these higher levels of cortisol cannot be produced, as in adrenal fatigue, the person cannot fully or appropriately respond to stress (see illustration "Cortisol Protects the Cells from Stress").

ADRENALS ROLE IN STRESS

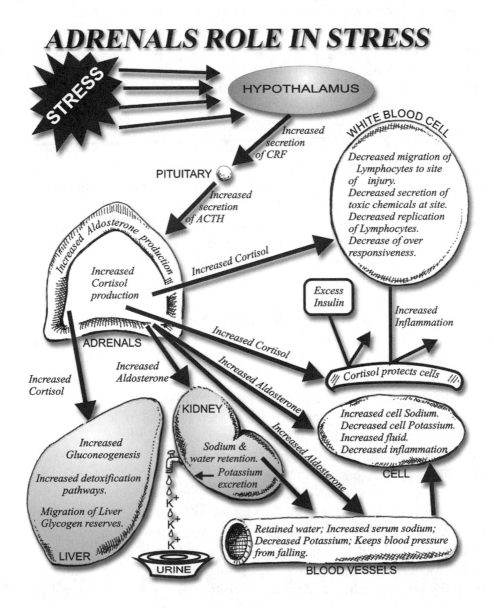

CORTISOL PROTECTS THE CELL FROM STRESS

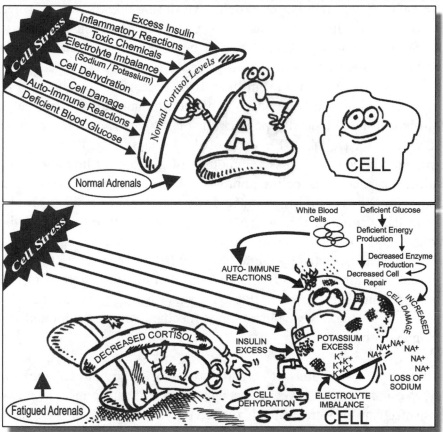

Even at normal levels, cortisol serves the very important function of priming the different mechanisms of your body so they can respond when called into action. During stress cortisol must simultaneously provide more blood glucose, mobilize fats and proteins for a back-up supply of glucose, and modify immune reactions, heartbeat, blood pressure, brain alertness and nervous system responsiveness. Without cortisol, these mechanisms cannot react adequately to a significant stress challenge. When cortisol levels cannot rise in response to these needs, maintaining your body under stress is nearly impossible. The more extreme the difference between the level of stress and the lack of cortisol, the more significant the consequences.

Cortisol can be viewed as sustaining life through two opposite but related kinds of regulatory actions: releasing and activating existing defense mechanisms of the body and shutting down and modifying the same mechanisms to prevent them from overshooting and causing damage or cell death. If this regulation is defective during stress, as it is when cortisol levels are low, an animal can be endangered or even die because its defense mechanisms cannot react or because they overreact. When your body is stressed cortisol is also needed to restrain various physiological mechanisms, to prevent them from damaging your body. For example, the elevation of blood sugar by the adrenals during stress helps control the insulin induced hypoglycemia that would occur if more blood glucose was not available. But cortisol also protects the cells against the detrimental effects of excessive amounts of glucose by helping create insulin resistance at the cell membrane to keep too much glucose from flooding into the cell. This damping down action of cortisol can also be seen in the way cortisol modifies the immune response to control the amount of inflammation in the involved tissues and suppress potentially toxic chemicals secreted by white blood cells, thus protecting the body from auto-immune processes and uncontrolled inflammation. Cortisol is so important that when the HPA axis cannot increase cortisol activity in response to stress, these unrestrained mechanisms overshoot and can damage your body.

In summary, these actions of cortisol have evolved to both enhance the body's response to stress, yet protect it from excessive responses to stress. These mechanisms were probably needed only occasionally in our distant ancestors' lives. However in modern life, with the myriad of physical, emotional and environmental stresses we face daily, our adrenals' capacity to rise to the occasion is challenged day after day. It is possible that we experience more stressful events in a year than our ancestors experienced in a lifetime. Yet your adrenal glands require some recovery time each time they are challenged. The constant "pedal to the metal" lifestyle leaves little room for an adequate adrenal response when the adrenal glands never get the chance to recoup and are already responding at their maximum capacity.

The more we understand about the physiology of stress, the more obvious it is that, unless we quickly evolve to have adrenal glands the size of footballs, we must learn to give our adrenals the opportunity they need to recover on a regular basis. This means using the information in Part III of this book to modify the effects that stress is most assuredly having on your body. Otherwise we will rapidly devolve into a society of the chronically sick and tired that even coffee, colas and other stimulants cannot rally.

The Interaction of Low Cortisol, Adrenal Fatigue and Hypoglycemia - Obviously there is a very close relationship between adrenal function and blood sugar levels (see illustration "Normal Adrenal Function and Blood Sugar"). We have known for almost a century that people who suffer from low blood sugar frequently suffer from adrenal fatigue. We also know that people who suffer from adrenal fatigue almost always have some form of irregular blood sugar pattern, of which hypoglycemia is the most common. With hypoglycemia there are usually cravings for sugar. There are real physiological reasons why these cravings exist. Let us take a closer look at these reasons.

NORMAL ADRENAL FUNCTION AND BLOOD SUGAR

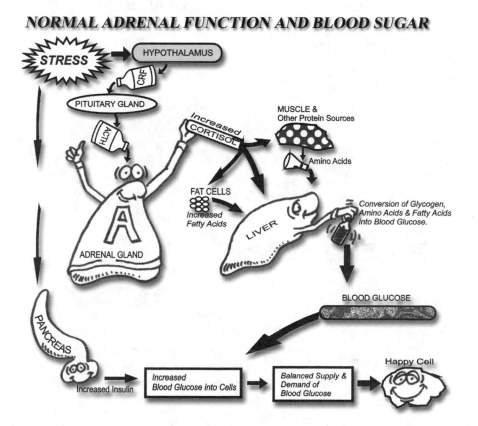

When your adrenals are fatigued, their cortisol output is diminished and you have lower levels of circulating blood cortisol (see illustration "Fatigued Adrenal Function and Blood Sugar"). With lowered blood cortisol, your liver has a more difficult time converting glycogen (stored blood sugar) into glucose (active blood sugar). Fats, proteins and carbohydrates, which normally can be converted into glucose, also cannot be as readily converted into glucose. These reserve energy pools controlled by cortisol are critical to achieving and maintaining normal blood sugar levels, especially during stress. Further complicating this matter is that during stress, insulin levels are increased because the demand for energy in the cells is greater. Insulin opens the cell wall membranes to take in more glucose in order to provide more energy to the cells. Without adequate cortisol levels to facilitate the conversion of glycogen, fats and proteins to new glucose supplies, this increased demand is difficult or impossible to meet. All this combines to produce low blood sugar.

FATIGUED ADRENAL FUNCTION AND BLOOD SUGAR

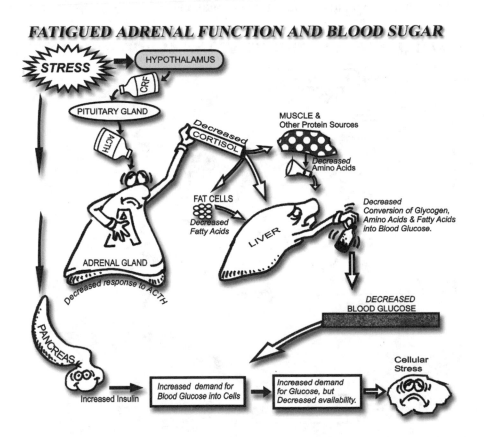

People with adrenal fatigue are in a real bind because when they are under stress (even a mild stress such as a math exam or an argument at home), demand for blood glucose increases, but their fatigued adrenals cannot produce enough cortisol to generate higher glucose levels from reserves. In the presence of increased insulin and decreased cortisol, blood sugar drops rapidly. When this happens at the same time as an increasing demand for glucose, the stage is set for tragedy. In a physical survival situation this might lead to death because response times slow down, thinking easily becomes confused, muscular strength is weakened, and other problems occur which render the individual too helpless to effectively defend themselves or escape.

Typically in our society in which physical survival is not usually a daily source of stress, people handle their low-adrenal related hypoglycemia symptoms with a double-edged sword; they eat something sweet with a cup of coffee or cola. This is a short acting emergency remedy that temporarily increases blood sugar with nearly immediate impact. They can almost feel it hit the back of their brain as their blood sugar moves out of the basement and shoots for the stars, relieving their hypoglycemic symptoms for about 45-90 minutes. However, this is inevitably followed by a precipitous plunge back to even lower blood sugar levels than they started with. Many individuals do this day in and day out, not realizing that hypoglycemia itself is a significant stress on the entire body, and especially on the adrenals.

To the body, hypoglycemia is a strong stressor, an emergency call to action that further drains already fatigued adrenals. People who treat their own hypoglycemia like the common example given above are on a constant roller-coaster ride throughout the day with their blood sugar erratically rising and then falling after each "sugar fix." This throws not only cortisol and insulin levels into turmoil, but also the nervous system and the entire homeostasis of the body. Therefore, by the end of the day, the person may feel nearly exhausted without having done anything. It might take an entire evening or weekend to recover from this daily/weekly roller coaster ride. It has sometimes been characterized as driving with both the brakes and the accelerator pushed to the floor at the same time.

Low blood sugar times are most likely to occur at around 10:00 AM, 2:00 PM, and between 3-4:00 PM. The old Dr. Pepper commercials had this pattern of hypoglycemia pegged when they created the slogan encouraging people to have a Dr. Pepper (high in sugar and caffeine) at "10, 2 & 4 each day." It is not by accident that work breaks are scheduled at about these times or that people typically have something sweet and/or caffeine during these breaks. We have a nation of hypoglycemics. 60% of people suffering from hypoglycemia go on to become diabetics. So is it any wonder that we have a nation suffering from diabetes in epidemic proportions.

Your brain also requires increased energy during times of stress and is especially affected by a lack of glucose. Although your brain uses several different fuels, when it is low on glucose, it often does not do well. In fact, most of the mechanisms involved in regulating blood sugar are designed to ensure that your brain always has adequate glucose with which to function. Many of the symptoms of adrenal fatigue and most of the symptoms of hypoglycemia are the result of insufficient glucose available to brain tissues.

Hypoglycemia, without proper snack and meal placement, also encourages overeating when food is available. The overeating causes rapid weight gain because the increased insulin is circulating in your blood, ready to usher that excess energy (glucose) from the extra food into your fat cells where it can be stored as fat. Even though you may not like its effects, this is a beautiful and savvy compensatory mechanism that has helped us survive.

Much of human history is a story of feast or famine; excess calories are a luxury in evolutionary terms. Therefore, after coming out of a situation of temporary famine (hypoglycemia) into a situation of excess calories (fat and sugary junk food), our evolutionary history urges us unconsciously to overeat and our bodies are designed to store that energy while it is available. In this way hypoglycemia creates a tendency to put on weight.

If you do not want to gain weight you should avoid those low blood sugar dips that not only make you so hungry you overeat, but also create a tendency in your body to store energy as fat. This means regular exercise and eating the kinds of meals and foods that control hypoglycemia.

It also means not eating those sugary foods and caffeine that send your blood glucose levels on a roller coaster ride and worsen your adrenal fatigue and hypoglycemia.

The Regulation of the Adrenal Sex Hormones

The manufacture of adrenal sex hormones in the zona reticularis of the adrenal cortex is primarily triggered by the same signal that initiates the production of aldosterone and cortisol in the other adrenal zones - the stimulation of the cell membrane by increased ACTH. This releases cholesterol to start the complicated cascade by which cholesterol is converted to pregnenolone and pregnenolone to various sex hormones. In the zona reticularis, unlike in the other adrenal zones, the cascade can follow a number of routes to produce various end product hormones. For example, pregnenolone can be converted to progesterone, which can then be converted to androstanedione, or pregnenolone can be converted to DHEA, which can then be converted to androstenedione. Androstenedione in turn can be converted to estrone or testosterone, either of which can then also be converted to estradiol. The sex hormone precursors such as DHEA are only somewhat diurnal, having small fluctuations throughout the day.

Actions of the Adrenal Sex Hormones and Their Precursors

Provides Supplementary Source of Sex Hormones - Both male and female hormones are made in the adrenals of each person, regardless of gender. In males, the adrenals provide a secondary source of testosterone and are the exclusive source of the female hormone estrogen. (Unless otherwise noted, estrogen refers collectively to the estrogens, i.e. estrone, estradiol, and estriol.) In females, the adrenals provide a secondary source of estrogen and progesterone, and are the nearly exclusive supplier of testosterone. Although we may not yet understand the exact role the adrenals play as a supplier of ancillary sex hormones, we do know that many women suffering from premenstrual syndrome (PMS) and difficult menopause have low adrenal function, and vice versa. We also know that when these women are given adrenal extracts, they often report their PMS or menopausal symptoms vanish or greatly improve. In boys entering puberty, low adrenal function is often associated with a lighter beard or less drive to achieve, with sparser hair on their arms and legs. Libido in both sexes is usually diminished by low adrenal function.

The Protective Effect of Adrenal Sex Hormones and Their Precursors - The adrenal sex hormones and their immediate precursors such as DHEA, pregnenolone and androstenedione do more than add to or balance other sex hormones. They also help balance the effects of cortisol and act as cellular anti-oxidants. Thus, the sex hormones and DHEA both limit cortisol's possible detrimental effects on cells and at the same time facilitate its actions by functioning as hormonal anti-oxidants. These precursors have their own actions as well as serving as raw material from which the sex hormones are made. For example, DHEA is exported to most cells and once inside the cells, it often becomes the resource material from which small amounts of local hormones can be created to carry out various specific tasks.

The Physiological Effects of Stress and Aging on Adrenal Sex Hormones - The more the adrenals are stimulated by stress and internal demands, the less responsive the zona reticularis becomes. Consequently, the adrenal output of sex hormones and their precursors decreases with chronic stress and adrenal fatigue. When less DHEA-S is manufactured in the zona reticularis, less DHEA-S and DHEA is available for export and use by other cells. This diminishes your ability to respond adequately to the demands placed on your body for increased DHEA-S and DHEA, thus, in turn, increasing the negative effects of chronic stress.

Loss of libido is commonly associated with adrenal fatigue, probably due in large part (in both men and women) to a drop in testosterone production by the adrenals. From your body's point of view, when you are in the midst of having to fight tigers and run for your life (i.e. when you are under a lot of stress), it is not a good time to feel amorous because your energy must be used for survival.

Output of adrenal sex hormones and their precursors also decreases with age. A decline in DHEA and testosterone levels accounts for many of the degenerative processes of aging. In fact, the levels of these two hormones in males track the progression of biological aging more closely than do any other markers. As we lose the available DHEA and testosterone, we become less able to counter the intense effects of cortisol in the cells. With age, cortisol levels remain relatively steady, while DHEA and testosterone decline and the other hormones range somewhere in between. In general as the levels of sex hormones and their precursors such as

DHEA and testosterone decrease because of age, stress and adrenal fatigue, their many and varied beneficial effects decrease as well.

The Regulation and Actions of Aldosterone
Adrenal Fatigue and the Craving for Salt

As mentioned in the "Anatomy" section, aldosterone is manufactured in the zona glomerulosa of the adrenal cortex.

Like cortisol, aldosterone follows a diurnal pattern of secretion with its major peak at around 8:00 AM and major low between midnight and 4:00 AM. Also like cortisol, its production and secretion increases and decreases in response to stimulation of the adrenal cortex by ACTH. This means that aldosterone levels generally rise in stressful situations. However, aldosterone is not part of the negative feedback loop controlling its release. Instead, it depends on the negative feedback loop in which cortisol levels trigger ACTH activity. This means that cortisol determines the amount of ACTH which controls production of both cortisol and aldosterone with aldosterone having no say in the matter. The only thing the cells that produce aldosterone can do to regulate production is to alter their sensitivity to ACTH. Therefore, after about 24 hours, the adrenal cells of the zona glomerulosa become less sensitive to the demands of ACTH and stop manufacturing more aldosterone. The amount of circulating aldosterone then begins to decrease, even though the ACTH levels are high and the need for increased amounts of aldosterone may continue. This decreased production continues until the cells of the zona glomerulosa recover their sensitivity to ACTH, but in the meantime the decreased aldosterone leads to many of the symptoms of adrenal fatigue.

Aldosterone is responsible for the maintenance of fluid (water) and the concentration of certain minerals (sodium, potassium, magnesium and chloride) in the blood, the interstitial fluid (area between the cells) and inside the cells. (See illustration – "The effects if Decreased Aldosterone in Adrenal Fatigue").Working with other hormones such as anti-diuretic hormone from the pituitary and renin and angiotensin I and II from the kidneys, aldosterone keeps the fluid balance and salt concentration intact, in roughly the same concentration as sea water. In the blood and interstitial fluid, sodium is the most dominant of the four minerals. Inside the cells, potassium has the highest concentration. These four minerals are called electrolytes because they carry minute electrical charges. These electrolytes are very important for proper cell function and fluid properties and they must remain in a relatively constant ratio to each other and to the body fluids. Small deviations in their ratios to each other or to their concentration in the body fluids means alterations in the properties of the fluid, the cell membrane and the biochemical reactions within the cell. In fact, most of the physiological reactions in the body depend in some way on the flow or concentration of electrolytes.

THE EFFECTS OF DECREASED ALDOSTERONE IN ADRENAL FATIGUE

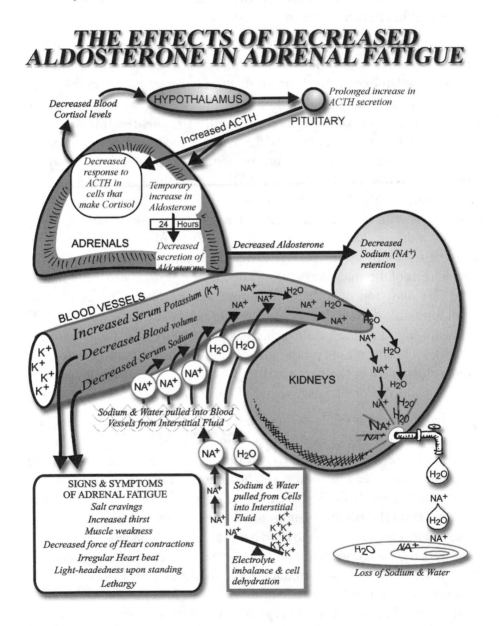

Aldosterone, in times of stress is the major director of these relationships by its influence on sodium and water concentrations. Although this interaction is somewhat complex, the overall process is easy to understand if you just keep an eye on the sodium in relation to aldosterone. As the concentration of aldosterone rises, the concentration of sodium rises in the blood and interstitial fluid. Wherever sodium goes, so follows water.

In adrenal fatigue, the craving for salt is a direct result of the lack of adequate aldosterone. As mentioned above, aldosterone controls sodium, potassium and fluid volumes in your body. When aldosterone secretions are normal, potassium, sodium and fluid levels are also normal. When aldosterone is high, sodium is kept high in the fluids circulating in your body.

However, as circulating aldosterone levels fall, sodium is removed from your bloodstream as it passes through the kidneys and is excreted in the urine. When sodium is excreted it takes water with it. Initially, there is some loss of volume of your body fluids but it does not become severe unless the condition worsens. Once your circulating sodium level drops to about 50% of its original concentration in body fluids, even a small loss of sodium or sodium restriction in your diet begins to have severe consequences. Tiny fluctuations in blood sodium concentration have a significant effect on blood volume when sodium is depleted to this level. When the sodium supply of the blood is not replenished by eating salt containing foods or liquids, sodium and water is pulled from your interstitial fluids into the blood to keep your blood sodium levels and water volume from getting too low. If too much salt or fluid is pulled from the interstitial fluids, the small amount of sodium in the cells begins to migrate out of the cells into the interstitial fluid. The cell does not have a great reserve of sodium because it needs to maintain its 15:1 ratio of potassium to sodium. As the sodium is pulled from the cell, water follows the sodium out.

This leaves the cell dehydrated as well as sodium deficient. In addition, in order to keep the sodium/potassium ratio inside the cell constant, potassium then begins to migrate out in small quantities. However, each cell has minimum requirements for the absolute amounts of sodium, potassium and water necessary for its proper function. When these requirements are not met cell function suffers, even if the proper ratio is maintained.

If you are suffering from moderately severe adrenal fatigue you must be careful how you re-hydrate yourself. Drinking much water or liquid without adequate sodium replacement will make you feel worse because it will dilute the amount of sodium in your blood even further. Also, your cells need salt to absorb fluids because sufficient sodium must be inside the cell before water can be pulled back across the membrane into the cell.

When you are already low on body fluids and electrolytes, as you are in this situation, you should always add salt to your water. Do not drink soft drinks or electrolyte rich sports drinks, like Gatorade™, because they are high in potassium and low in sodium, the opposite of what someone with low cortisol levels who is dehydrated needs. Commercial electrolyte replacement drinks are designed for people who produce an excess of cortisol when exercising, not people who are low on cortisol and aldosterone. Instead, you are much better off having a glass of water with ¼-1 teaspoon salt in it, or eating something salty with water to help replenish both sodium and fluid volume. In a nation of people suffering from adrenal fatigue, the fast food restaurants come to the rescue. Such restaurants use an excessive amount of salt in their foods; a custom leftover from the old road houses where lots of salt was used in the food to stimulate appetites and whet the thirst (for alcohol, the biggest profit item). Although not a good solution, it supplies "emergency" rations daily to people living in marginal health. It averts the crisis and replenishes their supplies for another few hours.

When your aldosterone levels are low and you are dehydrated and sodium deficient, you may also crave potassium because your body is sending you the message that your cells are low on potassium as well as sodium and water. However, after consuming only a small amount of potassium containing foods or beverages (like fruit, fruit juice, sodas and commercial electrolyte replacement drinks), you will probably feel worse because the potassium/sodium ratio will be further disrupted.

What you really need in this situation is a combination of all three, water, salt and potassium in the right proportions. One of the easiest ways to accomplish this is to drink small repeated doses of water accompanied by a little food sprinkled with kelp powder. Kelp powder contains both potassium and sodium in an easily assimilated form. Depending upon taste and symptoms, extra salt can be added. Sea salt is a better choice than regular table salt because it contains trace amounts of minerals in addition to the sodium. Another choice is to drink salted vegetable juice plus water.

Usually within 24-48 hours your hydration and electrolyte balance will have stabilized enough that you can proceed to the regular adrenal diet described in the chapter on food. You must continue to be careful to drink salted water 2-4 times during the day, varying the amount of salt according to your taste and you should avoid potassium-containing foods in the morning when your cortisol and aldosterone levels are low. Never eat or drink electrolyte depleting or diuretic foods and beverages such as alcohol and coffee, especially if you have been out in the sun or are otherwise dehydrated. One of the problems people with adrenal fatigue constantly deal with is a mild dehydration and sodium depletion.

But even in adrenal fatigue, the body is still wonderful, beautiful and incredibly wise. It is our society, our maladaptation to the stresses of modern life, and our poor judgment that need to change. We may not be able to change society but we can learn to use better judgment when it comes to taking care of ourselves and to respond to stress in healthier ways.

Chapter 23

The Stages of Adrenal Fatigue

Stress can kill. How do we learn to deal with it in a healthy way? To answer that, first let us look at the general adaptation syndrome and the role the adrenal glands and their hormones play in activating it. The general adaptation syndrome is the pattern of physiological adjustments your body makes in response to your environment (including your emotional environment). It has three phases: alarm, resistance and exhaustion which still function the same way in us as they did in primitive man, even though the stresses we face are very different. In this way our physical evolution has not kept pace with our social evolution. This means that our bodies create the same primitive response to a traffic jam on the way to work as early man's did to being in front of stampeding antelopes; cortisol levels rise to increase energy production for greater physical effort. In primitive man this is just what was needed to deal with the situation but in a traffic jam there is no increased physical demand and the extra energy turns into anger or other sideways emotions instead. Likewise, when you face an angry boss your body reacts the same way it would to a snarling tiger; it prepares to fight or run. Unfortunately neither of these responses is appropriate in the office, and therein lies the source of many of the health problems attached to modern stress. Recognizing this will help you to understand much better why your body responds the way it does to stress and how to help minimize its harmful effects.

The Alarm Reaction, a "Fight-or-Flight" Response
The initial response to the threat of a tiger or your boss is the alarm reaction, better known as the "fight-or-flight" response. This is your body's answer to any kind of challenge or danger; a complex chain of physical and biochemical changes brought about by the interaction of your brain, the nervous system and a variety of different hormones. Your body goes on full alert. Instantly, it responds to the stress chemicals released into the blood stream, such as adrenaline, by increasing blood pressure, heart rate, oxygen intake, and blood flow to the muscles.

Here is what happens, blow by blow:

- Your boss, or the tiger, triggers an immediate "red alert" arousal in your hypothalamus, a little cluster of specialized cells at the base of your brain that controls all automatic body reactions [see illustration "Selye's General Adaptation Syndrome (GAS)"]. The hypothalamus is part of the limbic system, the primitive brain that influences unconscious, instinctive behavior relating to survival and reproduction.

- Your hypothalamus signals your pituitary gland to release adrenocorticotrophic hormone (ACTH).

- ACTH instructs your adrenals to secrete epinephrine (adrenaline), norepinephrine (noradrenalin), cortisol and other stress related hormones. These hormones instantly mobilize your body's resources for immediate physical activity.

- Your breathing becomes faster and shallower to supply necessary oxygen to your heart, brain and muscles; blood in the intestines is shunted to areas of anticipated need.

- Your cortisol levels rise and convert increased amounts of stored glycogen into blood sugar in order to provide more energy for the increased work your cells are required to do during stress.

- Adrenaline and noradrenalin (from the adrenal medulla) are released directly into your bloodstream to produce a surge of energy for your body.

- Your heart rate increases, blood vessels dilate, and blood pressure rises (all due to increased cortisol and adrenaline).

- You sweat more (cortisol).

- Muscle tension increases (cortisol, adrenaline and testosterone) throughout your body.

- Your digestion shuts down as blood is diverted away from your skin and stomach (hypothalamus). Digestive secretions are severely reduced since digestive activity is not necessary for counteracting stress (hypothalamus).

- Your bladder and rectum muscles relax. (In extreme stress, such as in battle, they may void their contents, "dropping the ballast," so to speak).

SELYE'S GENERAL ADAPTATION SYNDROME (GAS)

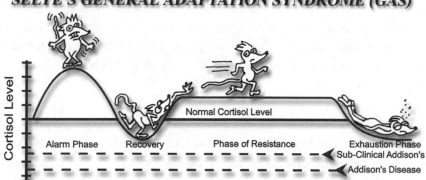

For a few brief moments during the "fight or flight" response you may experience nearly super-human power to deal with the situation. One of the most famous instances of the incredible power of adrenaline occurred in Seattle some 35 years ago, when a woman driving with her baby was hit on the freeway. The car flipped over, flinging her clear and breaking her right arm as it pinned the baby beneath it. Over a dozen people who had rushed over to help witnessed this extraordinary event. The woman jumped up, ran to the car, lifted it with her left arm *(that's right, the whole car with one arm)* and with her broken arm pulled the baby to safety. The baby, miraculously, was unharmed. The woman was admitted to a hospital with severe bruising on the left side of her body from the herculean feat and a broken right arm but she made a full recovery. The alarm stage is usually short lived. Typically the increased adrenaline level lasts a few minutes to a few hours and is followed by a drop in adrenaline, cortisol and other adrenal hormones that lasts a few hours to a few days, depending upon the magnitude of the stress.

After the alarm reaction is over, your body goes through a temporary recovery phase that lasts 24-48 hours. During this time there is less cortisol secreted, your body is less able to respond to stress, and the mechanisms over-stimulated in the initial alarm phase by the involved hormones become resistant to more stimulation. In this let down phase you feel more tired and listlessness, and have a desire to rest. This is a natural after-effect following the over-expenditure of energy during the alarm reaction.

After the recovery phase, if there is additional stress or a series of stressors, your body goes into another phase known as "the phase of resistance." This phase of resistance can last months or even up to 15-20 years. If there is no decrease in the amount of stress, or if there are suddenly new stresses, your body can go into the phase of exhaustion. Some people never experience the exhaustion phase; others visit it several times in their life.

The Resistance Reaction

Entering the phase of resistance reaction lets your body keep fighting a stressor long after the effects of the fight-or-flight response have worn off. The adrenal hormone cortisol is largely responsible for this stage. It stimulates the conversion of proteins, fats and carbohydrates to energy through a process called gluconeogenesis (gluco=glucose, neo=new, genesis=making or origin) so that your body has a large supply of energy long after glucose stores in the liver and muscles have been exhausted. Cortisol also promotes the retention of sodium to keep your blood pressure elevated and your heart contracting strongly.

The resistance reaction provides you with the necessary energy and circulatory changes you need to deal effectively with stress, so that you can cope with the emotional crisis, perform strenuous tasks and fight infection. Dr. Selye and subsequent researchers produced this GAS pattern over and over, resulting in hemorrhaged adrenal glands, atrophied thymus glands (the chief gland in immunity), and biochemically devastated bodies of animals exposed to repeated stress. The adrenals were the pivotal glands in the countless experiments involving stress.

If arousal continues, your adrenal glands will continue to manufacture cortisol. Cortisol is a powerful anti-inflammatory hormone that, in small quantities, speeds tissue repair, but in larger quantities depresses your body's immune defense system. A prolonged resistance reaction increases the risk of significant disease (including high blood pressure, diabetes, and cancer) because the continual presence of elevated levels of cortisol over-stimulates the individual cells and they begin to break down. Your body goes on trying to adapt under increasing strain and pressure. Eventually, if this phase goes on too long your body systems weaken in the final stage of the general adaptation syndrome, exhaustion. The resistance reaction phase can continue for years. But because each of us has a different physiology and life experience, the amount of time we can continue in the resistance reaction phase is unpredictable.

Exhaustion

In the exhaustion stage, there may be a total collapse of body function, or a collapse of specific organs or systems. Two major causes of exhaustion are loss of sodium ions (decreased aldosterone) and depletion of adrenal glucocorticoid hormones such as cortisol. In the resistance phase, with its increased levels of cortisol, there is also an increase in the level of aldosterone because both are stimulated during a normal response to stress. This keeps sodium high in the circulating blood and potassium low because it is excreted into the urine during times of high cortisol/aldosterone. However, the exhaustion phase can often begin so quickly that these electrolytes (sodium and potassium) are caught in the lurch. During this phase, lower levels of cortisol and aldosterone are secreted, leading to decreased gluconeogenesis, rapid hypoglycemia, sodium loss and potassium retention (for more detail, see the previous section on aldosterone "Adrenal fatigue and the craving for salt.") Body cells function less effectively in this condition as they rely heavily on a proper amount of blood glucose and the ratio of sodium to potassium. As a result, your body becomes weak. This means that during the exhaustion phase your body lacks the very things that would make you feel good and able to perform well.

When adrenal corticosteroid hormones are depleted, blood sugar levels drop because low cortisol levels lead to lower levels of gluconeogenesis. This means that your body is less able to produce its own blood glucose from stored fats, proteins, and carbohydrates, leaving you more dependent on food intake. Simultaneously, insulin levels are still high. The combination of low cortisol and high insulin levels leads to a slowing of glucose production and a speeding of glucose absorption into the cells. Hypoglycemia results because the body cells do not get the glucose and other nutrients they require. When energy is not available, every energy-requiring mechanism of the cell slows dramatically. This lack of energy combined with the electrolyte imbalance produces a cell in crisis. When energy and electrolytes once again become available and the cellular stress decreases, the damaged cell must be repaired or replaced. The reactivation of normal cell functions is an energy consuming series of events that uses up a greater amount of energy than is normally required.

Yet this has to take place in a situation in which your body is struggling just to produce enough energy to maintain some semblance of homeostasis.

Uninterrupted, excessive stress eventually exhausts your adrenal glands. They become unable to produce adequate cortisol or aldosterone. This combined effect on your kidneys of too little aldosterone, leads to collapse, and can even result in death in extreme cases.

Humans, although displaying many of the same physiological responses to stress, have their own unique pattern of adaptation and maladaptation. The next section is about how we respond to the various stresses of life.

Human Response Patterns to Stress

The general adaptation syndrome (GAS) described in the previous section is the model developed by Hans Selye to explain how animals adapt to stress. It is the paradigm commonly used to represent the generic physiological reaction to stress. In this model, the initial reaction that produces a large rise in cortisol is followed by a period of recovery in which the cortisol is low. As the stress is continued, the animal adapts to handle this stress and so produces higher levels of cortisol. This is called the phase of resistance. If the stress continues, eventually the adrenals give out and the animal plunges into the stage of exhaustion, unable to respond to stress. The GAS is an animal model that has many human variations. Humans however, being an odd kind of animal, do not necessarily respond in the same ways that laboratory animals do. In fact, humans have several additional patterns of responses to stress which vary in complexity and timing. The descriptions given below are brief snapshots of the most common patterns of adrenal fatigue I have seen clinically over the past twenty-four years. Any practicing physician who is aware of these patterns will notice them frequently in his practice. However, it is important to realize that each person suffering from adrenal fatigue has his or her own variation of the patterns of adrenal fatigue. Therefore individual profiles may not fit exactly any of the ones described below. The numbering is only for convenience sake and does not indicate the severity or importance. Despite the variety of forms adrenal fatigue can take individually, the Questionnaire and the other tools in this book are reliable ways of detecting its presence, no matter the individual pattern.

Pattern #1 - A long phase of resistance followed by adrenal fatigue

The first pattern is what is popularly referred to as the "iron man/woman." These are people who nothing seems to bother. They maintain a resistance stage most of their lives, being able to handle anything that life throws at them. Although stressors may get them down for a day or two, possibly even a week, they predictably bounce back as good as new. Usually these people remain in a resistance stage until late in life when old age diminishes their adrenal function. In some cases however, a major stressor, such as a very severe injury or emotional upset, precipitates adrenal fatigue. Sometimes they are still able to climb out and recover and will continue through life with ability to handle stress (see illustration "Human Response Pattern #1"). Clinically, these people would appear to have lost some of their previous ability to handle stress following a major life event (accident, illness, highly emotional situation, etc.). An example of this pattern is the guy who can handle anything at work, nothing ever bothers him. He takes on larger work loads and does whatever is demanded of him with no problem. Then one day an extremely stressful event occurs in his life, such as a major illness, surgery, or a marital break-up, and after that he seems much less able to handle the stresses of his job. Even after a time of recovery, he continues to work but is never the same person. If his salivary cortisol levels were checked carefully, they would probably be mildly elevated at first, but after the event, they would be mildly suppressed. If he took the questionnaire in this book he would show many of the indications of hypoadrenia or adrenal fatigue. However he probably started out in life with strong adrenals, otherwise he could not have endured stresses that his fellow workers were not up to. Chances are he did not experience the increased responsibilities or added work assignments he took on as stressors, but rather gladly accepted or even welcomed them. However, his added responsibilities were his undoing. This is a very common pattern. These people usually have an excellent chance of recovery, but must avoid the temptation to live on a constant "adrenal high"- the rush of continually pushing themselves to the brink, or to take on excessive responsibilities. If they continually push themselves, they can develop a pattern like the last part of this one or like #3. These are people born with strong adrenals and they are becoming more rare.

HUMAN RESPONSE PATTERN #1

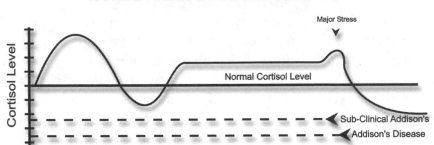

Suede was the top man in flight school. He was always the calm one, who remained even and good-natured no matter what challenges the flight instructor threw at him. He elected to be a tail gunner and was the best there was in any training school during World War II. No matter how much responsibility he was given, Suede could always be counted on. When he was assigned to a particular bomber, all his crew were happy to have him and considered him one of the strongest assets to their crew. During their first mission, they encountered unusually heavy anti-aircraft and enemy plane attacks. Suede was put on the spot almost immediately as the rear tail gunner. After suffering damage from gun fire to the rear of the plane, the Captain asked Suede if he was all right. Not getting any answer, he sent the radio operator back to check on him, fearing he might have been injured in the air battle. When the radio operator found Suede, he had both hands on the gun, starring straight ahead, frozen in one position. They had to pry his hand away from the gun and manually remove him from his perch. Once back on the ground, Suede was taken to the hospital and then to a recovery unit where he slept most of the day and could barely manage to dress or feed himself for several weeks. He was never to fly again.

This is a classic Pattern #1 response of adrenal overload and breakdown.

Reverend Little was a kind and caring man. He had been the pastor of his congregation for several years. Because it was a small church and unable to afford a full-time pastor, Reverend Little had a couple of side businesses in a larger town nearby to supplement his meager income.

He worked most nights when there wasn't any choir practice, prayer meeting or sermon to prepare. The number of his side jobs kept growing, as did his congregation. One night, Reverend Little went to sleep as usual, but the following morning he was unable to get out of bed. He had no fever, nausea or vomiting. He had no signs and symptoms of any typical illness. He just couldn't get out of bed. In fact, he lay there for three weeks before he was finally able to get up and return to work. After that he closed all but one of his businesses and shared the ministry with his oldest son. Reverend Little was never diagnosed with any ailment. He continued to operate on about one-quarter of the energy he had known, but he was able to manage by setting his sights lower and getting help from his family.

This is a classic example of a man who experienced a pattern #1 adrenal fatigue, yet never knew it and made the best adaptation he was able to make. Had his symptoms been diagnosed and treated, or better yet, had he seen that his lifestyle was placing him in jeopardy, he could have avoided much of what he suffered after his collapse. He could have remained extremely active, but in a more balanced way and thus avoided the period of debilitation caused by adrenal fatigue.

Pattern #2 – A single stressor followed by adrenal fatigue

There is a type of adrenal fatigue that can occur in people after only one stressful event. This pattern is similar to the first except there is no long phase of resistance. There is the typical alarm reaction and recovery phase, but only partial recovery is seen. These people never totally rebound from the recovery phase. Instead of progressing to the resistance phase, their cortisol levels remain below average, but at a level just high

HUMAN RESPONSE PATTERN #2

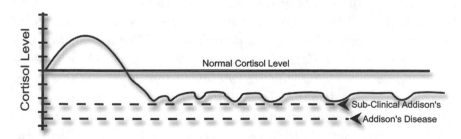

enough to allow them to function sub-marginally, with many of the symptoms of adrenal fatigue (see illustration "Human Response Pattern #2").

This pattern is turning up more frequently as more children are being born with weak adrenals and their diet does not provide enough of the nutrients needed to strengthen and rebuild their adrenals. Because the adrenal glands in these people do not have the resiliency to rebound after a severe stress, they have to function at a lower level with decreased adrenal output (as evidenced by the low cortisol levels). These people can recover, but they need to use the program in this book to do so, as well as avoid situations that constantly stress them. Rest and a calm, non-stressful lifestyle is essential if they are to be at their best.

Mrs. Ollert was a happy middle aged woman. Like most women, she was a dedicated mother and although divorced from her husband, had a good relationship with her 14-year old son, Robert. She had Robert later in life, when she was 35 and he was her pride and joy. One afternoon Robert and a friend of his were working out in the workshop on a science project. However, their curiosity had carried them way beyond the confines of their project. The two were constructing a homemade bomb when it exploded, killing both of them. Suprisingly, Mrs. Ollert took the news rather stoically. Even as saddened and disheartened as she was, she kept a cheerful front and carried on with life. On the anniversary of Robert's death, she decided to force herself to clean his room. When she got to his closet to clean out his clothes, something snapped. I saw Mrs. Ollert two days later. When no one came to the door and her car was still in the driveway, the neighbor became suspicious. Peeking through the windows, she could see Mrs. Ollert sitting in the living room with a box of chocolates open in front of her on the coffee table. Mrs. Ollert seemed to be awake, but did not respond to the knocks on the door or the yelling from the window. When I got there, she showed the same lack of response to my voice so we forced entry into the house. When I examined her, I found she was in a state of shock and fatigue and was quite dehydrated. After a brief hospital stay, during which her electrolytes were replenished and she was given intravenous nourishment, she became more conscious. At that point she broke down and sobbed for a long time as she experienced the sudden and severe emotional shock of confronting her son's death after hiding it from herself for a year. Her adrenals basically gave out temporarily. She was unable to care for herself. The only thing she could do was to sit on the couch and stare, eating an occasional chocolate. The chocolates, although giving her a temporary bit of energy, only worsened her low adrenal related hypoglycemia. Had care not intervened, she could likely have passed away. With a strong program of herbal, nutritional and other support, including counseling, Mrs. Ollert recovered. Nothing can replace the loss of a son, nor negate the traumatic shock of losing him so suddenly, but with time and care she was able to overcome the shock and grief enough to go on and live a good, normal life. She was careful to avoid unnecessary stress and regularly refresh herself.

This is an example of how one severe shock was enough to cause the adrenals to almost shut down. In pattern #2 adrenal fatigue, one intense episode of stress over-burdens already weak or strained adrenals causing a serious reduction in adrenal function. It can take many months or even years for these people to recuperate from such an event and, without proper treatment, many never regain normal adrenal function.

Pattern #3 – Repeated partial recovery followed by recurring adrenal fatigue

A third fairly common pattern of adrenal fatigue occurs when people experience a series of stressful events over time that keeps their adrenals continually over functioning until, finally, at some point in their lives their adrenals become fatigued and they do not rally. They go through repeated cycles of resistance and exhaustion after an initial shock or alarm reaction but each time they are able to return to a stage of resistance and function with above normal levels of cortisol. These people can carry on in a stage of resistance for several years until another major stressor or a series of stressors overwhelms them, after which there is another usually longer recovery phase that once again elevates them to the stage of resistance. The larger the stress, the longer the recovery. However in many of these patients, often in mid-life, there is a major stressor, after which they do not return to the high cortisol levels of the resistance stage but rather remain at the low cortisol levels of adrenal fatigue. This is illustrated in "Human Response Pattern #3."

HUMAN RESPONSE PATTERN #3

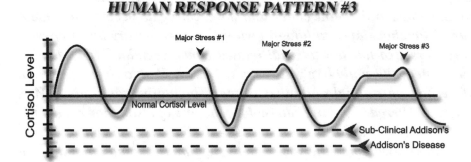

The people who follow this pattern usually have relatively strong adrenals but are unable or unwilling to change their continual encounters with stressful situations. Over time life beats them down, leaving them much less able to endure stresses that they previously would have handled with ease. These can be very willful individuals who refuse to change or they can also simply be people who unavoidably experience an unfortunate series of circumstances in life. It is possible for them to fully recover if they modify the problem areas in their life situation and follow the program in this book.

Perry was a gifted doctor. His understanding of physiology and pathology were beyond all of his peers. Perry was a person who needed to understand the entire picture. He could not rest until his understanding was complete. When he took a practice left by a retiring doctor in the woods of the North Country. Perry found that by using advanced nutritional techniques he could eliminate the rampant alcoholism prevalent in the community he served. When he tried to share how intravenous injections of Vitamin B and C complexes, consistently took away the compulsion to drink in his patients, none of his peers were interested and branded him a maverick. Eventually, one of his very ill patients died under his care. The medical board took the opportunity to penalize him for his progressive practices. After a kangaroo court inquiry, they found him guilty of medical malpractice and removed his license to practice medicine for life. The only other person given this harsh treatment was a serial killer Medical boards usually punish misconduct with a brief license suspension, a required remedial course or other such temporary measures. A 1-2 year suspension would have been a strong reprimand. Perry collapsed under the strain of their decision. However, with time and his understanding of physiology and nutrition, he was able to recover and was awarded a license by another health profession. Soon overburdened by patients due to his extraordinary approach, Perry began to buckle under the strain of treating very ill patients. He was a giver and he continually exhausted himself treating his patients. Luckily for him, Perry had a good ability to recover and could bounce back with rest and proper nutrition. However, when he was seeing patients, Perry did not incorporate rest or rejuvenating aspects into his lifestyle, and so he repeated the cycle of exhaustion and recovery until he closed his practice. It was only when he retired that Perry was able to recover and maintain his recovery. Perry is an excellent example of pattern #3 type of responses to stress.

Pattern #4 - Gradual decline into adrenal fatigue

This is a pattern of gradually decreasing resistance to stress (see illustration "Human Response Pattern #4). The people who exhibit this pattern experience many stresses over time but with each event their level of recovery diminishes. They are less and less able to return to high or even normal cortisol levels until, finally, their adrenals become so fatigued that they cannot handle anything more stressful than an uneventful routine day. Their cortisol levels may start out higher than normal but gradually drop below normal and then remain low, unless a concerted effort is made to help their adrenals recover. These people also can recover if they follow the program in this book, but it takes time and dedication.

HUMAN RESPONSE PATTERN #4

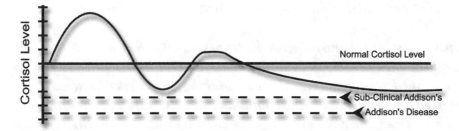

Michelle was a truly good woman, the kind you would like to have living next door. A mother of 5 who believed in trying to provide her children with everything, she was the dedicated mom other women

admired. As time went on, Michelle found herself lacking the energy she needed to give her children what she thought they needed. Five is a lot to take to music lessons, sports, play practices and birthday parties in between cooking, cleaning and the never ending demands of being a mom. Being on a low income, Michelle also suffered the stresses of trying to make ends meet and having to do things herself because they lacked the finances to hire someone to do or buy what she needed. Gradually, Michelle's spring wound down. Over time, she gradually slipped into a severe state of adrenal fatigue. When she first took my questionnaire she asked me, "How could you have been peeking in my windows when you didn't even know me? Answering your questionnaire was like seeing the story of my life." Seeing how her perfectionistic nature, religious convictions, and putting everyone else's needs first had driven her to adrenal exhaustion, Michelle was able to release her unreal expectations, let her children assume most of the household duties and develop a lifestyle that was both responsible and rewarding. Together with improved nutrition and dietary supplements, Michelle has entered into the best phase of her life.

Michelle is a good example of pattern #4. Without the change she implemented after seeing her state of adrenal health, recovery would not have been possible. This is a frequent pattern seen in strong willed perfectionistic people who constantly subjugate their own needs to "do their duty." It may be work, family or social demands that drive them, but the result is often the same. This is also a frequent pattern seen in single parents or in people who refuse to ask for help, trying to do it all themselves. Changing their physiology to recovery from adrenal fatigue is usually not the challenge. The challenge comes with changing the attitudes and beliefs that have driven them to adrenal fatigue.

Patty was a bright and athletic thirteen-year-old. She had all the right qualities to be a success in her present life and in her future. An accomplished soccer player, she was making top marks in school and enjoyed being one of the most popular students. Life was looking good for her. Then one day her soccer coach announced out of the blue that he was leaving the team. They were unable to find anyone else to replace him. There would be no more competitive soccer for her and her teammates. She was crushed because soccer had been her life; she had been practicing 25 hours per week, year round, for years and was hoping for a soccer scholarship to university. There was no other equivalent team for her to train with in town so Patty's world was suddenly turned upside down.

She went through a period of grief and depression that lasted over two years. In the middle of this difficult time she started attending a high school for the gifted and talented that required 3-5 hours of homework nightly. By the middle of the first term she was frequently getting sick and it was taking her longer to get over these bouts of flu and respiratory infections than normal. At the end of the first year she was asked to leave the school because her grades had fallen to unacceptable levels. But she appealed and was allowed to continue on probation for another year. Her sophomore year produced better marks, but the extreme stress of the previous two years had driven her into adrenal fatigue with many of the symptoms of hypoglycemia. This produced almost uncontrollable cravings for the quick energy of refined carbohydrates and resulted in unwanted weight gain.

Even though her Adrenal Questionnaire test score was extremely high, she initially resisted making any meaningful lifestyle changes, especially resting more and eating better. She continued at a school that pushed their students to the brink. The second year had nearly twice the homework as the first year, but she was unwilling to change schools, lessen her social life or do anything substantive about her hypoadrenia. Instead she continued to snack her way through life eating only occasional breakfasts, no lunches, grabbing something from the refrigerator after school, refusing to eat supper with her family on most occasions and keeping herself going with carbohydrate snacks late into the night. With her hypoadrenia also came problems sleeping, so she often was not able to go to sleep easily. On the surface she appeared to others to be managing well, still popular and active, but underneath, her health was being eroded by her insistence on pushing herself and refusal to change.

Patty was a person designing herself for pattern #4 hypoadrenia. Luckily, her youth and intelligence helped her recover and eventually have a life that was more enjoyable and less self demanding.

Bibliography

Chapter 1

McNulty J. New York Medical Journal xciii: 288, 1921.

Physicians Desk Reference (PDR). 53rd Edition, Medical Economics, Montvale NJ, p.1804, 2824, 1704, 2511; 1999.

Chapter 2

Addison T. On The Constitutional and Local Effects of Disease of the Suprarenal Capsules. London Highly, 1855.

Cutolo M, Villaggio, B., Foppiani, L., Briata, M., Sulli, A., Pizzorni, C., Faelli, F., Prete, C., Felli, L., Seriolo, B., Giusti, M. The hypothalamic-pituitary-adrenal and gonadal axes in rheumatoid arthritis. Ann NY Acad. Sci. 917: 835-43, 2000.

Harrower H, R. An Endocrine Handbook. Glendale, California: The Harrower Laboratory, Inc., p. 9, 14, 15, 16, 17, 19-22, 105, 109, 110, 111, 114, 115, 116, 120, 1939.

Hartman F, Brownell, KA., & Hartman, WE. The Hormone of the Adrenal Cortex. Am. J. Physiol. 72: 76, 1930.

Pottenger FJ, Pottenger, FM., Pottenger, RT. The Treatment of Asthma; with special reference to the oral use of the adrenal hormones and sodium chlorid. California & Western Medicine 43 (1): 1-15, 1935.

Pottenger FJ, and Pottenger, JE. Evidence of the Protective Influence of Adrenal Hormones Against Tuberculosis in Guinea Pigs. The Bulletin of the Association for the Study of Internal Secretions. 21 (4): 529-532, 1937.

Pottenger FJ. Non Specific Methods for the Treatment of Allergic States. The Journal of Applied Nutrition 17 (4): 49, 1964.

Pottenger FJ, & Krohn, Bernard. Emergency Treatment of the Asthmatic with Special Reference to Adrenal Cortex and Vitamin B-12. Rocky Mountain Medical Journal April, 1951.

Sergent E. Etudes cliniques sur l'insuffisance surrénale. Paris: A. Maloine et fils. Second Edition: 423-427, 1920.

Tintera JW. The Hypoadrenia Cortical State and its Management. New York State Journal of Medicine 55 (13): 1-14, 1955.

Chapter 5

Tintera JW. The Hypoadrenia Cortical State and its Management. New York State Journal of Medicine 55 (13): 1-14, 1955.

Chapter 6

Back JC, Casey, John, Solomon, S., Hoffman, MM. The Response of the Adrenal Cortex to Chronic Disease. In: GEW Wolstenholme aRP, ed. The Human Adrenal Cortex: Its function throughout life. Boston: Little, Brown and Company. pp. 94-119, 1967.

Bellometti SG, L. Function of the hypothalamic adrenal axis in patients with fibromyalgia syndrome undergoing mud-pack treatment. Int J Clin Pharmacol Res 19 (1): 27-33, 1999.

Bourne I. Local corticosteroid injection therapy. Acupuncture in Medicine 16 (2): 95-102, 1998.

Cowie DaB. JAMA xxiii: 363, 1919.

De Becker P, De Meirleir, K., Joos, E., Campine, I., Van Steenberge, E., Smitz, J., Velkeniers B. Dehydroepiandrosterone (DHEA) response to i.v. ACTH in patients with chronic fatigue syndrome. Hormone & Metabolic Research. 31 (1): 18-21, 1999.

Dessein P, Shipton, EA., Joffe, BI., Hadebe, DP., Stanwix, AE., Van der Merwe, BA. Hyposecretion of adrenal androgens and the relation of serum adrenal steroids, serotonin and insulin-like growth factor-1 to clinical features in women with fibromyalgia. Pain 83 (2): 313-319, 1999.

Feher I. Secretory function of adrenal cortex in chronic alcoholis. Med Pregl 52 (6-8): 221-225, 1999.

Feldman H, Johannes, CB., Araujo, AB., Mohr, BA., Longcope, C., McKinlay, JB. Low dehydroepiandrosterone and ischemic heart disease in middle-aged men: prospective results from the Massachusetts Male Aging Study. Am J Epidemiol 153 (1): 78-89, 2001.

Harrower HR. Practical Endocrinology. Second ed. Glendale, California: Pioneer Printing Company, p. 76-86, 265-277, 284-289, 308-309, 1932.

Harrower HR. Arthritis, p. 288, 1932.

Harrower HR. Burns. Practical Endocrinology: 308, 1932.

Harrower HR. Tb. Practical Endocrinology, 1932.

Heim C, Ehlert, U., Hellhammer, DH. The potential role of hypocortisolism in the pathophysiology of stress-related bodily disorders. Psychoneuroendocrinology 25 (1): 1-35, 2000.

Huysman M, Hokken-Koelega, AC., De Ridder, MA., Sauer, PJ. Adrenal function in sick very preterm infants. Pediatr Res 48 (5): 629-633, 2000.

Kuratsune H, Yamaguti, K., Sawada, M., Kodate, S., Machii, T., Kanakura, Y., Kitani, T. Dehydroepiandrosterone sulfate deficiency in chronic fatigue syndrome. Bioorganic & Medicinal Chemistry Letters. 1 (1): 143-146, 1998.

Lee S, Schmidt, ED., Tilders, FJ., Rivier, C. Effect of repeated exposure to alcohol on the response of the hypothalamic-pituitary-adrenal axis of the rat: I. Role of changes in hypothalamic neuronal activity. Alcohol Clin Exp Res 25 (1): 98-105, 2001.

Lucke B, Wright, T., Kime, E. Archives of Internal Medicine xxiv: 154, 1919.

Neeck G, Riedel, W. Hormonal pertubations in fibromyalgia syndrome. Ann N Y Acad Sci 876: 325-338; discussion 339, 1999.

Peebles RJ, Togias, A., Bickel, CA., Diemer, FB., Hubbard, WC., Schleimer, RP. Endogenous glucocorticoids and antigen-induced acute and late phase pulmonary responses. Clin Exp Allergy 30 (9): 1257-1265, 2000.

Pham-Huu-Chanh. The antagonistic effect of adrenal cortical extracts toward prostaglandin E2. C R Acad Sci Hebd Seances Acad Sci D 284 (16): 1601-1604, 1977.

Pottenger FJ, & Pottenger, FM. Adrenal Cortex in Treating Childhood Asthma: Clinical Evaluation of its use. California & Western Medicine 49 (4): 271-274, 1938.

Pottenger FJ, & Krohn, Bernard. Emergency Treatment of the Asthmatic with Special Reference to Adrenal Cortex and Vitamin B-12. Rocky Mountain Medical Journal April, 1951.

Pottenger F, Jr.,. The Use of Adrenal Cortex in the Treatment of the Common Cold. Medical Record: 1-5, 1938.

Pottenger FJ, Pottenger, FM., Pottenger, RT. The Treatment of Asthma; with special reference to the oral use of the adrenal hormones and sodium chlorid. California & Western Medicine 43 (1): 1-15, 1935.

Rivier CL, S. Effect of repeated exposure to alcohol on the response of the hypothalamic-pituitary-adrenal axis of the rat: II. Role of the length and regimen of alcohol treatment. Alcohol Clin Exp Res 25 (1): 106-111, 2001.

Roberts SE. Exhaustion; Causes and Treatment. Emmaus, Penna 18049: Rodale Books, Inc., p. 6, 16, 72-83, 1966.

Scott L, Teh, J., Reznek, R., Martin, A., Sohaib, A., Dinan, TG. Small adrenal glands in chronic fatigue syndrome: a preliminary computer tomography study. Psychoneuroendocrinology 24(7): 759-68, 1999.

Sergent E. Presse Med. xxix: 813, 1921.

Straub RC, M. Involvement of the hypothalamic—pituitary—adrenal/gonadal axis and the peripheral nervous system in rheumatoid arthritis: viewpoint based on a systemic pathogenetic role. Arthritis Rheum 44 (3): 493-507, 2001.

Tintera JW. The Hypoadrenia Cortical State and its Management. New York State Journal of Medicine 55 (13): 1-14, 1955.

Tintera J. Endocrine aspects of opthalmologic and otolaryngologic allergy. Presented before the 27th anniversary program of the American Society of Ophthalmologic and Otolaryngologic Allergy. Chicago, IL, 1969.

Tintera J. The Endocrine Approach to the Etiology and Effective Control of Functional Hypoglycemia. Scarsdale, NY: The Hypoglycemia Foundation, Inc., 1966.

Watterberg K, Scott, SM., Backstrom, C., Gifford, KL., Cook, KL. Links between early adrenal function and respiratory outcome in preterm infants: airway inflammation and patent ductus arteriosus. Pediatrics 105 (2): 320-324, 2000.

Chapter 10

Ackermann RJ. Adrenal Disorders: Know when to act and what tests to give. Geriatrics 49: 32-37, 1994.

Arroyo C. Med. Jour. and Rac. cxix: 25, 1924.

Harrower HR. Endocrine Diagnostic Charts. Glendale, CA: The Harrower Laboratory, Inc., p. 25-45, 79, 80-81, 1929.

Sergent E. Endocrinology. 1: 18, 1917.

Chapter 11

Fauci ASea. Harrison's Principles of Internal Medicine. 14th ed. New York: McGraw-Hill, p. 1965-1976, 1985-1986, 2003-2011, 2079-2087, 2035-2056, 1998.

Kos-Kudla B, Buntner, B., Marek, B., Ostrowska, Z., Swietochowska, E. Serum, salivary and urinary cortisol level in the evaluation of adrenocortical function in patients with bronchial asthma. Endocr. Regul. 30 (4): 201-206, 1996.

Chapter 12

Harrower HR. Practical Organotherapy. Third ed. Glendale, California: The Harrower Laboratory, p. 112-120, 1922.

Chapter 13

Downey DS. Balancing body chemistry with nutrition seminars; Cannonburg, MI. (3rd Edition): 158, 2000.

Erasmus U. Fats that Heal, Fats that Kill. Burnaby BC, Canada: Alive Books, p. 456, 1993.

Harrower HR. Practical Organotherapy. Third ed. Glendale, California: The Harrower Laboratory, p. 112-120, 1922.

Loeb R. Sodium Chlorid in Treatment of a Patient with Addison's Disease. Proc. Soc. Exper. Biol. and Med. 30: 808, 1933.

Roberts SE. Exhaustion; Causes and Treatment. Emmaus, Penna 18049: Rodale Books, Inc., p. 6, 16, 72-83, 1966.

Tintera JW. The Hypoadrenia Cortical State and its Management. New York State Journal of Medicine 55 (13): 1-14, 1955.

Tintera JW. Endocrine aspects of schizophrenia: hypoglycemia of hypoadrenocorticism. J Schizophr 1 (5): 150-181, 1967.

Tintera JW. Stabilizing Homostasis in the recovered alcoholic through endocrine therapy: evaluation of the hypoglycemic factor. J Am Geriatr Soc 14 (7), 1966.

Tintera J. Endocrine aspects of opthalmologic and otolaryngologic allergy. Presented before the 27th anniversary program of the American Society of Ophthalmologic and Otolaryngologic Allergy. Chicago, IL, 1969.

Tintera J. Hypoadrenocorticism: Endocrinologic approach to the etiology and treatment of functional hypoglycemia; non-surgical treatment of hypoglycemia states including those of alcoholism and drug addiction. The Hypoglycemia Foundation Inc. Scarsdale New York.: 15 pages, 1976.

Tintera J. The Endocrine Approach to the Etiology and Effective Control of Functional Hypoglycemia. Scarsdale, NY: The Hypoglycemia Foundation, Inc., 1966.

Chapter 15

Anbalagan K, Sadique, J. Withania somnifera (Ashwagandha), a rejuvenating herbal drug which controls alpha-2-macroglobulin synthesis during inflammation. Int. J. Crude Drug Res. 23 (4): 177-183, 1985.

Baron J, Nabarro, J., Slater, J., et al. Metabolic studies, aldosterone secretion rate and plasma renin after carbonoxolone sodium as biogastrone. Br. Med. J. 2: 793-795, 1969.

Bauer U. 5-month double-blind randomized clinical trial of ginkgo biloba extract cersus placebo in two parallel groups in patients suffering from peripheral arterial insufficiency. Aezneim Forsch 34: 716-721, 1984.

Brekhman I, Dardymov, IV. Pharmacological investigation of glycosides from ginseng and Eleutherococcus. Lloydia 32: 46-51, 1969.

Brekhman I, Kinillow, OI. Effect of Eleutherococcus on alarm-phase of stress. Life Sci 8 (3): 113-121, 1969.

Buittacharya S, Goel, Raj K., Kaur, Ravinder, and Ghosal, Shibnath. Anti-Stress ctivity of Sitoindosides VII and VIII, New Acysterylglucosides from Withania Somnifera. Phytotherapy Research. 1 (1): 32-37, 1982.

Chen M, Shimada, F., Kato, H, et. al. Effect of clycyerhigin on the pharmacokinetics f prednisolone following low dosage of prednisolone hemisuccinate. Endocrinol. Japan 37: 331-341, 1990.

Coburn S, Mahuren JD, Schaltenbrand WE, Wostmann BS, Madsen D. Effects of vitamin B-6 deficiency and 4'- deoxypyridoxine on pyridoxal phosphate concentrations, pyridoxine kinase and other aspects of metabolism in the rat. J Nutr 111 (2): 391-198, 1981.

Colloazo Jea. Experimental hypervitaminosis of rats caused by large doses of rradiated ergosterol. Biochem Ztschr. 204: 347-353, 1929.

DeFeudia F. Pharmacological activities and clinical applications. Elsevier; Paris, 1991.

Duke J. Handbook of medicinal herbs. Florida: CRC Press, p. 337-338, 1985.

Farnsworth N, Kindhorn, AD., Soejarto, D., Waller, DP. Siberian Ginseng: Current status as an adaptogen. Econ. Med. Plant Res. 1: 156-215, 1985.

Fidanza A. Therapeutic action of pantothenic acid. Int J Vitam Nutr Res Suppl. 24: 53-67, 1983.

Fidanaza A, Floridi, S., Lenti, L. Panthenol and glucocorticoids. Boll Soc Ital Biol Sper. 57 (18): 1869-1872, 1981.

Fidanza A, Bruno, C., De Cicco, A., Floridi, S., Martinoli, L. Effect of high doses of sodium pantothenate on the production of corticosteroids. (Article in Italian). Boll Soc Ital Biol Sper. 54 (22): 2248-2250, 1978.

Grandhi AM, AM; Patwardhan, Bhushan. A comparative pharmacological investigation of Ashwagandha and Ginseng. Journal of Ethno-pharnacology 44: 131-135, 1994.

Harris JM, T. Hypervitaminosis and vitamin balance: specificity of Vitamin D in irradiated ergosterol poisoning: pathology of hypervitaminosis. D. Biochem j. 23: 261-273, 1929.

Harris JM, T. On the problems of the development of hypervitaminosis D after the administration of synthetic Vitamin D preparations. Pediatrica. 40: 34-39, 1961.

Hindmarch I, Subhan, Z. The psychopharmacological effects of ginkgo biloba extract in normal healthy volunteers. Int. J. Clin. Pharmacol. Res. 4: 89-93, 1984.

Hornsby PJ, Harris, Sandra E. and Alern, Kathy A. The Role of Ascorbic Acid in the Function of the Adrenal Cortex: Studies in Adrenocortical Cells in Culture. Endocrinol. 117: 1264-1271, 1985.

Kosaka M, Kikui, S., Fujiwara, T., Kimoto, T. Action of pantetheine on the adrenal cortex; PMID: 4292291 [PubMed - indexed for MEDLINE]. Horumon To Rinsho. 14 (10): 843-847, 1966.

Krohn B, Pottenger, FM, Jr. Allergic Rhinitis: Tocopherol Therapy. Annals of Western Medicine and Surgery 6 (8): 484-487, 1952.

Kutsky R, J. Handbook of Vitamins, Minerals and Hormones. Second ed. Vancouver, Washington: Van Nostrand Reinhold Company, p. 411-413, 1981.

MacKenzie M, Janson, RW., Hoefnagels, WH., et al. The influence of glycyrrhetinic acid on plasma cortisol and cortisone in healthy young volunteers. J. Clin. Endocrinal Metab. 70: 1637-1643, 1990.

Mahuren J, Dubeski, PL., Cook, NJ., Schaefer, AL., Coburn, SP.
Adrenocorticotropic hormone increases hydrolysis of B-6 vitamers in swine
adrenal glands. J Nutr 129 (10): 1905-1908, 1999.

Mathias S, Mgbonyebi, OP., Motley, E., Owens, JR., Mrotek, JJ. Modulation of
adrenal cell functions by cadmium salts. 4. Ca(2+)-dependent sites affected by
CdCl2 during basal and ACTH-stimulated steroid synthesis. Cell Biology &
Toxicology. 14 (3): 225-236, 1998.

Meinig GE. Root Canal Cover-up. Second ed. Ojai, California: Bion Publishing, p.
220 pages, 1994.

Mgongo F, Gombe, S., Ogaa, JS. The influence of cobalt/vitamin B12 deficiency as a
"stressor" affecting adrenal cortex and ovarian activities in goats. Reprod Nutr
Dev 24 (6): 845-854, 1984.

Mitsuma T, Sun, DH., Nogimori, T., Ohtake, K., Hirooka, Y. Effects of calcium
hopantenate on the release of thyrotropin-releasing hormone from the rat
adrenal gland in vitro. Hormone & Metabolic Research. 19 (10): 475-477, 1987.

Murray MT, Pizzorno, Joseph E. Encyclopedia of Natural Medicine. Second ed:
Prima Publishing, 1998.

Ohuchi K, Kamada, Y., Levine, L., et al. Glycynhizin inhibits prostaglandin E2
formation by activated peritoneal macrophages from rats. Prostagland Med. 7:
457-463, 1981.

Oswald W, Raymond, GH., Glior, U. Obstruction and Distribution of Vitamin E in
the Tissues. Vitam-Horm. 20: 441, 1962.

Pietrzik K, Hornig, D. Studies on the distribution of (1-14C) pantothenic acid in rats.
Int J Vitam Nutr Res Suppl. 50 (3): 283-293, 1980.

Pietrzik K, Schwabeda, IP., Hesse, C., Bock, R. Influence of pantothenic acid
deficiency on the amount of CRF-granules in the rat median eminence. Anat
Embryol (Berl) 146 (1): 43-55, 1974.

Pyzhik T. The role of niacin in regulating the pentosophosphate pathway and
production of NADP-H in fatty tissue (Article in Russian). Vopr Pitan (5): 53-
55, 1989.

Roberts SE. Exhaustion; Causes and Treatment. Emmaus, Penna 18049: Rodale
Books, Inc., p. 6, 16, 72-83, 1966.

Rossier M, Burnay, MM., Maturana, A., Capponi, AM. Duality of the voltage-dependent calcium influx in adrenal glomerulosa cells. Endocrine Research. 24 (3-4): 443-447, 1998.

Sakensa A, Singh, SP., Dixit, KS., Singh, N., Seth, K., Seth, PK., Gupta, GP. Effect of Withania somnifera and panax ginseng on Dopaminergic receptors in rat brain during stress. Planta Medica 55: 95, 1989.

Schwabedal P, Pietrzik, K. , Wittkowsk, W. Pantothenic acid deficiency as a factor contributing to the development of hypertension. Cardiology, 72 Suppl (1): 187-189, 1985.

Sikora R, Sohn, M., Deutz, F., et al. Ginkgo biloba extract in the therapy of erectile dysfunction. Journal of Urology 141: 188A, 1989.

Spingen V, Beuge, JA., O'Neal, FO., Aust, SD. The Mechanism of NADPH-Dependent Lipid Peroxidation. J. Biol Chem 254: 5892, 1979.

Suzuki T. Physiology of Adrenocortical Secretion. Toyko, Japan: Karger Press, p. 1-4, 1983.

Takayanagi R, Kato, Ken-ichi, Ibayashi, Hiroshi. Relative Inactivation of Steroidogenic Enzyme Activities of Invitro Vitamin E-Depleted Human Adrenal Microsomes by Lipid Peroxidation. Endocrin. 119 (2), 1986.

Tarasov I, Sheibak, VM., Moiseenok, AG. Adrenal cortex functional activity in pantothenate deficiency and the administration of the vitamin or its derivatives. (Russian). Voprosy Pitaniia. (4): 51-54, 1985.

Taubold R, Siakotos, Ann, Perking, EG. Studies on Chemical Nature of Lipofuscin "H pigment", isolated from normal human brains. Lipids 10: 383, 1976.

Thenen S. Megadose effects of vitamin C on vitamin B-12 status in the rat. J Nutr 119 (8): 1107-1114, 1989.

Tully D, Allgood, VE., Cidlowski, JA. Modulation of steroid receptor-mediated gene expression by vitamin B6. FASEB J 8 (3): 343-349, 1994.

Umeda F, Kato, K., Ibayashih, Cogima, N., Shibatay, Yamamoto, T. Inhibitorial Effect of Vitamin E on Lipoperoxide Formation in Rat Adrenal Gland, Tohuku. J Exep Med.

Weglicki W, Reichel, W., Nair, PP. Accumulation of Lipofuscin-like pigment in the Rat Adrenal Gland as a Function of Vitamin E Deficiency. J. Gerontol. 23 (4): 469-475, 1968.

Windfeuer A, Mayerhofer, D. The effects of plant preparations on cellular functions in body defense. Arzneimittelforschung 44: 361-366, 1994.

Chapter 16

Britton SK, RF. The American Journal of Physiology. The Relative Effects of Desoxycortiosterone and Whole Cortico-adrenal Extract on Adrenal Insufficiency. 133 (3): 503-510, 1941.

Harrower HR. Practical Organotherapy. Third ed. Glendale, California: The Harrower Laboratory, p. 112-120, 1922.

Harrower HR. Practical Endocrinology. Second ed. Glendale, California: Pioneer Printing Company, p. 76-86, 265-277, 284-289, 308-309, 1932.

Pottenger F, Jr.,. The Use of Adrenal Cortex in the Treatment of the Common Cold. Medical Record: 1-5, 1938.

Pottenger FJ, and Pottenger, JE. Evidence of the Protective Influence of Adrenal Hormones Against Tuberculosis in Guinea Pigs. The Bulletin of the Association for the Study of Internal Secretions. 21 (4): 529-532, 1937.

Pottenger FJ. Non Specific Methods for the Treatment of Allergic States. The Journal of Applied Nutrition 17 (4): 49, 1964.

Pottenger FJ, & Krohn, Bernard. Emergency Treatment of the Asthmatic with Special Reference to Adrenal Cortex and Vitamin B-12. Rocky Mountain Medical Journal April, 1951.

Pottenger FJ, & Pottenger, FM. Adrenal Cortex in Treating Childhood Asthma: Clinical Evaluation of its use. California & Western Medicine 49 (4): 271-274, 1938.

Pottenger FJ, Pottenger, FM., Pottenger, RT. The Treatment of Asthma; with special reference to the oral use of the adrenal hormones and sodium chlorid. California & Western Medicine 43 (1): 1-15, 1935.

Roberts SE. Exhaustion: Causes and treatment. A new approach to the treatment of allergy. Emmaus, PA 18049: Rodale Books, Inc., p. 57, 62, 77-80, 1971.

Sergent E. Presse Med. xxix: 813, 1921.

Sergent E. Etudes cliniques sur l'insuffisance surrénale. Paris: A. Maloine et fils. Second Edition: 423-427, 1920.

Thorn GW. The Diagnosis and Treatment of Adrenal Insufficiency. Second ed. Springfield, Ill.: Charles C. Thomas, p. 86-91, 1951.

Tintera JW. Endocrine aspects of opthalmologic and otolaryngologic allergy. Presented before the 27th anniversary program of the American Society of Ophthalmologic and Otolaryngologic Allergy. Chicago, IL, 1969.

Tintera JW. The Hypoadrenia Cortical State and its Management. New York State Journal of Medicine 55 (13): 1-14, 1955.

Tintera JW. Endocrine aspects of schizophrenia: hypoglycemia of hypoadrenocorticism. J Schizophr 1 (5): 150-181, 1967.

Tintera JW. Stabilizing Homostasis in the recovered alcoholic through endocrine therapy: evaluation of the hypoglycemic factor. J Am Geriatr Soc 14 (7), 1966.

Tintera JW. The hypoadrenocortical state. Paper presented before the Annual Seminar of the Adrenal Metabolic Research Society of the Hypoglycemia Foundation, Inc., 1969.

Tintera J. Hypoadrenocorticism: Endocrinologic approach to the etiology and treatment of functional hypoglycemia; non-surgical treatment of hypoglycemia states including those of alcoholism and drug addiction. The Hypoglycemia Foundation Inc. Scarsdale New York: 15 pages, 1976.

Tintera J. The Endocrine Approach to the Etiology and Effective Control of Functional Hypoglycemia. Scarsdale, NY: The Hypoglycemia Foundation, Inc., 1966.

Chapter 19

Meinig GE. Root Canal Cover-up. Second ed. Ojai, California: Bion Publishing, p. 220 pages, 1994.

Chapter 22

Aptel HB, Johnson, Elizabeth IM., Vallotton, Michael B., Rossier, Michel F., Capponi, Alessandro M. Demonstration of an angiotensin II-induced negative feedback effect on aldosterone synthesis in isolated rat adrenal zona glomerulosa cells. Molecular and Cellular Endocrinology 119: 105-111, 1996.

Assenmacher IS, Alain; Alonso, Gerard; Ixart, Guy and Barbanel, Gerard. Physiology of Neural Pathways Affecting CRH Secretion. Annals of the New York Academy of Sciences 512: 149-158, 1987.

Boyd G, McNamara, B., Suckling, KE., Tocher, DR. Cholesterol Metabolism in the Adrenal Cortex. J. steroid Biochem. 19 (1): 1017-1027, 1983.

Bravo E, L. Physiology of the Adrenal Cortex. Urologic Clinics of North America 16
(3): 433, 1989.

Cherradits NR, Michel F; Vallottoni, Michel B; Timberg, Rina; Friedberg, Ido; Orlyl,
Joseph; Wang, Xing Jia; Stocco, Douglas M; Capponi, Alessandro M.
Submitochondrial Distribution of Three Key Steroidogenic Proteins
(Steroidogenic Acute Regulatory Protein and Cytochrome P450 and 3B-
Hydroxysteroid Dehydrogenase Isomerase Enzymes) upon Stimulation by
Intracellular Calcium in Adrenal Gomerulosa Cells. The Journal of Biological
Chemistry; The American society for Biochemistry and Molecular Biology, Inc.
272 (12): 7899-7907, 1997.

Collip J, Anderson, Evelyn M. Thyrotrophic Hormone of Anterior Pituitary.
J.A.M.A. 104 (12): 965-969, 1935.

Duncan WC, Jr. Circadian Rhythms and the Pharmacology of Affective Illness.
Pharmacol. Ther. 71 (1): 253-312, 1996.

Dupont E, Luu-The, V., Labrie, F., Pelletier, G. Ontogeny of 3B-hydroxysteroid
dehydrogenase/isomerase in human adrenal gland performed by
immunocytochemistry. Molecular and Cellular Endocrinology 74: R7-R10,
1990.

Fauci ASea. Harrison's Principles of Internal Medicine. 14th ed. New York:
McGraw-Hill, p. 1965-1976, 1985-1986, 2003-2011, 2079-2087, 2035-2056,
1998.

Harrop G, Soffer, LJ., Ellsworth, R., Tresher, H. Studies on the Suprarenal Cortex.
III. Plasma Electrolytes and Electrolyte Excretion During Suprarenal
Insufficiency in hte Dog. Jour. Exp. Med. 58: 17-38, 1933.

Hartman F, Brownell, KA., & Hartman, WE. The Hormone of the Adrenal Cortex.
Am. J. Physiol. 72: 76, 1930.

Jeffries WM. Safe Uses of Cortisol. Second ed. Springfield, Ill.: Charles C. Thomas,
Publisher Ltd., p. 35-65, 1996.

Jenkins JS. Biochemical Aspects of the Adrenal Cortex. London: Edward Arnold,
Ltd., p. 41-46, 1968.

Kendall E, Mason, HL., McKenzie, BF. Isolation in crystalline form of the hormone
essential to life from the suprarenal cortex—It's chemical nature and physiologic
properties. Proceedings, Mayo Clinic 9 (7): 245-250, 1933.

Labrie FG, Vincent; Meunier, Helene; Simard, Jacques; Gossard, Francis; Raymond, Vincent. Multiple Factors Controlling ACTH Secretion at the Anterior Pituitary Level. Annals of the New York Academy of Sciences 512: 97-114, 1987.

Loeb R. Sodium Chlorid in Treatment of a Patient with Addison's Disease. Proc. Soc. Exper. Biol. and Med. 30: 808, 1933.

Miesfeld RL. Biochemistry. Overview of Glucocorticoid Action at the Molecular Level.: 1656-1667, 1995.

Mortensen RMW, Gordon H. Aldosterone Action. Physiology 3rd edition: 1668-1710, 1995.

Palkovits M. Anatomy of Neural Pathways Affecting CRH Secretion. Annals of the New York Academy of Sciences 512: 139-148, 1987.

Pansky BahEL. Review of Gross Anatomy. Second ed. London: Macmillan Company, p. 344-345, 1969.

Quinn SJW, Gordon H. Regulation of Aldosterone Secretion. Second ed. New York: Raven Press, Ltd., p. 159-189, 1992.

Reichel W. Lipofuscin pigment accumulation and distribution in five rat organs as a function of age. J Gerontol. 23 (2): 145-153, 1968.

Roberts SE. The importance of being dehydroepiandrosterone sulfate (in the blood of primates): a longer and healthier life? Biochem Pharmacol. 57 (4): 329-346, 1999.

Rubel LL. The GP and the Endocrine Glands. Decatur, Ill: Louis L. Rubel Publisher, p. 104-122, 1959.

Rubin M, Kirch, EK. Effects of Adrenalectomy on Salt Metabolism in Rats. Proc. Soc. Exper. Biol. and Med. 31: 288, 1933.

Suzuki T. Physiology of Adrenocortical Secretion. Toyko, Japan: Karger Press, p. 1-4, 1983.

Timiras PS, Quay, Wilbur D., Vernadakis, Antonia. Hormones and Aging. New York: CRC Press, p. 29-35, 1995.

Vinson GaH, JP. Blood Flow and Hormone Secretion in the Adrenal Gland. In: James VHT, ed. The Adrenal Gland. Second ed. New York: Raven Press, Ltd., pp. 71-86, 1992.

Weglicki W, Reichel, W., Nair, PP. Accumulation of Lipofuscin-like pigment in the Rat Adrenal Gland as a Function of Vitamin E Deficiency. J. Gerontol. 23 (4): 469-475, 1968.

Wolfram J, Zwemer, RL. Cortex Protection Against anaphylactic Shock in Guinea Pigs. Jour. Exp. Med. 61: 9-15, 1933.

Chapter 23

Back JC, Casey, John, Solomon, S., Hoffman, MM. The Response of the Adrenal Cortex to Chronic Disease. In: GEW Wolstenholme aRP, ed. The Human Adrenal Cortex: Its function throughout life. Boston: Little, Brown and Company, pp. 94-119, 1967.

Holm R, R., Bjorntorp, P. Food-induced cortisol secretion in relation to anthropometric, metabolic and haemodynamic variables in men. Int. J. Obes Relat. Metab. Disord. 24 (4): 416-422, 2000.

Selye H. The Stress of Life. New York: The McGraw-Hill Companies, Inc., p. 29-38, 115, 486, 1984.

Appendix A

The Glycemic Index

The glycemic index (GI) is a way of systematically measuring how much a carbohydrate triggers a rise in circulating blood sugar. The higher the number, the more your blood sugar will rise in response to eating that food. Therefore, as a general rule, choose foods that have lower glycemic index numbers in preference to foods with higher ones. The GI given here is taken from information provided by Dr. Rick Mendosa, co-author of : *The Authoritative Guide to the Glycemic Index.* Marlowe & Company; New York on his website at www.mendosa.com/gilist/htm. and is a summary of over 80 studies. He updates this site regularly, so if you are interested in keeping up with the latest in GI information, this is a good source. The GI shown here compares the food in the left column with eating white bread (white bread has a value of 100 on the GI scale) The amounts of food consumed is assumed to be about 50 grams (a little less than 2 ounces). But the numbers here shouldn't be taken to be absolute numbers. They are only relative numbers so you can compare foods to each other using this scale.

Don't interpret this as 100 is OK and anything above 100 is high and anything below 100 is not. That is not the correct use of this index. One hundred (100) is too high. Try to choose foods in the 70s or lower and go by how your body feels with different foods. There are two lists given here. One is classified according to the category of food (breads, pasta, etc.), the other lists foods according to their GI value from lowest to highest. Some of these food you have probably never heard of. Don't worry. This list is a composite of all foods tested for their GI value to date.

If you are relatively sensitive to your body's reactions, you will soon learn which foods give you the right kind of energy, which ones drive you over the limit and which ones drag you down. So use this list as a general guideline, not as a rigid proclamation of carbohydrate foods.
No matter what the GI number, avoid foods you are sensitive or allergic to.

Glycemic Index

Food-based list: *White Bread =100*

Bakery Products

Cake, sponge	66
Cake, banana, made with sugar	67
Cake, pound	77
Cake, banana, made without sugar	79
Pastry	84
Pizza, cheese	86
Muffins	88
Cake, flan	93
Cake, angel food	95
Croissant	96
Crumpet	98
Donut	108
Waffles	109

Beverages

Soy milk	43
Cordial, orange	94
Soft drink, Fanta	97
Lucozade	136

Breads

Bürgen Soy Lin	27
Bürgen Oat Bran & Honey Loaf	43
Bürgen Mixed Grain	48
PerforMAX	54
Barley kernel bread	55
Bürgen Fruit Loaf	62
Holsom's	64
Rye Kernel bread	66
Fruit loaf	67
Ploughman's Loaf	67

Oat bran bread	68
Mixed grain bread	69
Pumpernickel	71
Bulger bread	75
Linseed rye bread	78
Pita bread, white	82
Hamburger bun	87
Rye flour bread	92
Semolina bread	92
Oat kernel bread	93
Barley flour bread	95
Wheat bread, high fiber	97
Wheat bread, wholemeal flour	99
Melba toast	100
Wheat bread, white	101
Bagel, white	103
Kaiser rolls	104
Whole-wheat snack bread	105
Bread stuffing	106
Wheat bread, Wonderwhite	112
Wheat bread, gluten free	129
French baguette	136

Breakfast Cereals

Rice Bran	27
Kelloggs' All Bran Fruit 'n Oats	55
Kelloggs' Guardian	59
All-bran	60
Porridge (oatmeal)	70
Red River Cereal	70
Bran Buds	75
Special K	77
Oat Bran	78
Kelloggs' Honey Smacks	78
Muesli	80
Kelloggs' Mini-Wheats (whole wheat)	81
Bran Chex	83
Kelloggs' Just Right	84

Life	94
Nutri-grain	94
Grapenuts	96
Sustain	97
Shredded Wheat	99
Kelloggs' Mini-Wheats (blackcurrant)	99
Cream of Wheat	100
Wheat Biscuit	100
Golden Grahams	102
Pro Stars	102
Sultana Bran	102
Puffed Wheat	105
Cheerios	106
Corn Bran	107
Breakfast bar	109
Total	109
Cocopops	110
Post Flakes	114
Rice Krispies	117
Team	117
Corn Chex	118
Cornflakes	119
Crispix	124
Rice Chex	127
Rice Bubbles	128

Cereal Grains

Barley, pearled	36
Rye	48
Wheat kernels	59
Rice, instant, boiled 1 min	65
Bulgur	68
Rice, parboiled	68
Rice, parboiled, high amylose	69
Barley, cracked	72
Wheat, quick cooking	77
Buckwheat	78
Sweet corn	78

Rice, specialty	78
Rice, brown	79
Rice, wild, Saskatchewan	81
Rice, white	83
Rice, white, high amylose	83
Couscous	93
Barley, rolled	94
Rice, Mahatma Premium	94
Taco shells	97
Cornmeal	98
Millet	101
Rice, Pedle	109
Rice, Sunbrown Quick	114
Tapioca, boiled with milk	115
Rice, Calrose	124
Rice, parboiled, low amylose Pelde	124
Rice, white, low amylose	126
Rice, instant, boiled 6 min	128

Cookies

Oatmeal cookies	79
Rich Tea cookies	79
Digestives	84
Shredded Wheatmeal	89
Shortbread	91
Arrowroot	95
Graham Wafers	106
Vanilla Wafers	110
Morning Coffee cookies	113

Crackers

Jatz	79
High Fibre Rye Crispread	93
Breton Wheat Crackers	96
Stoned Wheat Thins	96
Sao	100
Water Crackers	102
Rice Cakes	110

Puffed Crispbread   116

Dairy Foods

Yogurt, low fat, artifically sweet   20
Milk, chocolate, artifically sweet   34
Milk + 30 g bran   38
Milk, full fat   39
Milk, skim   46
Yogurt, low fat, fruit sugar sweet   47
Milk, chocolate, sugar sweetened   49
Yogurt, unspecified   51
Milk + custard + starch + sugar   61
Yakult (fermented milk)   64
Ice cream, low fat   71
Ice cream   87

Fruit And Fruit Products

Cherries   32
Grapefruit   36
Apricots, dried   44
Pear, fresh   53
Apple   54
Plum   55
Apple juice   58
Peach, fresh   60
Orange   63
Pear, canned   63
Grapes   66
Pineapple juice   66
Peach, canned   67
Grapefruit juice   69
Orange juice   74
Kiwifruit   75
Banana   77
Fruit cocktail   79
Mango   80
Sultanas   80
Apricots, fresh   82

Pawpaw	83
Apricots, canned, syrup	91
Raisins	91
Rockmelon (muskmelon, cantaloupe)	93
Pineapple	94
Watermelon	103

Legumes

Soya beans, canned	20
Soya beans	25
Lentils, red	36
Beans, dried, not specified	40
Lentils, not specified	41
Kidney beans	42
Lentils, green	42
Butter beans + 5 g. sucrose	43
Butter beans + 10 g. sucrose	44
Butter beans	44
Split peas, yellow, boiled	45
Lima beans, baby, frozen	46
Chick peas (garbanzo beans)	47
Kidney beans, autoclaved	49
Haricot/navy beans	54
Pinto beans	55
Chick peas, curry, canned	58
Black-eyed beans	59
Chick peas, canned	60
Pinto beans, canned	64
Romano beans	65
Baked beans, canned	69
Kidney beans, canned	74
Lentils, green, canned	74
Butter beans + 15 g. sucrose	77
Beans, dried, P. vulgaris	100
Broad beans (fava beans, fool, foul)	113

Pasta

Spaghetti, protein enriched	38

Fettuccine	46
Vermicelli	50
Spaghetti, wholemeal	53
Star pastina	54
Ravioli, durum, meat filled	56
Spaghetti, boiled 5 min	52
Spaghetti, white	59
Spirali, durum	61
Capellini	64
Macaroni	64
Linguine	65
Instant noodles	67
Tortellini, cheese	71
Spaghetti, durum	78
Macaroni and Cheese	92
Gnocchi	95
Rice pasta, brown	131

Root Vegetables

Yam	73
Sweet potato	77
Potato, white, not specified, boiled	80
Potato, new	81
Potato, white, Ontario	85
Potato, canned	87
Potato, Prince Edward Island, boiled	90
Beets	91
Potato, steamed	93
Potato mashed	100
Carrots	70
Swede (rutabaga)	103
Potato, boiled, mashed	104
French fries	107
Potato, microwaved	117
Potato, instant	118
Potato, baked	121
Parsnips	139

Snack Foods/Confectionaries

Peanuts	21
Mars M&Ms (peanut)	46
Mars Snickers Bar	57
Mars Twix Cookie Bars (caramel)	62
Mars Chocolate (Dove)	63
Jams and marmalades	70
Chocolate	70
Potato crisps	77
Popcorn	79
Muesli Bars	87
Mars Kudos Whole Grain Bars (choc chip)	87
Mars Bar	91
Mars Skittles	98
Life Savers	100
Corn chips	105
Jelly beans	114
Pretzels	116
Dates	146

Soups

Tomato Soup	54
Lentil soup, canned	63
Split pea soup	86
Black bean soup	92
Green pea soup, canned	94

Sugars

Fructose	32
Lactose	65
Honey	83
High fructose corn syrup	89
Sucrose	92
Glucose	137
Glucose tablets	146
Maltodextrin	150
Maltose	150

Vegetables

Peas, dried	32
Marrowfat, dried	56
Peas, green	68
Sweet corn	78
Pumpkin	107

INDIGENOUS FOODS

Pima Indian:

Acorns stewed with venison	23
Mesquite cakes	36
Yellow teparies broth	41
White teparies broth	44
Lima beans broth	51
Corn tortilla w/desert ironwood	54
Corn hominy (not modern corn)	57
Fruit leather	100
Cactus jam	130

South African:

Brown beans	34
M'fino wild greens	97
Maize meal porridge, unrefined	101
Maize meal porridge, refined	106

Mexican:

Nopal prickly pear cactus	10
Black beans	43
Brown beans	54

Asian Indian:

Bengal gram dal (chana dal)	12
Rajmah (red kidney beans)	27
Baisen (besan, chick pea flour) chapati	39
Green gram (mung beans)	54
Barley chapati	61

Black gram	61
Black gram dal with semolina	66
Horse gram	73
Bengal gram dal with semolina	77
Whole greengram	81
Bajra (millet)	82
Maize chapati	89
Green gram dal with semolina	89
Semolina	94
Varagu	97
Banana, unripe, steamed 1 hr.	100
Tapioca, steamed 1 hr.	100
Jowar	110
Green gram dal + paspalum scorbic.	111
Ragi (or Raggi)	123

Australian Aboriginal:

Mulga seed (Acacia aneura)	11
Blackbean seed	11
Cheeky yam	49
Macrozamia communis	57
Bush honey, sugar bag	61
Bread (Acacia coriacea)	66
Bunya nut pine	67
Castanospermum australe	106

Pacific Island Foods:

Sweet potato (Ipamoea batatas)	63
Taro	77
Breadfruit	97

Chinese Foods:

Lungkow bean thread	37
Rice vermicelli	83

Miscellaneous

Sausages	40

Vitari	40
So Good (Sanitarium)	43
Nutella spread(Ferrero)	46
Fish fingers	54
Ultracal	55
Sustagen Hospital Formula	61
VO2 Max Energy Bar (chocolate; Mars)	69
Power Bar (Powerfoods)	81
Tofu frozen dessert, non-dairy	164

*Glycemic Index-based list:*Listed from lowest to highest GI value

White Bread

Nopal prickly pear cactus	10
Mulga seed (Acacia aneura)	11
Blackbean seed	11
Bengal gram dal (chana dal)	12
Yogurt, low fat, artifically sweet	20
Soya beans, canned	20
Peanuts	21
Acorns stewed with venison	23
Soya beans	25
Rice Bran	27
Rajmah (red kidney beans)	27
Bürgen Soy Lin	27
Cherries	32
Fructose	32
Peas, dried	32
Milk, chocolate, artifically sweet	34
Brown beans (South African)	34
Barley, pearled	36
Grapefruit	36
Lentils, red	36
Mesquite cakes	36
Lungkow bean thread	37
Spaghetti, protein enriched	38
Milk + 30 g bran	38
Milk, full fat	39

Baisen (besan, chick pea flour) chapati	39
Beans, dried, not specified	40
Sausages	40
Vitari	40
Lentils, not specified	41
Yellow teparies broth	41
Kidney beans	42
Lentils, green	42
Black beans	43
Soy milk	43
Butter beans + 5 g. sucrose	43
So Good (Sanitarium)	43
Bürgen Oat Bran & Honey Loaf	43
So Good (Sanitarium)	43
Butter beans + 10 g. sucrose	44
Apricots, dried	44
Butter beans	44
White teparies broth	44
Split peas, yellow, boiled	45
Milk, skim	46
Lima beans, baby, frozen	46
Fettuccine	46
Mars M&Ms (peanut)	46
Nutella spread(Ferrero)	46
Yogurt, low fat, fruit sugar sweet	47
Chick peas (garbanzo beans)	47
Rye	48
Bürgen Mixed Grain Bread	48
Milk, chocolate, sugar sweetened	49
Kidney beans, autoclaved	49
Cheeky yam	49
Vermicelli	50
Yogurt, unspecified	51
Lima beans broth	51
Spaghetti, boiled 5 min	52
Pear, fresh	53
Spaghetti, wholemeal	53
Apple	54

Haricot/navy beans	54
Star pastina	54
Tomato Soup	54
Corn tortilla w/desert ironwood	54
Brown beans (Mexican)	54
Green gram (mung beans)	54
Fish fingers	54
PerforMAX	54
Barley kernel bread	55
Plum	55
Pinto beans	55
Ultracal	55
Kelloggs' All Bran Fruit 'n Oats	55
Ravioli, durum, meat filled	56
Marrowfat, dried	56
Corn hominy (not modern corn)	57
Macrozamia communis	57
Mars Snickers Bar	57
Apple juice	58
Chick peas, curry, canned	58
Wheat kernels	59
Black-eyed beans	59
Spaghetti, white	59
Kelloggs' Guardian	59
All-bran	60
Peach, fresh	60
Chick peas, canned	60
Milk + custard + starch + sugar	61
Spirali, durum	61
Barley chapati	61
Black gram	61
Bush honey, sugar bag	61
Sustagen Hospital Formula	61
Bürgen Fruit Loaf Bread	62
Mars Twix Cookie Bars (caramel)	62
Orange	63
Pear, canned	63
Lentil soup, canned	63

Sweet potato (Ipamoea batatas)	63
Mars Chocolate (Dove)	63
Pinto beans, canned	64
Capellini	64
Macaroni	64
Holsom's	64
Yakult (fermented milk)	64
Romano beans	65
Linguine	65
Rice, instant, boiled 1 min	65
Lactose	65
Cake, sponge	66
Rye Kernel bread	66
Grapes	66
Pineapple juice	66
Black gram dal with semolina	66
Bread (Acacia coriacea)	66
Cake, banana, made with sugar	67
Fruit loaf (bread)	67
Ploughman's Loaf (bread)	67
Peach, canned	67
Instant noodles	67
Bunya nut pine	67
Oat bran bread	68
Bulgur	68
Rice, parboiled	68
Peas, green	68
Mixed grain bread	69
Rice, parboiled, high amylose	69
Grapefruit juice	69
Baked beans, canned	69
VO2 Max Energy Bar (chocolate; Mars)	69
Porridge (oatmeal)	70
Carrots	70
Red River Cereal	70
Chocolate	70
Jams and marmalades	70
Pumpernickel	71

Ice cream, low fat	71
Tortellini, cheese	71
Barley, cracked	72
Yam	73
Horse gram	73
Orange juice	74
Kidney beans, canned	74
Lentils, green, canned	74
Bulger bread	75
Bran Buds	75
Kiwifruit	75
Cake, pound	77
Special K	77
Wheat, quick cooking	77
Banana	77
Sweet potato	77
Potato crisps	77
Bengal gram dal with semolina	77
Taro	77
Butter beans + 15 g. sucrose	77
Linseed rye bread	78
Oat Bran	78
Buckwheat	78
Sweet corn	78
Rice, specialty	78
Spaghetti, durum	78
Kelloggs' Honey Smacks	78
Cake, banana, made without sugar	79
Rice, brown	79
Oatmeal cookies	79
Rich Tea cookies	79
Jatz	79
Fruit cocktail	79
Popcorn	79
Muesli	80
Mango	80
Sultanas	80
Potato, white, not specified, boiled	80

Rice, wild, Saskatchewan	81
Potato, new	81
Whole greengram	81
Kelloggs' Mini-Wheats (whole wheat)	81
Power Bar (Powerfoods)	81
Pita bread, white	82
Apricots, fresh	82
Bajra (millet)	82
Honey	83
Bran Chex	83
Rice, white	83
Rice, white, high amylose	83
Pawpaw	83
Rice vermicelli	83
Pastry	84
Digestives	84
Kelloggs' Just Right	84
Potato, white, Ontario	85
Pizza, cheese	86
Split pea soup	86
Hamburger bun	87
Ice cream	87
Muesli Bars	87
Potato, canned	87
Mars Kudos Whole Grain Bars (choc chip)	87
Muffins	88
Shredded Wheatmeal	89
Maize chapati	89
Green gram dal with semolina	89
High fructose corn syrup	89
Potato, Prince Edward Island, boiled	90
Apricots, canned, syrup	91
Shortbread	91
Raisins	91
Beets	91
Mars Bar	91
Rye flour bread	92
Semolina bread	92

Macaroni and Cheese	92
Black bean soup	92
Sucrose	92
Cake, flan	93
Oat kernel bread	93
Couscous	93
High Fibre Rye Crispread	93
Rockmelon (muskmelon, cantaloupe)	93
Potato, steamed	93
Barley, rolled	94
Cordial, orange	94
Life	94
Nutri-grain	94
Rice, Mahatma Premium	94
Pineapple	94
Green pea soup, canned	94
Semolina	94
Cake, angel food	95
Barley flour bread	95
Arrowroot	95
Gnocchi	95
Croissant	96
Grapenuts	96
Breton Wheat Crackers	96
Stoned Wheat Thins	96
Soft drink, Fanta	97
Sustain	97
Taco shells	97
M'fino wild greens	97
Varagu	97
Breadfruit	97
Wheat bread, high fiber	97
Crumpet	98
Cornmeal	98
Mars Skittles	98
Wheat bread, wholemeal flour	99
Shredded Wheat	99
Kelloggs' Mini-Wheats (blackcurrant)	99

Melba toast	100
Cream of Wheat	100
Wheat Biscuits	100
Sao	100
Beans, dried, P. vulgaris	100
Potato mashed	100
Life Savers	100
Fruit leather	100
Banana, unripe, steamed 1 hr.	100
Tapioca, steamed 1 hr.	100
Millet	101
Maize meal porridge, unrefined	101
Wheat bread, white	101
Golden Grahams	102
Pro Stars	102
Water Crackers	102
Sultana Bran	102
Bagel, white	103
Watermelon	103
Swede (rutabaga)	103
Kaiser rolls	104
Potato, boiled, mashed	104
Whole-wheat snack bread	105
Puffed Wheat	105
Corn chips	105
Bread stuffing	106
Cheerios	106
Graham Wafers	106
Maize meal porridge, refined	106
Castanospermum australe	106
Corn Bran	107
French fries	107
Pumpkin	107
Donut	108
Waffles	109
Breakfast bar	109
Total	109
Rice, Pedle	109

Cocopops	110
Vanilla Wafers	110
Rice Cakes	110
Jowar	110
Green gram dal + paspalum scorbic.	111
Wheat bread, Wonderwhite	112
Morning Coffee cookies	113
Broad beans (fava beans, fool, foul)	113
Post Flakes	114
Rice, Sunbrown Quick	114
Jelly beans	114
Tapioca, boiled with milk	115
Puffed Crispbread	116
Pretzels	116
Rice Krispies	117
Team	117
Potato, microwaved	117
Corn Chex	118
Potato, instant	118
Cornflakes	119
Potato, baked	121
Ragi (or Raggi)	123
Crispix	124
Rice, Calrose	124
Rice, parboiled, low amylose Pelde	124
Rice, white, low amylose	126
Rice Chex	127
Rice Bubbles	128
Rice, instant, boiled 6 min	128
Wheat bread, gluten free	129
Cactus jam	130
Rice pasta, brown	131
Lucozade	136
French baguette	136
Glucose	137
Parsnips	139
Glucose tablets	146
Dates	146

Last modified: February 9, 2001

Appendix B

List of Vegetables

Below is a partial list of vegetables. Most of these vegetables are available from grocery stores, vegetable markets or oriental stores. This list is provided for you to see the variety of vegetables available and to invite you to try new ones regularly. To get the best quality with the most flavor and nutrients, but no sprays or irradiation, get organically grown vegetables. Find a local source if possible. The wider your food base, the more nutrients you will consume. Keep this list handy and refer to it often.

Vegetables:

Artichoke – globe, Jerusalem
Asparagus
Bamboo shoots
Beans (dried) – pinto, kidney, navy, black, lima, garbanzo (chick peas), soy, cow
    peas, white pigeon, azuki, mung, fava, etc.
Beans (green & wax)]
Bok choy
Breadfruit (unripe)
Broccoli
Brussels sprouts
Cabbage – nappa, Chinese
Carrots
Cauliflower
Celery
Celery root (celeriac)
Chard, Swiss
Chayote
Chervil
Chicory
Chive
Collards, many varieties of Green Leaves
Corn
Cress
Cucumber
Daikon
Dandelion
Dock

Eggplant
Endive
Escarole
Fennel
Garlic
Horseradish
Jicama
Kale
Kohlrabi
Leek
Lettuce – iceberg, bibb, romaine, butter, curly leaf, red curly
Mushrooms
Mustard greens
Mustard spinach
Okra
Onion
Parsley
Parsnip
Peas, snow, sugar snap
Peppers, bell – green, red, yellow, orange, white & purple
Peppers, Hot – jalapeno, Anaheim, banana, serrano
Potato, white, gold, blue, red
Pumpkin
Purslane leaves
Radish
Rhubarb
Rutabaga
Salsify
Seaweed
Shallot
Spinach
Sprouts (Almost any bean or seed can be easily sprouted. Common sprouts include
    mung bean, radish, sunflower seed and alfalfa.)
Squash, summer – zucchini, yellow, pattypan
Squash, winter – butternut, hubbard, acorn, buttercup, crookneck, kabocha, turban
    spaghetti, sweet dumpling, golden nugget, delicata,
Swamp cabbage
Sweet potato
Taro
Tomato
Turnip
Vine spinach
Yam
Yam bean

Appendix C

List of Fruits

Apple
Apricot
Avocado
Banana
Berries – blackberry, blueberry, elderberry, raspberry, gooseberry,
     loganberry, thimbleberry, strawberry, cranberry, etc.
Breadfruit (ripe)
Carambola (star fruit)
Carissa plum
Cherimoya (custard apple)
Cherry
Crabapple
Currant
Date
Durian
Fig
Granadilla
Grapefruit
Grapes
Groundcherry
Guava
Haw
Jackfruit
Jujube
Kumquat
Lemon
Lime
Loganberry
Longan
Loquat
Lychee
Mamey
Mango

Melon – muskmelon, cantaloupe, crenshaw, watermelon, honeydew, casaba, etc.
Nectarine
Olive
Orange
Papaw
Papaya
Peach
Pear
Persimmon
Pineapple
Pitanga
Plantain
Plum
Pomegranate
Prickly pear
Prune
Quince
Raisin
Rosehip
Sapodilla plum
Sapote
Soursop
Sweetsop (sugar apple)
Tamarind
Tangelo
Tangerine

Appendix D

How to Take Your Own Pulse and Blood Pressure

How to Take Your Own Pulse

Taking your own pulse is a simple procedure. The only equipment you will need is a watch with a second hand or a digital watch that displays seconds. Simply turn the inside of either wrist toward you and place the tips of the first three fingers of your other hand lightly on your upturned wrist so that they rest between the thumb side of your wrist and the tendons in the middle of your wrist. Your 4th finger should be resting on the inside crease of your wrist that is closest to your hand. Press down lightly and one of your fingers should feel a distinct pulse underneath it. If you do not feel it the first time, shift your fingers slightly to the side or to the middle of the wrist and keep trying until you can feel it. Everybody has a pulse, so if you are reading this book, you have one. When you are taking someone else's pulse, follow the same procedure, but be sure to place your fingers on the thumb side of their wrist. Do not use your thumb to take a pulse because your thumb's own pulse will interfere.

If, for some reason, you cannot take your pulse at the wrist, use the side of the neck instead. Press 2 to 3 fingers on either side of your Adam's apple. Feel for the pulse for 3-4 seconds. If you cannot feel it, shift your fingers slightly and try again until you do.

Once you find your pulse, start counting the beats. Begin when the seconds marker on your watch starts a new minute and continue for a full minute. The number of pulse beats in a full minute is your pulse rate. Many health professionals take the pulse for only 15 seconds and multiply by 4, but this is not as accurate. After you have determined your pulse rate, write it down to keep as a reference.

How to Take Your Own Blood Pressure

Taking your own blood pressure is also very simple. The only piece of equipment you will need is a sphygmomanometer with a digital readout. Place the cuff just above your elbow. Then either press the automatic inflation button or, if you have the bulb model, repeatedly press the bulb until the unit indicates you have sufficient pressure in the cuff for it to take your blood pressure. (Some of the bulb models require you to close a valve before beginning. If you have one of these models, be sure to close the valve before starting the procedure). After sufficient pressure has been reached, the sphyg will automatically deflate (most models), recording your blood pressure and pulse rate as it goes. It will keep this reading for several minutes allowing you to write it down before you turn it off. If the model you have does not release the pressure automatically, turn the valve near the bulb slowly to the left to deflate it. My suggestion is to get a model that does everything automatically.

Buying a sphygmomanometer
These are readily available on the Internet, at most medical supply houses, home health care centers, and at some drug stores and department stores. If you are buying it from a store, have the sales person show you how to use it and be comfortable with its use before you leave the store. To find one on the Internet, search using the word "sphygmomanometer". Be careful to select a unit that has a digital readout (not one with a gauge or mercury indicator). Get one that also gives a pulse readout as well. Some units have an automatic inflator and will pump up the cuff with a press of button. Others require you to inflate the cuff by repeatedly pressing an attached rubber bulb. Either one is fine. However, if you have arthritis, your hands cramp easily, or you lack normal hand strength, you will be happier with the self-inflating models. Although some models provide a paper printout of your blood pressure and pulse, you do not really need this feature. These models are more expensive and have more to go wrong. Generally, they are not worth the extra money. Most units come with at least a 1year warranty so check the warranty before you purchase it.

Glossary

Abscessed tooth – an infected tooth, usually with swelling and inflammation in the gum and surrounding tissue. Sometimes, as in root canals, it is too subtle to be detected on cursory examination.

Adaptogen – a substance, often an herb, that normalizes a biochemical process or tissue function, i.e. it brings the process or function back towards normal, no matter if it is too high or too low. Adaptogens are usually non-toxic and often have other beneficial effects.

Addison's disease – adrenal failure or severe adrenal insufficiency, usually caused by an auto-immune process but can be induced by stress, direct infection, destruction, or other causes.

Adrenal glands – two glands that sit over the kidneys, primarily responsible for governing the body's adaptations to stress of any kind.

Adrenal cascade – the bio-chemical process in the adrenals involved in changing cholesterol to the various adrenal hormones.

Adrenal cell extracts – dietary supplements containing the extracts of the adrenal glands, usually from beef.

Adrenal cortex – the outer portion of the adrenal gland comprising about 80% of the adrenal gland. The cortex is divided into three and possibly four zones. It is responsible for producing over 50 hormones including cortisol, aldosterone, DHEAS and is a secondary producer of the sex hormones. (See adrenal zones).

Adrenalcorticotrophic hormone (ACTH) – a hormone secreted by the pituitary gland to stimulate the production of cortisol and other adrenal hormones.

Adrenal fatigue – a term used to denote a syndrome due to the decreased ability of the adrenal glands to respond adequately to stress.

It affects the daily life of those suffering from it. Adrenal fatigue is a less severe condition than Addison's disease.

Adrenal medulla – the inner part of the adrenal gland responsible for producing epinephrine (adrenaline) and norepinephrine (noradrenalin).

Adrenal reserves – the untapped but available capacity of the adrenal glands to respond to stress.

Adrenal zones – the three (probably 4) zones of the adrenal cortex, including the zona fasciculata, from which cortisol is produced; zona glomerulosa, that produces aldosterone; zona reticularis, that produces DHEA & DHEAS; and in humans an interface zone between the zona fasciculata and the zona reticularis, probably responsible for producing the sex hormones, along with the zona reticularis.

Adrenalfatigue.org – the website dedicated to helping people who are suffering from adrenal fatigue.

Adult onset diabetes – often referred to as "adult onset non-insulin dependent diabetes," or Type II diabetes. This is the most common type of diabetes and is caused more from insulin resistance of the cell rather than lack of production of insulin.

Alarm reaction – the first of three stages of the general adaptation syndrome (GAS) of Hans Selye.

Aldosterone – a hormone produced by the Zona Glomerulosa of the adrenal cortex, responsible for sodium and potassium levels in the blood and individual cells throughout the body, greatly influencing the fluid volume.

Androgens – male sex hormones. The adrenal glands are the chief auxiliary source in males and the only main source in females.

Anti-inflammatory – hormones such as cortisol and other substances that decrease inflammation of tissues (heat, redness, swelling).

Antioxidants – substances produced by the body or dietary supplements that prevent chemical oxidation in the body from happening too rapidly and/or prevent the accumulation of oxygen with unpaired electrons within the cell.

Apoptosis - programmed cell death

Ashwagandha – an East Indian herb known for its beneficial effects on the adrenal glands, as well as other properties.

Asthenia – Weakness, lack of strength to do normal tasks.

Atherosclerosis – hardening of the arteries.

Auto-immune disorders – a process where the immune system attacks one or more parts of the body. Auto-immune disorders are greatly enhanced in people with adrenal fatigue.

Basophils – one of the white blood cells. Basophils are responsible for secreting IgE immunoglobulins that cause histamine reactions in allergies and produce inflammation of tissue.

Bioflavinoids – substances found in conjunction with Vitamin C in all vegetables and fruits containing vitamin C. Bioflavinoids enhance the activity of Vitamin C and have independent beneficial functions of their own in the human body.

Blood pressure, postural – blood pressure taken in reference to what position the body is in at the time the blood pressure is taken; sitting, standing or lying down.

Bronchitis – inflammation of the bronchial tree, the passageways to the lungs, caused by irritation or infection.

Burn-out – a term used to denote the signs and symptoms of someone who has totally depleted their energy reserves by driving themselves to the point of exhaustion.

Carbohydrates – that portion of food composed of carbon, hydrogen and oxygen. Carbohydrates can be divided into unrefined (whole grains), refined (processed grains, white flour and sugar products), and fiber. Most carbohydrates can be burned for energy, except for fiber, and are the major source of energy in most diets.

Cellular metabolism – the work done inside the cells to manufacture energy and make new chemical and physical products.

Central nervous system (CNS) – that part of the nervous system that includes the brain and spinal cord.

Central obesity – central obesity, also called abdominal fat, is a term used to describe the accumulation of fat around the abdomen (spare tire). It is an indication of high cortisol levels, and/or an over-consumption of refined carbohydrates that is also seen in some cases of adrenal fatigue.

Cerebral allergies – a term used to denote allergies or sensitivities to foods or inhalants that affect the central nervous system (brain and spinal cord). Cerebral allergies often produce changes in behavior or thought processes.

Cholesterol – a four-ring carbon chain manufactured by the liver and consumed in the diet, used in the manufacturing of steroid hormones including all hormones from the adrenal glands.

Chromium – a mineral in trace elements important in helping to regulate blood sugar and necessary for the manufacture of insulin.

Chronic fatigue syndrome – persistent debilitating fatigue of recent onset, with reduction of physical activity to less than half of usual, accompanied by some combination of muscle weakness, sore throat, mild fever, tender lymph nodes, headache, and depression, with the symptoms not attributable to any other known cause.

Circadian rhythm – the cyclic fluctuations of hormones or other substances within a 24-hour cycle.

Colloidal silver – minute particles of silver suspended in water by an electrical process, used to kill over 300 microorganisms.

Corticosteroids (also known as adrenal cortical hormones and corticoids) - steroid hormones (excluding the sex hormones) secreted by the adrenal cortex. Corticosteroids are divided into two major groups: glucocorticoids, which affect fat, carbohydrate and protein metabolism, and mineral corticoids, which affect the regulation of electrolyte and water balance. Cortisol is a major glucocorticoid and aldosterone is the major mineral corticoid.

Corticoids – See Corticosteroids

Corticotrophin releasing factor (CRF) – the hormone secreted by the hypothalamus that directs the pituitary to create adrenal corticotrophic hormones (ACTH). CRF is the major regulator of the production of cortisol.

Cortisol – the hormone produced by the zona fasciculata of the adrenal cortex that is necessary for life.

Cushing's disease – a disease of excessively high levels of circulating cortisol. The most common cause of Cushing's disease is the use of prescription steroids, It can also be caused by excessive secretion of ACTH from the pituitary.

Cytokines – substances secreted by white blood cells, especially lymphocytes. Cytokines include interferons, interlukins, and transfer factors.

Cytosol – the liquid inside of the cell.

Detoxification – the process of removing poisons and other toxic substances from the cells, tissues, interstitial fluid, blood, or body as a whole.

Dehydroepiandosterone (DHEA) – a hormone secreted in the adrenal cascade serving as a precursor to sex hormones in the adrenal cortex and in several other tissues of the body.

Diabetes Mellitus – a chronic syndrome of impaired fat, carbohydrate and protein metabolism owing to insufficient secretion of insulin or to insulin resistance at the target tissue.

Electrolyte drink – a beverage containing high amounts of electrolytes (potassium, magnesium, chloride and sodium). Most of the commercial electrolyte drinks are high in potassium and low in sodium, and also contains refined carbohydrates as an energy source.

Electrolyte homeostasis – the balance of electrolytes (sodium, potassium, magnesium, chloride) within the cells and in the blood.

Endocrine Glands – ductless glands that secrete hormones directly into the bloodstream, influencing metabolism and other body processes. The endocrine glands include the hypothalamus, pituitary, thyroid, pancreas, parathyroid, adrenals, thymus, pineal and gonads (ovaries and testicles).

Endocrinologist – a doctor who specializes in treating disorders of the endocrine glands of the body.

Energy suckers – usually people, but sometimes situations, which cause a drop in energy of the person experiencing them.

Environmental toxins – toxic substances encountered by touching, inhaling, or some other method of contact.

Eosinophils – one of the white blood cells often elevated in adrenal fatigue, allergies and parasitic infections.

Epinephrine – one of the two hormones secreted by the adrenal medulla, also known as adrenaline.

Essential fatty acids – the two fatty acids that are necessary for human life and health; alpha-linolenic acid and linoleic acid.

Fats – one molecule of glycerin, serving as a backbone to three fatty acid molecules. Fats can be solid or liquid.

Fats, hydrogenated – a fat in which one or more of the double bonds normally occurring in that fat has been replaced by a hydrogen molecule. Hydrogenated fats increase shelf life, but are responsible for many conditions of ill health.

Fats, monounsaturated – a fatty acid in which there is only one unsaturated double bond.

Fats, unsaturated – fats in which there are one or more double bonds in their fatty acids. The essential fatty acids are unsaturated.

Fats, saturated – fats in which there are no unsaturated double bonds. All are filled with hydrogen molecules.

Fatty acids – strings of carbon from 4-27 carbons long that serve as key building blocks of all fats and oils in our foods and bodies. Fatty acids play key roles in the construction of maintenance of all healthy cells.

Fiber – indigestible or partially digestible carbohydrates, an abundance of which is important for proper intestinal and overall health. Unrefined grains, vegetables, seeds, nuts and some fruits are high in fiber. Fiber includes cellulose, hemi-cellulose and pectins.

Fibromyalgia – A group of rheumatic disorders not involving the joints characterized by pain, tenderness, and stiffness of muscles, areas of tendon insertions and adjacent soft tissue. Fibromyalgia may be primary or secondary to another underlying condition. It may be generalized or localized

General adaptation syndrome (GAS) – a term coined by Dr. Hans Selye to describe the three phases of stress; the alarm phase, the resistance phase, and the exhaustion phase.

Ginger root – a herb commonly used as an adaptogen in adrenal fatigue, also for nausea and intestinal upsets.

Glucocorticoids – steroids secreted by the adrenal cortex affecting blood sugar, the most common by far is cortisol.

Gluconeogenisis – the making of blood sugar by converting fatty acids or amino acids into glucose.

Glucose intolerance – sensitivity to increases in glucose by the cells, often producing symptoms known as hyperglycemic reactions.

Glycemic index – an index describing the effects of various foods on circulating blood glucose levels.

Glycolysis – the process used by cells to break down glucose into pyruvic acid, and finally into the Krebs (tricarboxylic acid) cycle for metabolism that creates energy.

Herbal extracts – the end product of extracting the ingredients from herbs using alcohol, water, or another solvent.

Holistic (wholistic) medicine – a term to denote the consideration of the whole person in the treatment process.

Homeostasis – the balance of the internal body mechanisms and processes.

Hormone replacement – taking hormones created outside the body, either orally or by injection, to replace a lack of the hormone circulating the body.

Hydrocortisone – a name in medicine, given to the synthetic pharmaceutical preparation of cortisol. In physiology, hydrocortisone is the name of one of the hormones in the adrenal cascade.

Hydrogenated oils – see fats, hydrogenated

Hypertension – high blood pressure

Hypoadrenia – low adrenal function

Hypoglycemia – low blood sugar

Hypotension – low blood pressure

Hypothalamus – an endocrine gland situated in the brain below the thalamus and above the pituitary gland. The hypothalamus regulates most of the functions of the endocrine system and many other automatic functions of the body.

Hypotonia – lack of muscle tone.

International Classification of Disease (ICD) Codes – the use of various numbers to represent all disease states and health conditions. It is used by all hospitals, physicians and insurance companies.

Immunoglobulins – "y" shaped proteins secreted by the B-lymphocytes, one of the white blood cells, used to protect the body against infections and other foreign substances.

Indian ginseng – see Ashwagandha

Individual biochemical variation (also known as biochemical individuality) – recognition that each person has unique biochemistry and often can't be classified within a group and must be considered alone, as a unique process. This is in opposition to assuming that people are biochemically the same.

Inflammatory reaction – reactions of the body that involve redness, swelling, heat, and sometimes pain and loss of function.

Insomnia – the inability to sleep

Insulin resistance – lack of response of cells to the presence of insulin, often seen in non-insulin dependent diabetes and syndrome X.

Lactose – milk sugar

Lethargy – A clinical term used to denote a condition of listlessness, drowsiness, apathy and indifference.

Lymphocytes – one of the white blood cells. Lymphocytes are divided into two broad classifications of B and T lymphocytes, both of which are greatly involved in the immune process.

Lipolysis – the breakdown of fat into fatty acids and often further into glucose through gluconeogenesis.

Magnesium – one of the minerals used by the body and often deficient in people with adrenal fatigue. Magnesium is important in creating energy from blood sugar in several biochemical reactions and several functions of the body.

Manganese – a metal used by the body in some key biochemical reactions, such as the manufacture of insulin and some functions of the hypothalamus. It is also a critical component in the structure of tendons, ligaments and joint tissue.

Marmite – a commercial vegetable paste.

Metabolism – the breakdown or creation of chemical and structural elements in the body.

Millet – a round yellow whole grain used as a staple in some parts of the world.

Miso – a soup base composed of fermented soy beans and rice or barley. Used as a staple in Japanese cooking, rich in minerals, trace minerals and protein.

Mitochondria – the power plant of the cell that manufactures most of the energy used by the cell to carry out its functions.

Monocytes – one of the white blood cells, especially active in recovering from infections.

Nicotinamide Adenine Dinucleotide (NAD) – a niacin containing coenzyme present in many of the steps in the adrenal cascade.

Neurons – nerve cells in the human body, sometimes many inches or even feet long.

Niacin – one of the B vitamins. Niacin is very important in helping people recover from adrenal fatigue and is essential in the reactions involving NAD in the adrenal cascade.

Noradrenalin (also known as norepinephrine) - a hormone secreted by the adrenal medulla.

Norepinephrine – see noradrenalin

Nutrient – any food or substance that nourishes the cell or the body.

Orthostatic blood pressure – blood pressure taken in the standing position.

Pantothenic acid – one of the B vitamins. Although occurring in all cells, pantothenic acid is especially essential for the adrenal glands and is used in high amounts in the rehabilitation from adrenal fatigue.

Partially hydrogenated oils – unsaturated oils that have had one or more hydrogens replace the normal double bond, but still have at least one double bond free. These are oils that have usually been synthetically manipulated and interfere drastically with your health and should be avoided.

Pectin – a type of soluble fiber appearing in many fruits.

Potassium – one of the macronutrients. Potassium is the most abundant mineral inside the cell. During adrenal fatigue, potassium levels can be abnormally high.

Pro-oxidants – a substance that encourages oxidation within the cell, sometimes to the detriment of the cell.

Pyridoxine – one of the B-vitamins. It has a significant role as a co-factor in many metabolic pathways, including the adrenals. Pyridoxine is available in two forms, pyridoxine hydrochloride (HCl) and pyridoxine 5 phosphate (P5P). P5P is a natural form that appears in your body.

Refined carbohydrates – starches and sugars that have been refined and in doing so, have had the nutrition removed, leaving only the energy portion. This includes all white sugar and white flour products, white rice, and most pasta.

Reframing – the ability of the mind to shift its perception of a situation and to see it from a different perspective. A classic example of reframing would be to shift from seeing a glass half full to seeing a glass half empty. Reframing is a powerful psychological tool.

Sandwich stress – the stress created when one is caught in the middle position of different demands and lacks the power or the authority to resolve the situation. Typical example of this is a middle executive in a corporation.

Selenium – one of the natural elements of the earth. It is important in several aspects of human metabolism, especially those involving immunity.

Siberian ginseng – the popular herb that is not from Siberia and not ginseng, but acts somewhat like ginseng in its effects on the body. Siberian ginseng is valuable in helping adrenal fatigue and re-establishing normal hormone levels, especially in females.

Sodium – one of the natural elements used extensively in the body to balance electrolytes. Sodium is probably the most critical element in adrenal fatigue. It's deficiency in the blood and inside the cell causes many of the symptoms of adrenal fatigue.

Steroids – steroids are hormones or hormone like substances formed from cholesterol in the body and created synthetically by many drug companies. The balance of steroid hormones are extremely important in balancing body chemistry. The adrenals use approximately 50 steroid hormones, of which about a dozen go out to effect the entire body.

Stressor – anything that causes a disruption in the body balance (homeostasis of the body). Stress can be physical, emotional, psychological, environmental or of an infectious source.

Suprarenals – an older term used for adrenals glands.

Syndrome – a collection of signs and/or symptoms occurring together in a disease or medical disorder.

Synthetic Corticosteroids – manufactured steroids imitating the actions of the adrenal cortex. These often have serious side effects that can include liver damage, immune shut down and even death. Synthetic steroids must be used very cautiously and monitored judiciously to prevent destruction.

Trace Minerals – those minerals occurring naturally needed in small amounts for the body to maintain health. Examples of trace minerals include zinc, manganese, selenium, chromium, and copper.

Triglycerides – three fatty acids attached to glycerol that normally circulate in the blood. Fatty acids are elevated by consumption of refined carbohydrates or carbohydrate metabolism impairment.

Vena cava – the largest vein in the body going from the liver to the heart that carries blood back to the heart.

Index